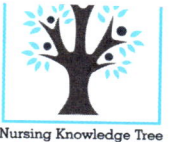

Textbook of
Nursing Management & Services for BSc Nursing

[*As per the Syllabus of Indian Nursing Council & KUHS for BSc Nursing Students*]

Beena MR MSc (N), PhD
Associate Professor
Government College of Nursing, Government Medical College
Thiruvananthapuram, Kerala

Hari Krishna GL MSc (N), MHA, MPA, PGDHSR, PGDHHA, CDM, PhD Scholar
Assistant Professor and In-service Education Coordinator
Department of Psychiatric Nursing
Sree Gokulam Nursing College, Sree Gokulam Medical College and Research Foundation
Thiruvananthapuram, Kerala

Kiruba JC MSc (N), PhD Scholar
Professor
SSNMM College of Nursing
Varkala, Thiruvananthapuram, Kerala

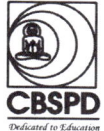

CBS Publishers & Distributors Pvt Ltd
• New Delhi • Bengaluru • Chennai • Kochi • Kolkata • Lucknow
• Mumbai • Hyderabad • Nagpur • Patna • Pune • Vijayawada

Textbook of
Nursing Management & Services for BSc Nursing

ISBN: 978-93-88178-62-4

Copyright © Publishers

First Edition: 2020

All rights are reserved. No part of this book may be reproduced or transmitted in any form or by any means, electronic or mechanical, including photocopying, recording, or any information storage and retrieval system without permission, in writing, from the publishers.

Published by **Satish Kumar Jain** and produced by **Varun Jain** for

CBS Publishers and Distributors Pvt Ltd

4819/XI Prahlad Street, 24 Ansari Road, Daryaganj, New Delhi 110 002, India.
Ph: +91-11-23289259, 23266861, 23266867   Website: www.cbspd.com
Fax: 011-23243014
e-mail: delhi@cbspd.com; cbspubs@airtelmail.in.

Corporate Office: 204 FIE, Industrial Area, Patparganj, Delhi 110 092
Ph: +91-11-4934 4934   Fax: 4934 4935
e-mail: feedback@cbspd.com; bhupesharora@cbspd.com

Branches

- **Bengaluru:** Seema House 2975, 17th Cross, K.R. Road, Banasankari 2nd Stage, Bengaluru 560 070, Karnataka
  Ph: +91-80-26771678/79   Fax: +91-80-26771680   e-mail: bangalore@cbspd.com
- **Chennai:** 7, Subbaraya Street, Shenoy Nagar, Chennai-600 030, Tamil Nadu
  Ph: +91-44-26680620, 26681266   Fax: +91-44-42032115   e-mail: chennai@cbspd.com
- **Kochi:** 68/1534, 35, 36-Power House Road, Opp. KSEB, Cochin-682018, Kochi, Kerala
  Ph: +91-484-4059061-65   Fax: +91-484-4059065   e-mail: kochi@cbspd.com
- **Kolkata:** Hind Ceramics Compound, 1st floor, 147, Nilganj Road, Belghoria, Kolkata-700056, West Bengal
  Ph: +033-2563-3055/56   e-mail: kolkata@cbspd.com
- **Lucknow:** Basement, Khushnuma Complex, 7-Meerabai Marg (Behind Jawahar Bhawan), Lucknow-226001, Uttar Pradesh
  Ph: +0522-4000032   e-mail: tiwari.lucknow@cbspd.com
- **Mumbai:** PWD Shed, Gala No. 25/26, Ramchandra Bhatt Marg, Next to J.J. Hospital Gate No. 2, Opp. Union Bank of India, Noor Baug, Mumbai-400009, Maharashtra
  Ph: +91-22-66661880/89   Fax: +91-22-24902342   e-mail: mumbai@cbspd.com

Representatives

- **Hyderabad** +91-9885175004
- **Pune** +91-9623451994
- **Patna** +91-9334159340
- **Vijayawada** +91-9000660880

Printed at: Magic International Pvt. Ltd., Greater Noida, UP, India

Reviewers' List

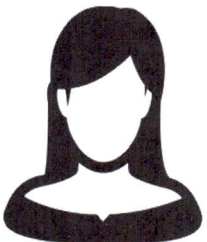

Meera K Pillai
Principal
Sree Gokulam Nursing College
Thiruvananthapuram, Kerala

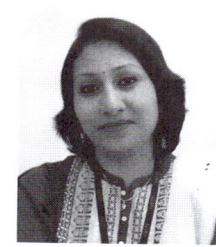

Sheuli Sen
MSc (Child Health Nursing)
Pursuing PhD
Professor
Amity College of Nursing
Amity University, Gurugram, Haryana

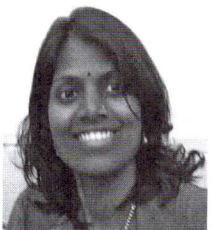

Prema Balusamy
MSc (Community Health Nursing)
PhD (N)
Principal
Muzaffarnagar Nursing Institute
Muzaffarnagar, Uttar Pradesh

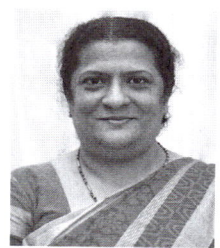

Shirley Prakash
MSc (Community Health Nursing)
Pursuing PhD
Principal
Westfort College of Nursing
Thrissur, Kerala

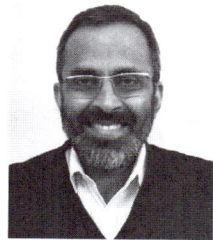

Roy K George
MSc (Psychiatric Nursing)
Pursuing PhD
Professor and Principal
College of Nursing
Academic Director
Baby Memorial Hospital (BMH)
Kozhikode, Kerala

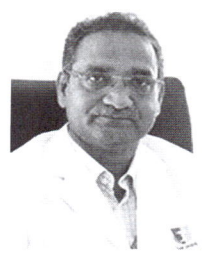

Suresh KN
MSc (N), Pursuing PhD
Professor/Principal
NS Memorial College of Nursing
Kollam and SIMET College of Nursing
Palluruthy, Kochi, Kerala

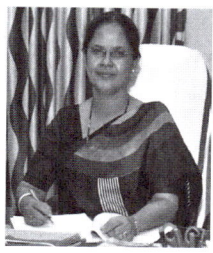

Saleena Shah
MSc (Medical Surgical Nursing), PhD
Registrar
Kerala Nurses and Midwives Council
Thiruvananthapuram, Kerala

The names of the reviewers are arranged in an alphabetical order.

Preface

"Strength and growth come only through continuous efforts and struggle"

—*Napoleon Hill*

Nurses play an integral role in the healthcare industry, like providing care to the patients and filling leadership roles at hospitals, health systems and other organizations. However, being a nurse comes with its own challenges. The profession demands a lot of dedication and commitment. Therefore, the student nurses, who are the future nurse leaders, nurse managers or nurse educators, need to be equipped with management skills to meet the challenges ahead.

Graduates from today's nursing education have great opportunities for professional practice and today's nursing students must learn more, do more and be more.

The aim of the book is to provide concise presentation of contents of nursing management with emphasis on effective responsive strategy.

This book is designed to address the knowledge thirst of undergraduate students with the student's experience in mind and to prepare them for university examinations. This textbook provides concise presentation of the essential nursing management content, providing ample opportunities to test the mastery over the subject. Care has been taken to appeal all learning styles. The student friendly writing style ensures that students will comprehend and retain information with consistent and cohesive learning experience. The consistency followed within the chapters ensures that the text is easy to understand. This book is being written according to curriculum prescribed by Indian Nursing Council and will also cater the needs of the students belonging to various other Indian Universities. The authors recognize the need of switching to the new strategies of nursing management.

Along with preparing the students for examination, this book also serves as a guide for future reference.

We appreciate suggestions for the improvement of this textbook in future editions and we welcome it with gratitude. We wish all the best for the future nurse managers.

Beena MR
Hari Krishna GL
Kiruba JC

Acknowledgements

Our profound gratitude to God Almighty for the guidance, strength and wisdom bestowed upon us on every step of the preparation and completion of the book.

We would like to thank our teachers for making us capable of writing this book.

We convey our sincere thanks to our parents, family members and friends for the exemplary help throughout the preparation of the book.

We would like to express our thanks to students and colleagues who have given their time, knowledge and understanding of what is required to promote nursing profession.

We would like to thank **Mr Satish Kumar Jain** (Chairman) and **Mr Varun Jain** (Managing Director), M/s CBS Publishers and Distributors Pvt Ltd for providing us the platform in bringing out the book. We have no words to describe the role, efforts, inputs and initiatives undertaken by **Mr Bhupesh Arora,** (Vice President - Publishing and Marketing, PGMEE and Nursing Division) for helping and motivating us.

We sincerely thank the entire CBS team for bringing the book colourful with utmost care and presentation. I thank Dr Mrinalini Bakshi (Editorial Head and Content Strategist) for her editorial support and Ms Nitasha Arora (Production Head & Content Strategist), Dr Anju Dhir (Senior Scientific Coordinator/Editor), Mr Nitish Dubey (Senior Editor) and all the production team members Mr Ashutosh Pathak, Mr Chaman Lal, Mr Prakash Gaur, Mr Phool Kumar, Mr Bunty Kashyap, Ms Tahira Parveen, Ms Babita Verma, Mr Chander, Mr Raju Sharma, Mr Manoj Chaudhary, Mr Vikram Chaudhary, Mr Manoj Malakar, Mr Arun Kumar and Ms Manorama for devoting laborious hours in designing and typesetting of the book. We also thank Ms Vasantha Chitra for her critical analysis of the manuscript which has helped us to strengthen the content of the book.

How to Make the Most Out of this Book?

The prime motto of writing this textbook is to make concepts of management easy to understand and comprehend by undergraduate students. Solved samples for correct application of concepts are incorporated in this book, which makes this textbook a unique one.

- **Unit 1:** **Introduction to Management in Nursing** introduces managerial concepts, difference between administration and management, principles, functions and theories of management.
- **Unit 2:** **Management Process** explains in detail about POSDCORB functions of management. It emphasises on planning—its types, principles and planning hierarchy, **Organization**—its principles, types, organizational structure, organizational chart, planning a hospital, **Staffing**—Recruitment, norms, staff development, **Controlling**—Quality control, quality assurance-objectives, models, approaches, tools etc. **Reporting and budgeting**—Principles, types and planning budget proposal for college and hospital. Also planning methods like PERT and Gantt Chart is explained using illustrations.
- **Unit 3:** **Management of Nursing Services in the Hospital and Community** explains about organization of hospital, nursing department, hospital planning and various departments, patient classification system, methods of patient assignment, job analysis, material management, delegation, supervision, standards, manuals, quality assurance, reporting and various records and reports in nursing service department, telemedicine, telenursing, electronic medical records, performance appraisal and nursing audit.
- **Unit 4:** **Organizational Behavior and Human Relations** focuses on various concepts related to organizational behavior (OB) like communication, leadership, motivation, transactional analysis, group dynamics, human relations and collective bargaining and unionization.
- **Unit 5:** **In-service Education** explains about types of ISE, components, approaches, principles of adult learning and standards.
- **Unit 6:** **Management of Nursing Educational Institutions** discusses about essentials of nursing institution, guidelines and minimum requirements of school/college of nursing, staffing, job description, staff and student welfare, staff development program, discipline and guidance.
- **Unit 7:** **Nursing as a Profession** explains about regulatory bodies, issues and challenges in nursing management, ethical principles, Consumer Protection Act, legal aspects and legal responsibilities in nursing.
- **Unit 8:** **Professional Development** discusses on career development, scope, informatics and management information system.

Overall, this book is intended to be accessible to the undergraduate (UG) students who are studying basics of nursing management.

Special Features of the Book

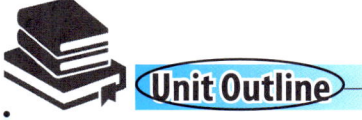

Unit Outline → Every unit contains an outline to give a brief view of the contents covered in it.

- Introduction
- Definitions of Management
- Nature of Management
- Importance of Management
- Concepts of Management
- Levels of Management
- Functions/Elements of Management
- Principles of Management
- Theories of Nursing Management
- Administration
- Role and Functions of Nurse as a Manager
- Management Roles
- Managerial Skills

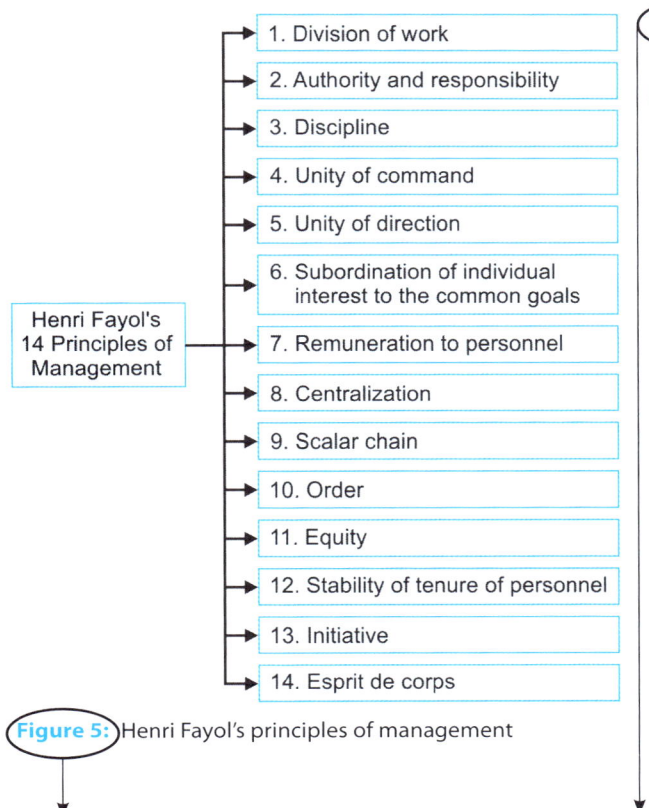

Figure 5: Henri Fayol's principles of management

The book is well illustrated with relevant figures.

Table 2: Differences between administration and management

Area	Administration	Management
Nature	It is a determinative or thinking function	It is an executive or doing function
Level of activity	It is mainly top level function	It is largely middle level or lower level
Function	Planning and control	Directing and organizing
Skills	Conceptual skill	Technical skill
Activity	Administration is concerned with the formation of objectives, plans and policies	Management is getting things done through and with people
	It is often associated with government policies	It is widely used in the business world
	It is more administrative rather than a technical activity	It needs more technical rather than administrative activity

Numerous tables have been used in the chapters to facilitate learning in a quick way.

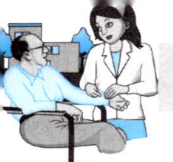

Box: 2

FAYOL'S Six Functions of Management
- Technical (production)
- Commercial (buying and selling)
- Financial (use of capital)
- Security (protection of property)
- Accounting (keeping financial records)
- Managerial skills

→ Boxes are used to highlight the important facts in the chapter wherever required.

Suggested Reading

→ Additional reading sources to enhance the knowledge bed are enlisted in suggested reading.

- Edythe L Alexander. Nursing Service Administration – Principles and Practice. The C V Mosby Company, New York.
- Harold Koontz, Heinz Weihrich. Essentials of Management – An International Perspective. Tata McGraw Hill Publishing Company Ltd. 2005, Delhi.
- Barret Jean. Ward Management and Teaching. Konark Publishers, Delhi.
- BT Basavanthappa. Nursing Administration. Jaypee Brothers Medical Publishers Pvt Ltd. Second edition 2009.
- CM Francis, Mario C Desouza. Hospital Administration 3rd edition. Jaypee Brothers Medical Publishers Pvt Ltd. New Delhi, 2000.
- Dr Sreeranganadhan and GG Mathews. Styles of Management in the Industries in Kerala, New Delhi Serial Publications.
- Satyasaran Chatterjee. An Introduction to Management, its Principles and Technique. The World Press Private Ltd. 1993, Calcutta.
- Patricia Kelly RN. Leadership and Management in Nursing. Cengage Learning India Ltd. 2000, New Delhi.

Assess Yourself

→ Important university level questions are enlisted at the end of every chapter to help students to assess their learning.

LONG ANSWERS

1. Define administration. Describe significance and scope of administration in modern society.
2. Discuss principles of management in detail with suitable examples.

SHORT NOTES

1. Trends and issues in nursing administration
2. Principles of administration
3. Functions/Elements of administration
4. Qualities of a good manager
5. Explain the role of a nurse as a manager
6. Concepts of management
7. Scope of management
8. Theories of management
9. Levels of management
10. Elements of administration

Contents

Unit 1 Introduction to Management in Nursing   1–16

- Introduction 2
- Definitions of Management 2
- Nature of Management 2
- Importance of Management 3
- Concepts of Management 3
- Levels of Management 3
- Functions/Elements of Management 4
- Principles of Management 6
- Theories of Nursing Management 7
- Administration 13
- Role and Functions of Nurse as a Manager 14
- Management Roles 15
- Managerial Skills 15

Unit 2 Management Process   17–55

- Planning 18
- Organizing 23
- Centralization and Decentralization 33
- Organizational Charts 33
- Staffing 35
- Human Resource Management 36
- Staffing Process 37
- Retention 40
- Separation 42
- Directing 42
- Control in Management/Controlling 44
- Planning Methods 46
- Bench Marking 49
- Budget 50

Unit 3 Management of Nursing Services in the Hospital and Community   57–126

- Nursing Service Administration 58
- Organization of a Hospital 60
- Hospital Planning 62
- Elements/Divisions of a Hospital 66
- Hospital Departments 66
- Hospital Ward 68
- Patient Classification Systems 70
- Progressive Patient Care 72
- Factors Influencing the Quality Patient Care 72
- Duty Roster 73

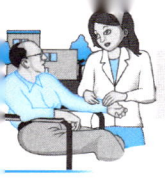

- Job Analysis 73
- Job Responsibilities of Different Categories of Nursing Personnel 74
- Steps in Budgetary Process 80
- Material Management 81
- Inventory Control 83
- Delegation 85
- Supervision 88
- Standards in Nursing 91
- Nursing Manuals 93
- Role of Head Nurse in Clinical Teaching 93
- Nursing Rounds 94
- Bedside Clinic 94
- Nursing Care Conference 95
- Ward Management Role of Head Nurse 96
- Accountability 97
- Quality Assurance 97
- Continuous Quality Improvement 104
- Total Quality Management 104
- Patient Record System/Documentation 105
- Documentation 105
- Records and Reports of the CNO Office 108
- Telemedicine/Tele Health 109
- Telenursing 110
- Electronic Medical Records 111
- Performance Appraisal 112
- Nursing Audit 117
- Conclusion 120
- Disaster Management 120
- Phases of Disaster 120
- Disaster Nursing: Role of Nurse Administrator 123

Unit 4 Organizational Behavior and Human Relations 127–154

- Organizational Behavior 128
  - Definition 128
  - Concepts of Organizational Behavior 128
  - Elements/Factors Affecting Organizational Behavior 128
  - Approaches to Organizational Behavior 129
  - Organizational Behavior Models 129
  - Dependent and Independent Variables in Organizational Behavior 130
  - Challenges for Organizational Behavior 131
  - Communication 131
  - Transactional Analysis 132
  - Johari Window 134
  - Leadership 135
  - Motivation 142
  - Group Dynamics 147
- Human Relations 150
  - Public Relations 150
  - Union 152
  - Collective Bargaining 152

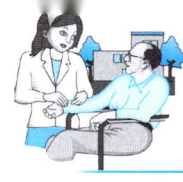

Unit 5 In-service Education   155–163

- Staff Development 156
- Types of Staff Development Program 156
- In-service Education 156
  - Definition of In-service Education 156
  - Objectives of In-service Education 156
  - Aims of In-service Education 156
  - Concept of In-service Education 156
  - Scope of In-service Education 156
  - Components/Organization/Types of In-service Education 157
  - Approaches/Types of In-service Education 158
  - Factors Affecting In-service Education 158
  - Characteristics of a Good
    In-service Education Program 159
  - Principles for Developing an In-service Education Program 159
  - Problems of In-service Education Program 159
  - Benefits of In-service Education Program 159
  - Planning of In-service Educational Program 159
  - Steps in Developing In-service Program 159
  - Conditions for Success of In-service Program 160
  - Methods of In-service Educational Program 160
  - Evaluation of In-service Program 160
  - Sample In-service Education Plan 160
  - Conclusion 161
- Adult Learning 161
  - Principles of Adult Learning 161
  - Knowles' 5 Assumptions of Adult Learners 162
  - Knowles' 4 Principles of Andragogy 162
  - Characteristics of Adult Learners 162
  - Adult Learning Cycle 162
  - Factors Affecting Adult Learning 162
- Standards of Staff Development Program According to American Nurses Association 163

Unit 6 Management of Nursing Educational Institutions   165–192

- Introduction 166
- Organization of Nursing Educational Institutions 166
- Essentials of Educational Institutions as per INC Norms 166
- Guidelines and Minimum Requirements to Establish School of Nursing 166
- Minimum Requirement to Establish General Nursing and Midwifery Program 167
- Teaching Faculty—Qualifications and Experience in School of Nursing 170
- Budget 171
- Affiliation 171
- Distribution of Beds 171
- Staffing 172
- Admission Terms and Conditions 172
- Health Services 173
- Institutional Records 173
- Transcript 173

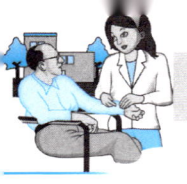

- Credit System 173
- Guidelines and Minimum Requirements to Establish BSc (N) College of Nursing 173
- Recognition, Affiliation and Accreditation 178
- Management of Faculty 180
- Job Description of Faculty College of Nursing..180
- Staff Welfare..182
- Staff Development Program 183
- Administration of Students..184
- Discipline in Educational Institutions...188
- Administration of Curriculum..189

Unit 7 Nursing as a Profession   193–210

- Profession..194
- Nursing as a Profession..194
- Regulatory Bodies..196
- Issues and Challenges in Nursing Management 197
- Ethical and Legal Aspects in Nursing 198
  - Ethical Principles 198
  - Code of Ethics...200
  - Standards for Nursing Practice/Code of Professional Conduct 202
  - Patient's Bill of Rights 203
  - Consumer Protection Act 204
  - Redressal Agency..204
  - Legal Aspects in Nursing 205
  - Legal Safe Guards in Nursing Practice..207
  - Ethical and Legal Issues in Nursing 208
  - Legal Responsibilities of Nurses 208
  - Hospital Ethics Committee...209

Unit 8 Professional Development   211–220

- Career Development in Nursing..212
- Career Opportunities in Nursing 212
- Scope of Nursing Career 213
- Membership With Professional Organization: National and International...................................214
- Professional Organization at National Level 215
- Nursing Informatics 217
- Management Information System 218
- Application of Nursing Informatics 220

Index..*221*

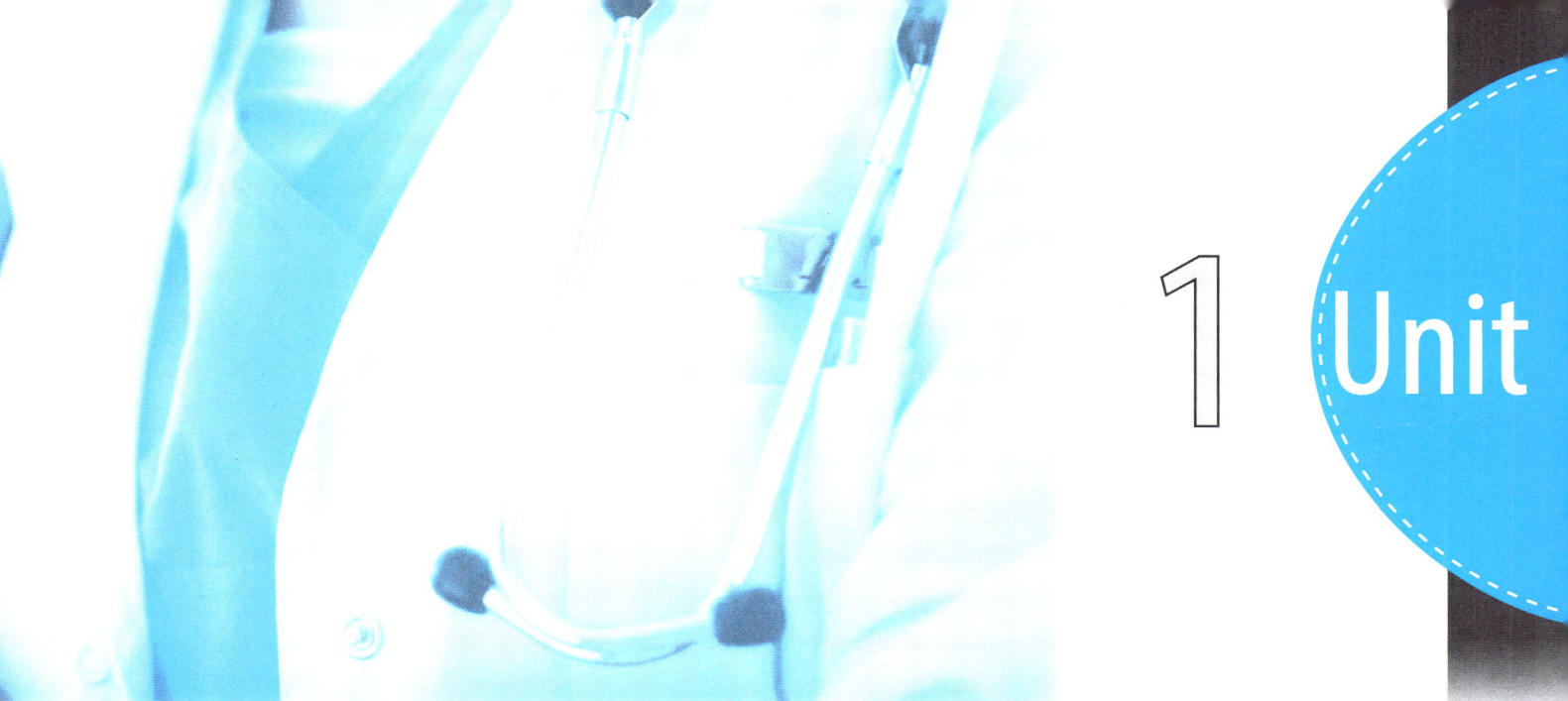

Unit 1

INTRODUCTION TO MANAGEMENT IN NURSING

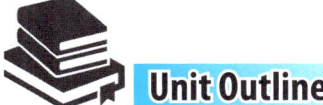

Unit Outline

- Introduction
- Definitions of Management
- Nature of Management
- Importance of Management
- Concepts of Management
- Levels of Management
- Functions/Elements of Management
- Principles of Management
- Theories of Nursing Management
- Administration
- Role and Functions of Nurse as a Manager
- Management Roles
- Managerial Skills

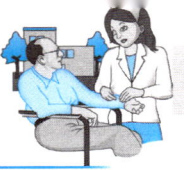

INTRODUCTION

Management is essential for life and is necessary to run all types of organizations. People began forming groups to accomplish aims they could not achieve as individuals and here came the role of management so as to accomplish the tasks in an organized manner. Traditional authors defined management as an art of getting things done and modern authors view management as a process to achieve objectives through utilization of resources. Management involves making plans and decisions about the future needs of business. Management is about making cost effective use of resources through efficient organization and control on overall process. Good management is essential for the success of an organization.

Today, management has become a theory jungle due to various theories put forth by contributions of scholars and writers from different disciplines of sciences, like sociology, psychology, social psychology, cultural anthropology, political science, economics, statistics and others. These contributions have created a diversity in understanding the concepts of management. **Health management** is a process with interpersonal and technical aspects through which the objectives of health service organizations are specified and accompanied by utilizing human and physical resources and technology.

DEFINITIONS OF MANAGEMENT

Management is the process of designing and maintaining an environment in which individuals working together in groups, efficiently to accomplish selected goals.
—*Heinz Weihrich and Harold Koontz*

Management is defined as the art of securing maximum results with minimum of efforts so as to secure maximum prosperity and happiness for both employer and employee and give public the best possible evidence. —*John Mee F*

Management is the creation and maintenance of an internal environment in an enterprise where individuals working in groups can perform efficiently and effectively toward the attainment of group goals. —*Koontz and Donnel*

Management is an organ of society specifically charged with making resources productive. —*Ducker*

Management is a problem-solving process of effectively achieving organizational objectives through the efficient use of scarce resources in a changing environment.
—*Robert Kreitner*

Management is the coordination of all resources through the process of planning, organizing, directing and controlling in order to attain stated objectives. —*FW Taylor*

NATURE OF MANAGEMENT

Management is an activity or process composed of some basic functions for getting the objectives accomplished through a team and with the focused efforts of its personnel. As human, aims and beliefs are mostly realized through the establishment of diverse institutions in our society, management is usually needed for operating all such organizations. Management acts as a creative and invigorating force in the organization. It provides new ideas, imaginations and visions for the group functioning and integrates its efforts in such a manner as to account for better results. Management involves plans and decisions about the future needs to run an organization successfully.

Management is always concerned about productivity. It enables the organization to survive in changing environment. Management is the core of an organization. Its main aim is to get maximum achievement through minimum resources. The main features of management are given below:

- *Management is a universal process*: The process of management can be noticed in all spheres of life.
- *Management is goal oriented*: The most important goal of management is to achieve objectives of the organization in an efficient and cost effective manner.
- *Management determines and accomplishes the goals of an organization*.
- *Management is universal in character*: The principles of management are equally applicable in various fields like business, education, military, etc.
- *Management is a group activity*: For efficient achievement of objectives, all human and physical resources are efficiently coordinated.
- *Management is a distinct process*.
- *Management is an integrated force*: It integrates human and other resources.
- *Management is intangible*: It cannot be seen but its presence can be felt.
- *Management is a continuous and ongoing process*.
- *Management is a process*: The process is primarily concerned with achievement of goals of management.
- *Management is multi-disciplinary in nature*: Management is multi-disciplinary as it has drawn contributions from various disciplines like economics, sociology, psychology, anthropology, philosophy and statistics. etc.
- *Management as science, art and a profession*.

In a nutshell, we can say that:

Management is an art as well as a science (Box 1).

Box: 1

As a science, management has:
- Systematic body of knowledge
- Scientific method of observation
- Universally accepted principles
- Predictability of results based on cause-effect relationship

As an art management has:
- Practical knowledge
- Personal skill and creativity
- Tangible results
- Constructive objectives
- Perfection through practice

IMPORTANCE OF MANAGEMENT

Management is beneficial to the society. It raises the standard of living of people and promotes peace and prosperity in the society. Management is an essential component of all social organizations.

According to Peter F Drucker, the significance of management is:
- Management determines and accomplishes the goals of an organization.
- Management ensures effective utilization of resources as man, material and money.
- Management has vision for recognition.
- Management directs the organization.
- It helps to establish team spirit.
- Management helps to establish sound organizational structure.
- Management provides innovation.
- Management is the crucial factor to economic and social development.

CONCEPTS OF MANAGEMENT

General Concepts

Manager is a formal, specifically designated position within the organization. To be a good manager, it is absolutely necessary to be an effective leader. In fact all nurses should at times assume some leadership roles.

Sub Concepts

- **Authority:** Authority is the legitimate right given to a manager by an organization in order to command subordinates and to act in the interest of an organization to achieve its goals.
- **Power:** Power is capacity to influence others to act, and it is the most important ingredient of a manager in an organization.
- Effectiveness and efficiency

Specific Concepts

Different scholars have their own specific way of describing specific concepts on management. The selective concepts are as follows:

According to Raymond Gi Leon

- **Management by communication:** According to this concept, the success of management depends upon the successful communication.
- **Management by systems:** This refers to recognizing the problems, analyzing it and defining the objectives. It is more concerned with experimentation and analysis.
- **Management by results:** This concept states that the end results are significant. Management is result oriented. Success and strength of management is determined by the results.
- **Management by participation:** This concept takes worker into confidence, helps to create a sense of involvement among the workers.
- **Management by motivation:** It is among the chief tasks of the general management to keep team motivated.
- **Management by exception:** It is a special skill of managing by attending only to exceptionally important matters and taking vital decisions.
- **Management by objectives:** It is a dynamic system which seeks to integrate the company's need to clarify and achieve its profit and growth goals with the manager's needs to contribute and develop himself. It is a demanding and rewarding style of managing a business.

According to Dr C B Gupta

- **Management as an economic resource:** Management is a vital factor of production.
- **Management as a team:** As a team, management consists of all personnel having managerial responsibility.
- **Management as an academic discipline:** Management implies a branch of knowledge. It comprises management theory and principles.
- **Management as a process:** Management is described in terms of what managers do? It involves organizing, directing and controlling human efforts to accomplish predetermined goals.
- **Management as a human process:** According to this concept, manager get things done through and with the help of people. The study of management should be centered around the workers and their interpersonal relations.
- **Management is the effective utilization of human and material resources**
- **Management is concerned about ideas, things and people:**
  - **Management of ideas:** It is the job of management to generate, organize and articulate creative ideas and transform these into operating results.
  - **Management of things:** Refers to mobilization and allocation of material, machinery, technology and other facilities to connect ideas into results and performance.
  - **Management of people:** Refers to procurement, development, maintenance and integration of human beings working in the organization. It is the most important task of a manager.

LEVELS OF MANAGEMENT (FIG. 1)

The levels of management determines chain of command, amount of authority and status enjoyed by any managerial position.

The different levels of management include: Top Level Management (Administrative level), Middle level (executory level) and Low level (supervisory/operative/first-line).

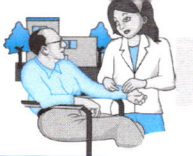

Figure 1: Levels of management

Top level management:
Involved in delegation, leadership, empowerment, change management

Middle level management:
Talent development, team building, problem solving

Low level management:
Emotional intelligence and mentoring

Table 1: Level of skills in different levels of management

Skills	Top level	Middle level	Low level
Intellectual skills	+++++++	++++	+++
Human skills	+++	++++++	+++++
Technical skills	+++	+++	++++++++

Top Level Management

Top level management is constituted by chairman, head of organization, directors, etc. They are responsible for day to day decisions according to changing scenario. The main functions of 'Top Level Management' are:

Levels of skills in different levels of management is depicted above in Table 1.

- Make an outline of planning through formation of basic objectives and policies of service.
- Arrange staffing of the department.
- Prepare overall budget for operation.
- Plan policies and programs
- Effective coordination of all activities.
- Ensure continuity of services focusing changing technology.
- Maintain public relations with all beneficiaries.
- Ensure documentation that is accountable.
- Plan activities for development of manpower.

Middle Level Management

The level of management between top level and operational level management is called as middle level management. It is constituted by divisional and departmental heads. The main functions of 'middle level management' are:

- Develop objectives and policies based on aims of the institution.
- Formulate departmental budget.
- Execute programs through orders, instructions and advice.
- Develop standards and criteria for evaluation.
- Assess adequate utilization of resources.
- Proper coordination between top level and operative level management.

Low Level Management

It is the lowest level management constituted by administrative officers or section charges. They are managers who coordinate and supervise the activities of employees. The main functions of this category are:

- To translate plan into action
- To assign work to subordinates
- Provide a favorable environment for workers
- Provide adequate facilities, supplies and equipment
- To ensure control and coordination of all functions
- Supervision of subordinates
- Ensure quality service
- Maintain good human relations

FUNCTIONS/ELEMENTS OF MANAGEMENT

Luther Halsey Gullick (1892–1993) was born in Osaka, Japan and he was the first Director of the National Institute of Public Administration, USA (Fig. 2). He summed up functions of management in the acronym '**POSDCORB**' (Fig. 3):

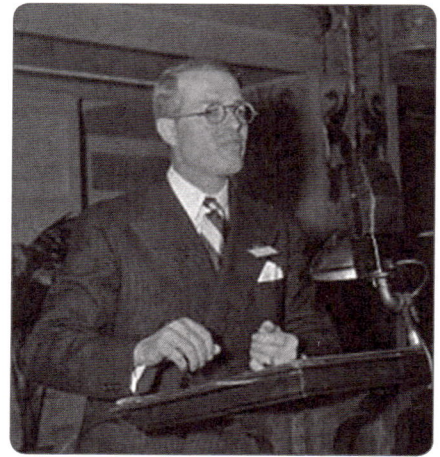

Figure 2: Luther Halsey Gullick

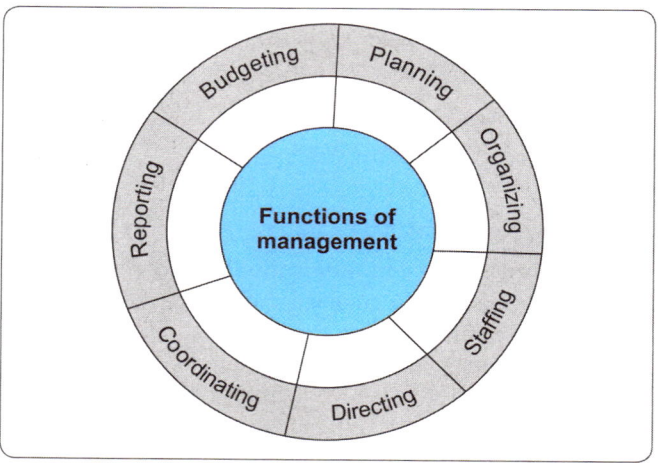

Figure 3: Functions of management – POSDCORB

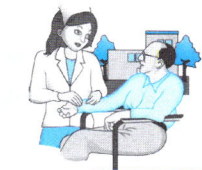

- **P**lanning
- **O**rganizing
- **S**taffing
- **D**irecting
- **Co**ordination
- **R**eporting
- **B**udgeting

We will discuss them now in detail.

Planning

It is the basic function of management. It deals with chalking out a future course of action and deciding in advance the most appropriate course of actions for the achievement of pre-determined goals. According to Koontz, "Planning is deciding in advance—what to do, when to do and how to do. It bridges the gap from where we are and where we want to be?"

A plan is a future course of actions. It is an exercise in problem solving and decision making. Planning is determination of courses of action to achieve desired goals. Thus, planning is a systematic thinking about ways and means for accomplishment of predetermined goals. Planning is necessary to ensure proper utilization of human and nonhuman resources. It is all pervasive, it is an intellectual activity and it also helps in avoiding confusion, uncertainties, risks, wastages etc. Planning is a systematic way of making decisions. It is rational and orderly thinking about ways and means for realization of certain goals. During this phase the manager ascertain what the work is, how and when the work is to be done, and who is to do the work. Planning is an ongoing process. Planning involves:

- Identification of the present situation
- Formulation of aims and objectives
- Identification of alternative plans
- Selection of the best alternative
- Preparation of action plan
- Implementation
- Follow up and review

Organizing

Organizing is an activity by which managers bring together the resources for action. It provides the mechanism for purposive, integrated and cooperative action by two or more persons to implement a plan which includes determination of activities and assigning the jobs for employees. Organization process involves:

- Find out the tasks that must be performed in the organization and grouping them in a logical pattern
- Assigning tasks to the workers
- Delegating authority and responsibility
- Coordinate the activities

Staffing

It is the function of manning the organization structure and keeping it manned. Staffing has assumed greater importance in the recent years due to advancement of technology, increase in size of business, complexity of human behavior etc. The main purpose of staffing is to put right man on right job, i.e. square pegs in square holes and round pegs in round holes.

According to Kootz and O'Donell, "Managerial function of staffing involves manning the organization structure through proper and effective selection, appraisal and development of personnel to fill the roles designed and the structure". Staffing involves:

- Manpower planning (estimating man power in terms of searching, choose the person and giving the right place)
- Recruitment, selection and placement
- Training and development
- Remuneration
- Performance appraisal
- Promotions and transfer

Directing

Directing is largely a function of human relations and motivation. The managers direct the employees through the medium of leadership, supervision, communication, motivation, guidance and counseling. The employees are inspired and motivated to do the job with team spirit. Directing involves guiding and overseeing the personnel at work with a view to secure their cooperation through maintenance of their interpersonal and group relations. Directing is concerned with issuing of orders, assignments and instructions that permit the subordinates to contribute effectively and efficiently to achieve goals. Direction has following elements:

- Supervision
- Motivation
- Leadership
- Communication

Supervision

It implies overseeing the work of subordinates by their superiors. It is the act of watching and directing work and workers.

Motivation

It means inspiring, stimulating or encouraging the subordinates with zeal to work. Positive, negative, monetary, nonmonetary incentives may be used for this purpose.

Leadership

It may be defined as a process by which manager guides and influences the work of subordinates in desired direction.

Communication

It is the process of passing information, experience, opinion etc. from one person to another. It is a bridge of understanding.

Controlling

It implies measurement of accomplishment against the standards and correction of deviation if any to ensure

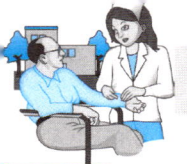

achievement of organizational goals. The purpose of controlling is to ensure that everything occurs in conformities with the standards. An efficient system of control helps to predict deviations before they actually occur.

According to *Theo Haimann*, "Controlling is the process of checking whether or not proper progress is being made toward the objectives and goals and acting if necessary, to correct any deviation". According to Koontz and O'Donell "Controlling is the measurement and correction of performance activities of subordinates in order to make sure that the enterprise objectives and plans desired to obtain them are being accomplished".

Controlling has following steps:
- Establishment of standard performance
- Measurement of actual performance
- Comparison of actual performance with the standards and finding out deviation if any
- Corrective action

Coordination

Coordination is the unification, integration, synchronization of the efforts of group members so as to provide unity of action in the pursuit of common goals. It is a hidden force which binds all the other functions of management. According to Mooney and Reelay, "Coordination is orderly arrangement of group efforts to provide unity of action in the pursuit of common goals". According to Charles Worth, "Coordination is the integration of several parts into an orderly hole to achieve the purpose of understanding".

Reporting

It refers to keeping those to whom the executive is responsible, informed as to what is going on.

Budgeting

Budget is the heart of administrative management. It is based on expected income and expenditure and is expressed in monetary terms. Budget should be flexible, and be a synthesis of past, present and future.

Functions of Management by Henri Fayol (Fig. 4)

Henri Fayol (1841-1925) was a French manager and industrialist. He was one of the first theorists to define functions of management in his book "Administration Industrielle et Generale". He is known as 'Father of Modern Operational Management'. Henri Fayol identified functions of management: **forecasting and planning, organizing, commanding, coordinating and controlling**. Henri Fayol theorized that these functions were universal and that every manager performed these functions in their daily work.
- **Forecasting and planning**
- **Organizing**

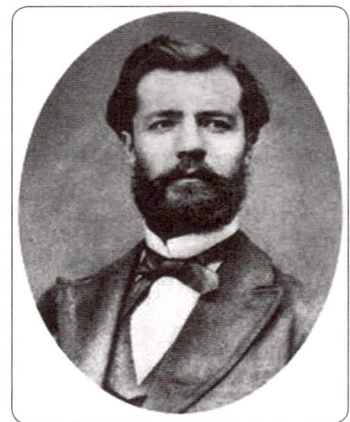

Figure 4: Henri Fayol

- **Commanding**
- **Coordinating**
- **Controlling**

PRINCIPLES OF MANAGEMENT

Henry Fayol has suggested 14 principles of management. According to him there is nothing rigid or absolute in management affairs, it is all a question of proportion. Thus these principles are flexible and capable of adaptation to every need. Principles of management summarized by the Father of functional management that is Henri Fayol are (Fig. 5):

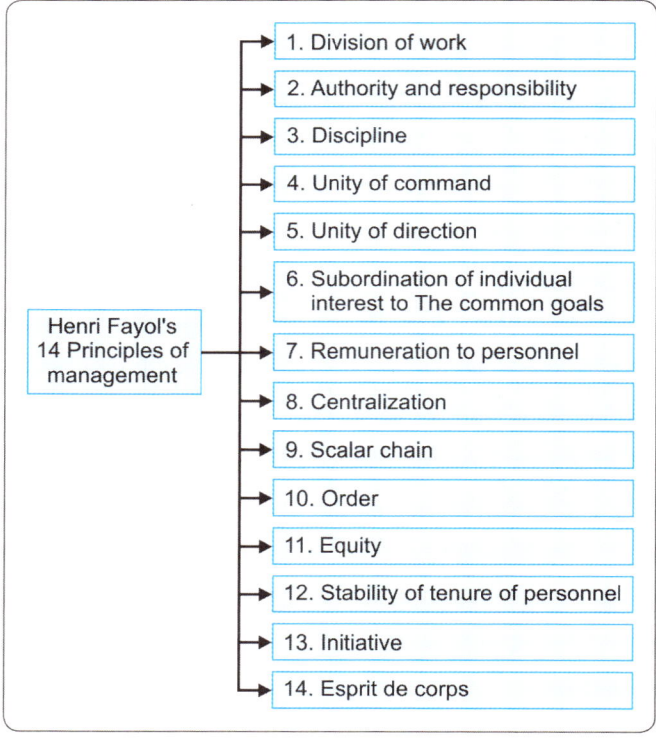

Figure 5: Henri Fayol's principles of management

- **Division of work:** According to Henri Fayol, works of all kinds must be divided and subdivided and allotted to workers. Work should be divided among individuals and groups to ensure that efforts and attention are focused on special portions of the task.
- **Authority and responsibility:** Fayol defined authority as the right to give orders and power to extract obedience. Authority means certain rights, powers and permission to act for the organization, give orders to subordinates and to control and coordinate all functions. The concept of authority and responsibilities are closely related. Responsibility involves being accountable or the duty which subordinates are expected to do.
- **Discipline:** Each employer and employee must maintain discipline. This principle suggests that the organization is required to have a set of clearly defined rules and regulations.
- **Unity of command:** An employer should receive orders from only one superior at a time which is necessary to avoid confusion and conflict regarding roles and responsibility. Dual command confuses employees and disturbs stability.
- **Unity of direction:** The organization should be moving toward a common objective. All similar activities are grouped together and should be supervised by one supervisor and have one plan of action. According to Fayol for the accomplishment of a group of activities having the same objectives, there should be one head and one plan.
- **Subordination of individual interest to the common goals:** The interest of one person should not take priority over the interest of the organization as a whole.
- **Remuneration to personnel:** Remuneration to employee should be fair and satisfactory to both the parties. The remuneration is just and equitable for both employee and employer.
- **Centralization:** Fayol defined centralization as lowering the importance of the subordinate role. He mentioned everything which goes to increase the importance of subordinator's role is decentralization.
- **Scalar chain:** Scalar chain is the line of authority from the highest executive to the lowest employer, especially for the purpose of communication. The existence of scalar chain and adherence to it is necessary if the organization has to be successful.
  Scalar chain states superior subordinate relationship throughout the concern. It is essential in an organization to ensure unity of command and effective communication. But there are some limitations to scalar chain.
    - The communication takes more time as the order flows from top level managers to bottom level.
    - There is also chances of distortion of messages during the flow of transmission. However, a gang plank may be created by passing the established line of authority to allow quick communication.

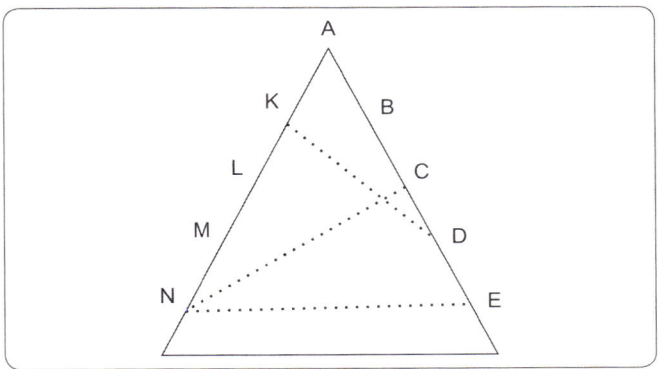

Figure 6: Scalar chain of command

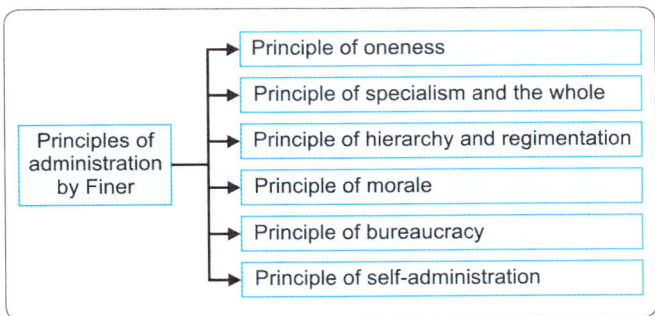

Figure 7: Finer's principles of administration

In the Figure 6 any communication from N to E will flow upward to A through M, N, L, K and downward through B, C, D, E. In order to minimize the delay in communication a 'gang plank' between K to D, N to C or N to E etc. may be created as shown using dotted line in the Figure 6.

- **Order:** Fayol pointed out that there should be a place for everything and everyone. All equipment and materials related to a specific kind of work should be in proper order.
- **Equity:** Equity means justice and kindness. All employees should be treated as equally as possible.
- **Stability of tenure of personnel:** Retaining productive employees should always be a high priority of management.
- **Initiative:** Initiative means freedom to think and implement plan.
- **Esprit de corps:** Esprit de corps means the spirit of loyalty and devotion which unites the workers in an enterprise. Management should ensure harmony and general good feeling among employees.

THEORIES OF NURSING MANAGEMENT

Theory is a set of interrelated concepts, statements, propositions and definitions which have been derived from philosophical beliefs of scientific data and from which questions or hypotheses can be deducted, tested and verified. There are several theories of management. Concept of management has attracted the attention of psychologists, sociologists, anthropologists, mathematicians, political scientists, economists and so on. They have given different theories, based on management in later part of the 19th century and early 20th centuries. Some of these theories have been discussed here:

Classification of nursing theories

Based on the field of vision that is contained in a theory, nursing theories can be classified as:

- **Meta theory:** It focuses on major issues related to philosophy, methods of generating knowledge and development of theory.
- **Grand theory:** These are macro theories that focus on broad concepts and are applied to a general area within a particular discipline.
- **Middle range theories:** They lie between nursing models and practice theories.
- **Practice theories:** They are micro theories, more specific than middle range theories.

Basic theories which explain the management of nursing are:

- Classical theory
- Neoclassical theory
- Behavioral science theory
- Modern theory

Classical Theory

The term classical means something traditionally accepted or long-established.

It does not mean that classical views are static and time bound that must be dispensed with.

Some of the elements of classical theory are still with us, in one form or other. The features of classical theory are:

- **Interrelated functions:** Management consists of several inter-related and interdependent functions (planning, organizing, staffing, directing and controlling) which are exercised in a sequential form. This is repeated over and over again to bring a systematic order out of chaos.
- **Guiding principles:** In order to increase the knowledge there are certain principles based on practical experience.
- **Bureaucratic structure:** For maximum efficiency, this theory specified that the work must be logically divided into simple, routine and repetitive tasks. These tasks should then be grouped according to similar work characteristics and arranged in the form of departments. Work must be assigned to individuals based on job demands and the individual's ability to do the job. The organization has complex mechanisms, rules, regulations and procedures. The whole structure takes the shape of a pyramid. As the organization grows and develops in—operation grows in size. It would inevitably acquire a bureaucratic, pyramidal structure, as shown in Figure 8.
- **Reward and punishment nexus:** Follow the rules, obey the orders, show the results and get the rewards. If you lag behind in the race, you will become a second-class citizen and not entitled to receive extra benefits. Great emphasis is put on efficient use of resources while producing results.

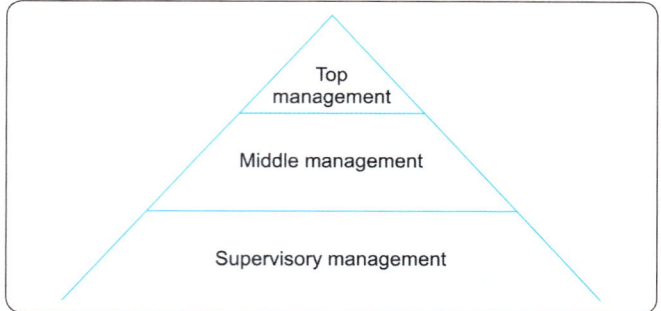

Figure 8: Pyramid structure of classical theory

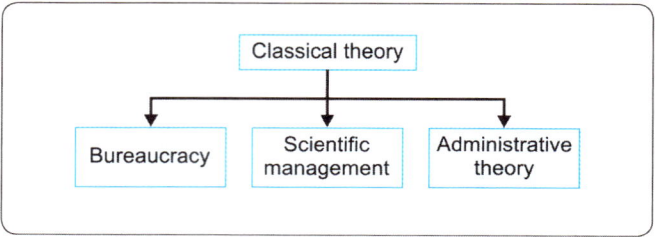

Figure 9: Parts of classical theory

Parts of Classical Theory (Fig. 9)

Bureaucracy

Classical organization especially was developed by FW Taylor. The word 'bureaucracy' implies an organization characterized by rules, procedures, impersonal relations and elaborate and fairly rigid hierarchy of authority-responsibility relationships. Persons with proper qualifications are selected so that the work is done efficiently.

Main elements of bureaucracy

- **Hierarchy:** Hierarchy is a way of ranking various positions in descending order from top to bottom of an organization. Ultimately, no office is left uncontrolled in the organization.
- **Division of work:** The total work is divided into specialized jobs. Each person's job is broken down into simple, routine and well-defined tasks. Each employee knows his boundaries.
- **Rules, regulations and procedures:** The behavior of employees is regulated through a set of rules. Employees are expected to follow these rules strictly.
- **Records:** Proper records have to be kept for everything. Files have to be maintained to record the decisions and activities of the organization on a day to day basis for future use.
- **Impersonal relationships:** Everything should proceed according to rules. There is no room for personal involvement, emotions and sentiments. If an employee comes late, whether he is a manager or a peon, the rules must be same for all.
- **Administrative class:** Bureaucracies generally have administrative class responsible for coordinating the work.

These officials are selected on the basis of their competence and skills. They are paid salary, which increases according to age and experience and they receive a pension when retire. Promotion is based on seniority and achievement, decided by judgment of senior officials.

Advantages of a bureaucratic structure

- **Specialization:** People can specialize in their respective fields and show improved performance.
- **Rationality:** Bureaucracy brings rationality to an organization. Judgments are made according to an objective and these are generally based upon criteria. Logical structuring of activities brings about orderly execution of assigned tasks.
- **Predictability:** The rules, regulations, training, specialization, structure and other elements of bureaucracy enable it to provide predictability and stability of an organization.
- **Democracy:** In bureaucratic organizations, decisions are arrived at, according to an acceptable criteria. People are selected on the basis of merit. Patronage and favoritism are not given weightage. Because the opportunity to train, apply and be selected for a job is open to every citizen, a significant degree of democracy is achieved.

Disadvantages of bureaucratic structure

- **Rigidity:** Critics of bureaucracy claim that it is rigid, static and inflexible. Strict adherence to rules produces timidity, conservatism and techniques. In the name of following rules, people may even shirk away from their responsibilities.
- **Impersonality:** Bureaucracy emphasizes mechanical way of doing things. Rules and regulations are glorified, in place of employee's needs or emotions.
- **Displacement of objectives:** Specialists may concentrate on their own finely toned goals and forget their goal area meant for reaching the broader objectives of the organization.
- **Compartmentalization of activities:** Strict categorization of work, restricts people from performing tasks that they are capable of doing.
- **Red tape:** Bureaucracies are paper mills. Everything is recorded on paper. Files move through endless official channels, resulting in inordinate delays.

Scientific Management

Frederick Winslow Taylor (1856–1915) has given the concept of scientific management. He is known as Father of 'Scientific Management'. Scientific management is an approach that emphasizes the scientific study of work in order to improve worker efficiency.

Basics of scientific management

It is based on 4 basic principles:
1. Each task must be scientifically designed so that it can replace the old.
2. Workers must be scientifically selected and trained so that they can be more productive on their jobs.
3. Bring the scientifically designed jobs and workers together so that there will be a match between them.
4. There must be division of labor and cooperation between management and workers.

> **Taylor's philosophy in a nutshell**
> - Based on science, not rule of thumb
> - Attained by harmony and not discard
> - Can yield maximum output, in place of restricted output
> - Maximum prosperity of employer, coupled with maximum prosperity of each employee

Limitations of scientific management

- **Exploitative device:** Emphasis on productivity rather than sharing the benefits with workers.
- **Depersonalized work:** Scientific management supply standardized jobs to workers. They continue with the same job throughout their career which leads to boredom and monotony, so workers do not like the ideas of becoming glorified machines.
- **Un-psychological:** Because there is no accurate information as to how the wages are to be given, it is not based on psychological results.
- **Undemocratic:** Because it overshadows the workers independence and treats workers as unthinking animals.
- **Antisocial:** Because workers are treated as glorified economic tools only which is antisocial element.
- **Unrealistic:** Only concentrated on physical and financial needs and completely ignoring the social as well as ego needs of people.

Administrative Theory: Henry Fayol (1841-1925)

This is an approach that focuses on principles that can be used by managers to coordinate the internal activities of an organization. According to Fayol the functions of management are: *Forecasting and Planning, Organizing, Commanding, Coordination*, and *Controlling*.

Fayol emphasized that managers should have certain skills in order to carry on their work efficiently and these are:
- Good physical health
- Mental ability to understand, learn and judge a situation
- Moral strength (energy, initiative, loyalty, tact and dignity)
- Educational background (acquaintance with matters)
- Technical skills (specialized knowledge relating to one's area of specialization)
- Experience related to the work being carried out (Box 2)

> **Box: 2**
>
> **FAYOL'S SIX Functions of Management:**
> - Technical (production)
> - Commercial (buying and selling)
> - Financial (use of capital)
> - Security (protection of property)
> - Accounting (keeping financial records)
> - Managerial skills

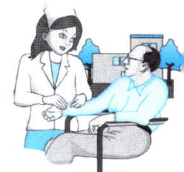

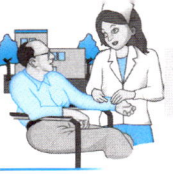

Management functions

Forecasting and Planning, Organizing, Commanding, Coordination, Controlling

Principles of management

Fayol gave certain principles of management which are given below:
- Division of work
- Authority and responsibility
- Discipline
- Unity of command
- Unity of direction
- Subordination of individual interest to the common goal
- Remuneration of personnel
- Order
- Centralization
- Scalar chain
- Equity
- Stability of tenure
- Initiative
- Esprit de corps

Limitations of fayol's theory

- **Lack of empirical evidence:** For example, the principle specialization does not tell us the way to divide the tasks.
- **Neglect of human factor:** Human attributes such as emotion, attitude and creativity have been totally ignored.
- **Pro-management bias:** It suffers from pro-management bias. It is more concerned with what managers should know and do rather than with a more general understanding of managerial behavior.

Neoclassical Theory

It is also known as 'Human Relations Theory'. Neoclassical theory is the modification of classical theory including insights from behavioral sciences like psychology, sociology and anthropology. Human relations movement began with Hawthorne studies, which were conducted from 1924 to 1933 at Hawthorne Plant of Western Electric Company in Cicero by Elton Mayo and Chester Bernard.

It is defined as movement in management thinking and practice that emphasized satisfaction of employees basic needs as the key to increased worker productivity.

Characteristics of Neoclassical Theory

- Structural organization is a social system.
- Behavior is a product of feelings, sentiments and attitudes.
- Primary focus is on small groups, on emotional and human qualities of employees.
- Emphasizes personal, security and social needs of workers while achieving organizational goals.
- Democratic practices, participation of employees in decision making in order to improve morale and happiness of employees. It recognizes the importance of human dignity and values.
- Happy employees trying to produce more.

Behavioral Science Theory

It includes theories of leadership and motivation.

Theories of Leadership

Trait Theory of Leadership

'Trait' is defined as *a relatively enduring quality of an individual*. The trait approach seeks to determine 'what makes a successful leader' from the leader's own personal characteristics. Research on leadership traits suggests that some factors differentiate leaders from non-leaders. The most important traits are a high level of personal drive, desire to lead, personal integrity and self-confidence. Cognitive (analytical) ability, knowledge, charisma, creativity and flexibility are also desired. The various traits can be classified into innate and acquirable traits, on the basis of their source. These qualities are natural and often known as God-gifted. The individuals cannot acquire these qualities. Major innate qualities in a successful leader are:

- *Physical features:* Physical features of a man are determined by heredity factors. Heredity is the transmission of the qualities from ancestor to descendent. Physical characteristics and rate of maturation determine the personality formation which is an important factor in determining leadership success.
- *Intelligence:* For leadership, higher level of intelligence is required. Intelligence is generally expressed in terms of mental ability. Intelligence, to a very great extent, is a natural quality in the individuals because it is directly related to the brain.

Acquirable qualities of leadership are those which can be acquired and increased through various processes. Many of these traits can be increased through training programs. Following are the major qualities essential for leadership:
- *Emotional stability:* A leader should have high level of emotional stability. He should be free from bias, consistent in action and refrain from anger. He is well adjusted and believes that he can meet most situations successfully.
- *Human relations:* A successful leader should have adequate knowledge of human relations. An important part of a leader's job is to develop people and get their voluntary cooperation for achieving work. He should have intimate knowledge of how human beings behave and how they react to various situations.
- *Empathy:* Empathy relates to observing the things or situations from other's points of view. The ability to look at things objectively and understanding them from others' point of view is an important aspect of successful leadership. Empathy requires respect for the rights, beliefs, values and feelings of others.

- *Objectivity:* Objectivity implies that what a leader does should be based on relevant facts and information. He should make an objective diagnosis and implement the action required.
- *Motivating skills:* A leader should be self-motivated and have the requisite quality to motivate his followers. There is an inner drive in people for motivation to work. The leader can play an active role in stimulating the inner drives of his followers.
- *Technical skills:* The ability to plan, organize, delegate, analyze, seek advice, make decisions, control and win cooperation requires the use of important abilities which constitute technical competence of leadership.
- *Communicative skills:* A successful leader knows to communicate effectively. A leader uses communication skilfully for persuasive, informative and stimulating purposes.
- *Social skills:* A successful leader has social skills. He understands people and knows their strengths and weaknesses. He has ability to work with people so that he gains their confidence and loyalty.

Behavioral Theory

According to this theory, a leader behaves according to the role expectations of the group. Strong leadership is the result of effective role behavior. To operate effectively, group needs someone to perform two major functions: (a) Task related or problem solving functions and (b) Group maintenance or social functions.

Assumptions

- Leaders can be made, rather than are born.
- Successful leadership lies in definable, learnable behavior.

Behavioral theories of leadership do not seek inborn traits or capabilities. Rather, they look at what leaders actually *do*. This leadership theory focuses on the actions of leaders, not on mental qualities or internal states.

This theory failed to explain why a particular leadership behavior is effective in one situation, but fails in another situation. Thus, situational variables are not considered.

McGregor Theory

Douglas McGregor categorized leadership style into two brand categories in his management theories, i.e., theory X and theory Y, having two different beliefs and assumptions about subordinates. McGregor (1906–1964) postulated that managers tend to make two different assumptions about human nature (Box. 3).

> **Box: 3**
>
> **Theory X**
> - The average human being has an inherent dislike of work and will avoid it, if he or she can.
> - Because of this human characteristic, most people must be coerced, controlled, directed and threatened with punishment to get them to put forth adequate efforts toward the achievement of organizational objectives.
> - The average human being prefers to be directed, wishes to avoid responsibility, has relatively little ambition and wants security above all.
>
> **Theory Y**
> - The expenditure of physical and mental effort in work is as natural as play or rest.
> - External control and threat of punishment are not the only means for bringing out efforts towards organizational objectives. People will exercise self-direction and self-control in the service of objectives to which they are committed.
> - Commitment to objectives is a function of the rewards associated with their achievement.
> - The average human being learns, under proper conditions, not only to accept responsibility but to seek it too.
> - The capacity to exercise a relatively high degree of imagination. Ingenuity and creativity in the solution of organizational problems is widely, not narrowly, distributed in the population.
> - Under the conditions of modern industrial life, the intellectual potentialities of the average human beings are only partially utilized.

Motivational Theories

Abraham Maslow's Need Hierarchy Theory

One of the most popular theories of motivation is the hierarchy of needs theory put forth by psychologist Abraham Maslow (Fig. 10). Maslow saw human needs in the form of a hierarchy, ascending from the lowest to the highest, and he concluded that when one set of needs are satisfied, people will go for the next set of needs. He classified the human needs into five, which are:
- Physiological needs
- Safety needs
- Social needs
- Esteem needs
- Self-actualization needs
- Maslow later refined his model to include a level between esteem needs and self-actualization: the need for knowledge and aesthetics.

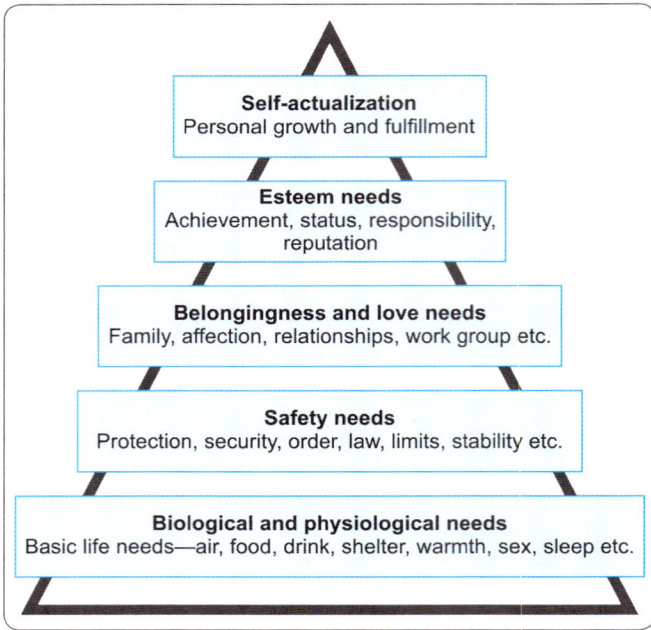

Figure 10: Maslow's Hierarchy of needs

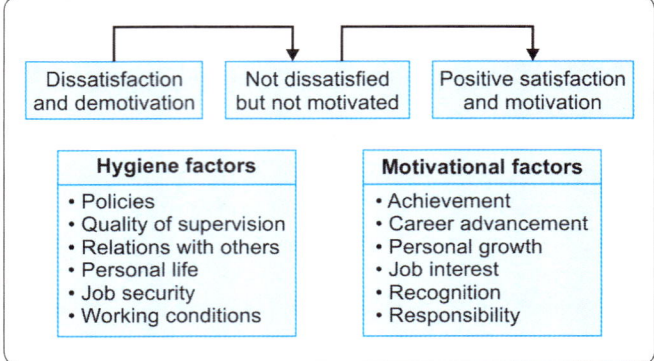

Figure 11: Herzberg's two-factor theory

The two factors identified by him are:
1. **Hygiene factors**—which can demotivate when not present. For example, security, status, relationship with subordinates, personal life, salary, work conditions, relationship with supervisor and administration.
2. **Motivational factors**—Which will motivate when present. For example, growth prospects, job advancement, responsibility, challenges, recognition and achievements.

Herzberg states that presence of certain factors like security, status, relationship with subordinates, personal life, salary, work conditions, relationship with supervisor and administration in the organization does not lead to motivation. However, their absence leads to dissatisfaction. These are called 'Hygiene factors (or) Dissatisfiers'.

Similarly the absence of certain factors like growth prospectus, job advancement, responsibility, challenges, recognition and achievement causes no dissatisfaction, but their presence has motivational impact. These are called 'Motivational factors or Satisfiers'.

Implications

In order to motivate employees, the manager must ensure to provide the hygiene factors and then motivating by the motivational factors. So, if we want to motivate employees on their jobs, it is suggested to give much importance on those job content factors such as opportunities for personal growth, recognition, responsibility and achievement. These are the factors of intrinsic motivation.

Herzberg model sensitizes that managers should utilize the skills, abilities and talents of workers.

Modern Theory

In this, modern management thought (MMT) combines the valuable concepts of classical theory with the social and natural sciences. The source of inspiration of MMT is the system analysis.

Implications for management

Maslow's theory has some important implications for management. This model helps the managers to understand and deal with issues of employee motivation at work place. Managers who understand the need patterns of their staff, can help the employees the kinds of work activities. Some of the implications to be met are:

- **Physiological needs:** Provide lunch periods, rest breaks and wages that are sufficient to purchase the essentials of life.
- **Safety needs:** Provide a safe working environment, retirement benefits and job security.
- **Social needs:** Create a sense of community via team-based projects and social events.
- **Esteem needs:** Recognize achievements to make employees feel appreciated and valued. Offer job titles that convey the importance of the position.
- **Self-actualization:** Provide employees a challenge and the opportunity to reach their full career potential.

Frederick Herzberg's Motivation-hygiene Theory or Herzberg's Two Factor Theory

Herzberg stated that there are certain 'satisfiers and dissatisfiers' for employees at work. They are intrinsic factors that are related to job satisfaction and extrinsic factors which are associated with dissatisfaction (Fig. 11). Removing dissatisfying characteristics from a job does not necessarily make the job satisfying.

Characteristics of MMT

- **Open system view:** It treats the organization as an open system. Because it interacts with the environment continually, in order to survive and flourish. It receives input from the environment, processes them into meaningful services and offers to the environment.
- **Dynamic and adaptive:** Modern theory is dynamic. Changes according to change in outer environment.
- **Multilevel and multidimensional:** MMT is both micro and macro. It is macro when considered with respect to the entire nation or industry; it is micro with respect to internal parts of the organization.
- **Multimotivated and multidisciplinary:** MMT recognizes that the behavior is the product of multifarious factors. A worker can be motivated with good salaries, extra incentives and benefits. Similarly, it is multidisciplinary as other disciplines too embrace it like economics, sociology, engineering, psychology etc.

This applies system theory and contingency theories.

System Theory

It tries to solve problems by diagnosing them within the framework of input, transformations processes, output and feedback (Fig. 12).

Relevance and usefulness of system's theory

- In a system, a manager operates with a view to complete all tasks which would give relevant results to the organization.
- He thinks before he acts, evaluates works before and after implementation.
- It makes a good balance between various parts of the organization and goals.

Contingency Theory: (Situational Approach)

It argues that appropriate managerial action depends on the particular parameters of the situation. Important elements in contingency theory are:

- According to it, effective management varies with the organization and its environment.
- Spells out the relationship of organization to its environment clearly.

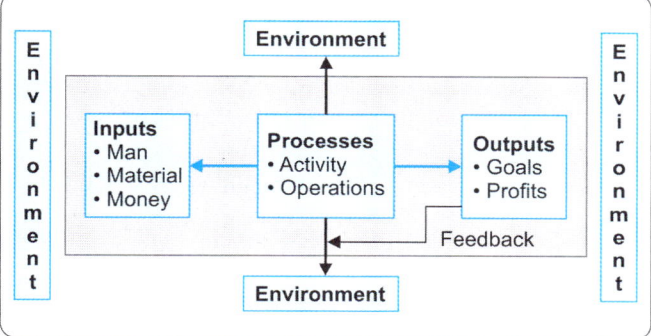

Figure 12: System theory

- Each organization is unique.
- It is more pragmatic and action-oriented.
- It tries to identify nature of interdependence between various parts of an organization and their impact on various things.

ADMINISTRATION

The word **"administer"** is derived from the Latin word **"ad+ministraire"** which means to care for or to look after people to manage affairs. The meaning is suggestive enough, as it insists on the administrator to regard himself as servant, not as the master to look after and perform all functions.

Administration means the overall determination of policies, setting of major objectives, the identification of general purposes and laying down of broad programs and projects.
—*Theo Haimann*

Administration is direction, coordination and control of many persons to achieve same purpose or objectives.
—*LD White*

Administration is the organization and direction of human material resources to achieve desired ends.
—*Pfiffer and Presthus*

Hospital administration is highly complex and the administrator has to bring about harmony and ensure smooth, efficient and comprehensive working of the entire hospital to achieve its objective.

Nursing service administration is a coordinate system of activities which provides all the facilities necessary for rendering nursing care services to patients.

Nursing service administration is a coordinated system of activities concerned with providing holistic care to patients and include the establishment of objectives and policies within the aims of health agency and provision for organization, personnel and facilities to accomplish these goals in the most effective and economical manner through cooperative efforts of all members of the staff.

Administration Versus Management

Administration is a function concerned with determination of policies, coordination of finance, production, distribution and structure under the ultimate control of the executive.
—*Oliver Sheldon*

Management is the process concerned with the implementation of plans through direction and guidance of personnel and optimum use of the required resources to attain the predetermined objectives. It is a process concerned with determining goals, objectives policies and plans for operation of health organization.

Administration is concerned with decision making and management do execution of policies. According to American School of Thoughts, administration is superior to management.

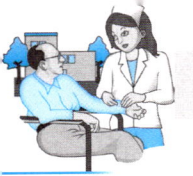

Table 2: Differences between administration and management

Area	Administration	Management
Nature	It is a determinative or thinking function	It is an executive or doing function
Level of activity	It is mainly top level function	It is largely middle level or lower level
Function	Planning and control	Directing and organizing
Skills	Conceptual skill	Technical skill
Activity	Administration is concerned with the formation of objectives, plans and policies	Management is getting things done through and with people
	It is often associated with government policies	It is widely used in the business world.
	It is more administrative rather than a technical activity	It needs more technical rather than administrative activity.

According to views of Henri Fayol and Newman management and administration are the same and can be used interchangeably. Every manager spends part of his time in performing administrative/management functions and the remaining time on operative management function.

The term 'Administration' is more commonly used in Government departments, educational institutions, non-business organizations, but management is commonly used in business enterprises.

Difference between administration and management is depicted in Table 2

Philosophy of Administration

- Cost effectiveness
- Effective execution and control of work plans
- Delegation of responsibility and authority
- Human relations and good morale
- Effective communication
- Flexibility in work situation

ROLE AND FUNCTIONS OF NURSE AS A MANAGER

The role of nurse administrators are changing according to changing health care scenario and they are responsible to meet issues and challenges in the field of nursing care, thereby providing optimum services to patients and there families. For that, they should keep in acquainted with the changing health scenario and coordinate as well as direct nursing service department with challenge. They are responsible for planning, organizing, staffing, directing and evaluating nursing services. The role and functions of nurse manager are summarized below:

- Establish goals and objectives for each area and communicate them to persons who are responsible for attaining them.
- Formulate standards, policies, rules and regulations of the organization.
- Organize and analyze the activities, decisions and relations needed to work in a healthcare setting and divides them in to manageable tasks.
- Organize and direct nursing service.
- Formulate nursing policies to ensure quality care to patients.
- Establish a good system for economical and proper use of hospital finances and develop adequate financial controls.
- Ensure recruitment of staff for proper functioning of the hospital.
- Delegate responsibility and authority to subordinates.
- Provide scientific and quality nursing care in a coordinated way.
- Coordinate nursing service department with other allied departments.
- Ensure adequate supplies and equipment for care of patients and take all measures to ensure 'Standards of Nursing Service' and see whether materials and supplies are available for providing patient care services.
- Create a favorable organizational climate, resolve major organizational conflicts, promote high employee morale and job satisfaction.
- Responsible for health employer-employee relations and negotiations with employee union.
- Motivates and communicates with the people responsible for various jobs through team work
- Maintain good order and discipline in nursing service department.
- Monitor infection control practices and biomedical waste management regularly.
- Conduct staff development program regularly and encourage staff to participate in updated courses and continuing educational program.
- Promote and maintain effective communication and inter-personal relations between departments and among staff.
- Arrange orientation programs to newly joined staff.
- Organize and conduct monthly staff meeting, encourage educational activities and publications.
- Ensure quality service through conduct of nursing audit and evaluation of nursing service.
- Identify issues and challenges in nursing care delivery system and recommend for policy changes.
- Build image of hospital and maintain good public relations
- Ensure proper maintenance of records and maintain confidentiality of medical records and documentation.

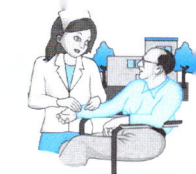

- Provide guidance and counseling services as and when needed.
- Analyzes, appraises and interprets performance of staff along with communicating it to them.
- Encourages evidence-based practice and ensures professional improvement by continuing education and research.
- Nurse manager acts as a role model. Develop professional and technical knowledge by attending conferences and participating in professional organizations.

MANAGEMENT ROLES

Mintzberg proposed **management roles** that a manager has to perform and they are:

Interpersonal Role

- **Figure head role:** The manager performs a role as symbolic head and accordingly is obliged to perform a number of routine duties of a legal and social nature.
- **Leader role:** As a leader, the manager gives directions to his employees and other subordinates. Some of the activities include goal setting, providing guidance, an so on.
- **Liaison role:** The manager is required to maintain contact with external sources that provides valuable information for example acknowledging mail, doing external board works and so on.

Informational Roles

- **Monitor:** Manager seeks and receives variety of special information to develop through understanding of organization and environment.
- **Disseminator:** Manager acts as conduits of information to organizational members. He is expected to transmit information received from outside or from subordinates to member of organization by holding meetings and so on.
- **Spokesman:** The manager transmits information to outside people on organization's plans, policies, results and achievements and so on.

Decisional Roles

- **Entrepreneur role:** The manager initiates and oversees new methods that will improve organization's performance.
- **Disturbance handler:** Manager is responsible for corrective action when organization faces important, unexpected disturbances.
- **Resources allocator:** Manager is responsible for the allocation of organizational resources as man, money and material.

MANAGERIAL SKILLS

Managers need to possess skills for accomplishment of goals in an institution. The skills are:

- **Managerial skill:** It is the ability of manager to utilize resources to achieve objectives. A manager must be skilled in effective utilization of all resources.
- **Technical skills:** Technical skills are skills needed to accomplish the specific kinds of work being done in an organization. These skills involve use of knowledge, methods and techniques in performing a job effectively.
- **Conceptual skills:** Conceptual skills are mental ability to analyze and diagnose complex situations. It is the manager's ability to think in abstract. Conceptual skill is crucial for top level management.
- **Interpersonal skills:** It is the ability to communicate and motivate employees. It involves understanding, patience, trust and genuine involvement in interpersonal relationships. These skill are necessary to all levels of management.
- **Communication skills:** Communication skill is the ability to convey ideas and information effectively to others and receive information from others. Good communication is necessary in an organization to avoid misunderstanding, confusion and conflicts.
- **Decision making skills:** It is the ability to choose an action between alternatives.
- **Human skills:** Human skills are the ability to work with a good understanding of people and motivating other people. Without the cooperation of employees, managers cannot control organization smoothly. The human skills are the most important assets of manager.

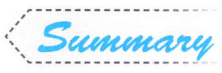

Management is a process of designing and maintaining an environment for efficient accomplishment of selected aims. Management is an essential activity at all levels; however managerial skills required vary with organizational levels.

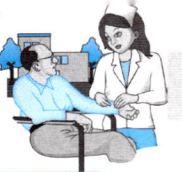

Suggested Reading

- Edythe L Alexander. Nursing Service Administration – Principles and Practice. The C V Mosby Company, New York.
- Harold Koontz, Heinz Weihrich. Essentials of Management – An International Perspective. Tata McGraw Hill Publishing Company Ltd. 2005, Delhi.
- Barret Jean. Ward Management and Teaching. Konark Publishers, Delhi.
- BT Basavanthappa. Nursing Administration. Jaypee Brothers Medical Publishers Pvt Ltd. Second edition 2009.
- CM Francis, Mario C Desouza. Hospital Administration 3rd edition. Jaypee Brothers Medical Publishers Pvt Ltd. New Delhi, 2000.
- Dr Sreeranganadhan and GG Mathews. Styles of Management in the Industries in Kerala, New Delhi Serial Publications.
- Satyasaran Chatterjee. An Introduction to Management, its Principles and Technique. The World Press Private Ltd. 1993, Calcutta.
- Patricia Kelly RN. Leadership and Management in Nursing. Cengage Learning India Ltd. 2000, New Delhi.

Assess Yourself

LONG ANSWERS

1. Define administration. Describe significance and scope of administration in modern society.
2. Discuss principles of management in detail with suitable examples.

SHORT NOTES

1. Trends and issues in nursing administration
2. Principles of administration
3. Functions/Elements of administration
4. Qualities of a good manager
5. Explain the role of a nurse as a manager
6. Concepts of management
7. Scope of management
8. Theories of management
9. Levels of management
10. Elements of administration

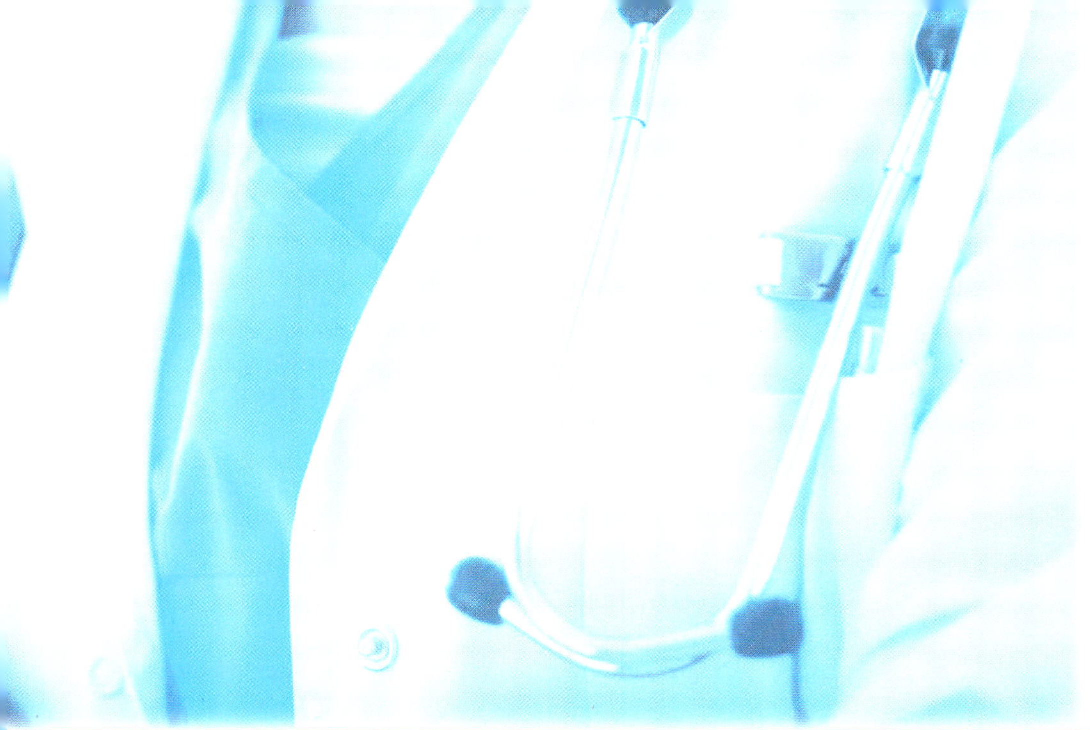

Unit 2

MANAGEMENT PROCESS

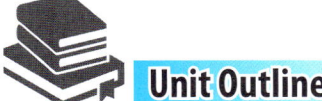

Unit Outline

- Planning
- Organizing
- Centralization and Decentralization
- Organizational Charts
- Staffing
- Human Resource Management
- Staffing Process
- Retention
- Separation
- Directing
- Control in Management/Controlling
- Planning Methods
- Bench Marking
- Budget

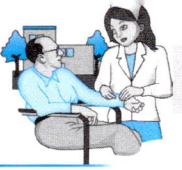

PLANNING

Introduction

Planning is an essential process of making choices between available alternatives at all levels of decision making. It is the exercise of intelligence to deal with facts and solutions and find a way to solve problems. Planning is an organized, conscious and continual attempt to select the best available alternative to achieve specific goals.

Plan is a forecast for accomplishment. Planning is one of the major fundamental elements of administration. It is predetermined course of action. It is a today's projection for tomorrow's activity.

Definitions

Planning is defined as pre–determining a course of action in order to achieve a designed result —*Venzon*

Planning is a process of determining the objectives of administrative efforts and devising the means calculated to achieve them. —*Millet*

Planning is an intellectual process, the conscious determination of courses of actions, the basis of decisions on purpose, acts and considered estimates. —*Koonts O' Donnel*

Planning means the determination of what is to be done, how and where it is to be done, who is to do it and how results are to be evaluated. Planning bridges the gap between where we are to and where we want to go. —*James Lundy*

Planning is a continuous process of making present entrepreneurial decisions systematically and with best possible knowledge of their futurity, organizing systematically the efforts needed to carry out these decisions and measuring the results of these decisions against expectation through organized systematic feedback. —*Peter Drucker*

Examples of Questions that form the Basis of Planning

Planning is deciding in advance what to do, how to do it and who is to do it. It bridges the gap from where we are to where we want to go. It is the function that answers four basic questions.

- **Where we are now?** This question is concerned with making a realistic assessment of the current situation and forecasting how the picture may change in the future.
- **Where do we want to be?** This is concerned with finding out the desirable objectives, keeping the present as well as future requirements in mind.
- **Gap?** What is the amount of difference between where we are now and where we want to be?
- **How can we get there from here?** This is a question of deciding in the present what has to be done in the future that is planning. Planning is concerned with future implications of current decisions, not with decisions to be made in the future.

Importance of Planning

- Planning is a goal oriented element of management that leads to achievement of goals and objectives.
- Planning pervades all management functions/element and is basic to all functions. Planning process is the basis for organizing, staffing, directing and controlling functions.
- Planning provides for effective use of available resources and facilities.
- It is based on facts and events.
- Planning is an intellectual process of thinking in advance. It is forward looking futuristic process and encourages innovations and creativity.
- Planning is a process that involves selection of suitable course of action from alternative choices.
- It is based on past and future activities.
- It gives meaning to work and helps manager to express his/her creativity.
- Planning is cost effective.
- It is a continuous activity which provides facilities to achieve coordination between different departments of organization.
- Planning process is flexible to meet the new challenges and changing situations.
- It provides a basis for control.
- It leads to the realization of the need for change.
- Planning involves the ability to foresee the effects of current actions in the future.

Purposes and Objectives of Planning

- Planning leads to more effective and faster achievement of objectives.
- Planning helps to anticipate issues and problems.
- It makes optimum utilization of all available resources.
- Planning provides direction. Through planning all employees get proper information, correct instructions and guidance regarding the activities of organization.
- Planning helps in decision making about future activities.
- Planning facilitates effective control of an organization. Planning helps to control a situation by furnishing standards of performance.
- Planning facilitates delegation of authority in a better way.
- It helps to deal with uncertainties. Planning is always done for future and future is uncertain. Through proper planning, manager is able to anticipate possible changes in future and plan activities accordingly.
- Planning promotes coordination.
- Planning is the element that basically decides the function of management.
- Planning provides unique contribution to the efficacy of other functions of management.

Principles of Planning

- Planning should focus on purposes and it should be based on clearly defined objectives.

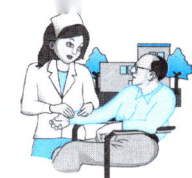

- Planning should be realistic in its scope.
- In planning, provision should be made to use all resources that are available.
- Continuity and flexibility should be maintained in planning.
- It must be precise, simple and concise.
- Planning should be flexible so that organization could cope up with changing social needs.
- Principle of coordination must be followed. Plans should be communicated to employees to achieve organizational goals.
- Planning should always be documented.

Characteristics of Planning

- **Planning is goal oriented:** Planning identifies the action that would lead to desired goals quickly and economically. Planning is made to achieve the desired objective.
- **Planning is looking ahead:** Planning requires forecasting, analyzing and predicting. Planning is based on forecasting and synthesis of forecast.
- **Planning is an intellectual process:** Planning is a mental exercise involving creative thinking, sound judgement and imagination.
- Planning is the primary function of management.
- Planning serves as a guide for organizing, staffing, directing and controlling. All functions of management are performed within the framework of plans laid out. Therefore, planning is the basic or fundamental function of management.
- Planning is a continuous process. Planning involves: where we are now? Where we want to go? How we will reach there?
- Planning is pervasive. Planning process is needed at all levels, like top level, middle level and lower level of management. Top level may be involved in planning the organization as a whole, middle level in planning departmental roles and lower level is involved in execution of work plans.
- Planning is designed for efficiency. Planning is concerned with productivity with optimum utilization of resources.
- Planning is flexible so that it could be adapted according to the needs of the time.

Components of Planning

Objectives

Objectives are the basic plans which determine goals or end results of the projected action of an enterprise. By setting goals, objectives provide the foundations upon which structure of a plan can be built.

Policies

Policies are written statements or oral understandings. They are general terms for governing actions in repetitive situations. Realization of objectives is made easy with the help of policies, as policies provide standing solutions to problems.

Procedures

Procedures indicate the specific manner in which a certain activity is to be performed. They are more definite and specific guides to action, but only for fulfillment of objectives.

Program

Program welds together different plans for implementing them into complete and orderly course of action. Programs are both repetitive (routine planning) and non-repetitive (creative planning) course of action.

Budget

Budget is pre-estimation of income, expenditure and material resources.

Steps of Planning Process

Preparing a plan is a step by step exercise (Fig. 1). Generally the following steps are involved in planning:

- **Analyzing and understanding the system:** Administrators or managers needs to understand the system, where he/she is working and consisting of their subordinates, communities and higher authorities.
- **Formulation of operational goals and objectives:** These set the pattern of the proposed course of action and shape, the structure of other subsidiary objectives in the organization. This implies the establishment of goals for the whole organization. Objectives must be specific, informative and clear to indicate what is to be done.

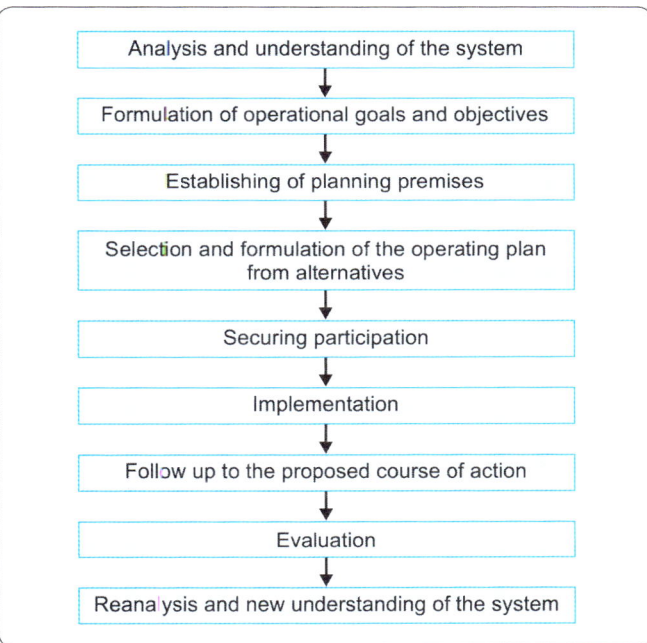

Figure 1: Steps of planning process

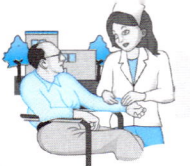

- **Establishment of planning premises:** Premises refers to the factors in the environment that affect the achievement of goals. They are assumptions about the future understanding of the expected situation. These premises may be internal or external premises. Internal premises include organizational policies, resources as capital investment etc and external premises include economic, cultural and technological conditions. Once the objectives are clear, there is need to assess the resources available to reach the goals.
- **Selection of alternative course of action:** The next step of planning process is to determine different courses of action. These course of action have to be evaluated in terms of effectiveness and efficiency.
- **Formulation of derivative plan:** From alternative course of action, select the best course of action after evaluation. The managers must formulate plans and programs and the sequence of tasks to accomplish goals and objectives.
- **Securing participation:** Subordinate's participation has been found to be extremely essential for effective implementation of the program. Plans must be communicated for proper implementation of the plan.
- **Implementation:** Implementation is the key step in planning process. Special attention is needed for the use of strategy. Strategy means a set of decisions taken to achieve the objectives. It dictates some adjustment and adaptation of the plan in accordance with changing situation or events.
- **Follow-up of the proposed course of action:** There should be a prior provision for follow up of the proposed program when it is put into action. So there should be regular feedback in both ways that is written records and reports as well as by direct observation.
- **Evaluation:** Evaluation is measuring what has been done against what was planned to do in the past. Any deviation has to be explained and necessary action has to be initiated.
- **Reanalysis and new understanding of the system:** Here managers can take an overview of the plan of the work and visualize what has been achieved.

Types of Planning

Planning must be done at several levels and each has its own particular problem and configuration of the planners and methods may be different too. Planning may be classified as: long range, medium range and short range or directional planning, administrative planning and operational planning.

Directional Planning

It is often called policy planning and is concerned with the broad general direction of the program—as setting the framework of intent and philosophy—within which the program will proceed and with relating the program to the broad planning of the community in which the program will function.

Administrative Planning

It is concerned with the overall implementation of the policies developed with mobilization and coordination of the personnel and material available in the administrative unit. Medical superintendent of major hospitals or district surgeon of district hospital are responsible for administrative planning.

Operational Planning

Operational plans are everyday working management plans. They are plans developed from both long range objectives or strategic planning process and short range or tactical plans.

Operational planning is concerned with the actual delivery of the services to the community. Usually operational and short range planning is undertaken by middle level or supervisory level personnel. This involves:
- Formulating objectives
- Activities to be delivered
- Quality standards
- Desired outcomes
- Staffing and resource requirements
- Implementation
- Evaluation

The characteristics of strategic and operational planning are given in Table 1.

Strategic Planning

Usually the strategic and long range planning is undertaken by the top level management and it involves the following activities:
- Detailed analysis of strength, weakness, opportunities and threats (SWOT) of organization: Both internal and external environment.
- Developing philosophy and formulation of policies and objectives on the basis of analysis of the organization
- Allocation of resources on the basis of priority
- Evaluation of activities to increase efficiency
- Providing proper direction to avoid duplication of services

Table 1: Characteristics of strategic and operational plans

Feature	Strategic	Operational
Time horizon	5 years or more	Under 1 year
Purpose	Adapt to external environment based on internal strength	Implement internal goals
Activity controlled	Total institutional performance	Internal tasks and operations
Decision range	Relatively enduring	Short term
Organizational level involved	Top management	Middle and lower management
Basis for planning	Primary judgmental	Exact data and standards used

Contd…

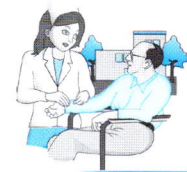

Feature	Strategic	Operational
Predictability	Uncertain	Highly certain
Anticipated accuracy	Within 25 percent	Within 2 or 3 percent
Management functions involved	Planning and forecasting dominant	Control primarily
Management control of outcomes	Slight contingency plans required	Almost complete, slight option plans used

Table 2: Long range Vs short range planning

Long range planning	Point of distinction	Short range planning
5 years or more	Time factor	Upto one year
Mission, long term goals and strategies	Deals with	Current operations of an organization
Demands changes in the structure, resource allocation	Impact	Operates within the existing structure and resources
It goes too far into the future, the risk and uncertainty level is high	Uncertainty	The time horizon is limited and the risk associated with uncertainty level is low
Top management	Prepared by	Lower level executives

Among the benefits of strategic planning, main benefit is giving sense of direction to all managers and practitioners of nursing within the organization. The strategic plan deals concretely with complex projects or programs in multistage time sequences (Table 2).

Advantages of Planning

- Planning leads to more effective and faster achievements of goals of organization. It replaces random operation by orderly and meaningful action.
- Planning gives a competitive edge to the organization as it forecasts and plans. As planning foresees the future and makes provision for it, planning gives an added strength to the business for its continuous growth and steady prosperity.
- Planning secures and ensures unit of purpose, direction and effort by focusing attention on objectives. It avoids duplication of services.
- Planning has unique contribution towards the efficiency of other managerial functions.
- Planning provides the basis for control in an organization.
- Planning serves as an integral part of other administrative functions (POSDCORB). It ensures order and control and determines appropriateness and feasibility of action in terms of cost effectiveness and quality control. It eliminates chances of uncertainty and avoids arbitrary decisions. It provides flexibility and makes provision for future growth and development.

Disadvantages of Planning

- Planning may lead to internal inflexibilities and procedural rigidities.
- It is time consuming and expensive process (fault may lie with the planner)
- Unplanned operation produces chaos and disorder everywhere without exception—changing the situation, immediate action is not possible

Planning Hierarchy (Fig. 2)

Vision

The vision of an organization depicts where the organization wants to go and what it will look like when it reaches there. The vision describes the future goal of an organization and it reflects what the organization wants to be. It is the end result of what the organization wants to achieve. It is an image of the desired future and/or a vision from which individual department later creates its own statement and implementation of the mission. Vision also provides direction for the employees regarding the area in which it operates and the services it offers to the community. It reflects the consistency, ethics, principles and standards of practice of an organization.

Mission Statement

Mission of an organization shows what an organization do to achieve vision. It describes the goals, purposes and the primary objectives. The mission statement provides a primary focus. It also provides direction regarding how the organization acts and by whom it acts. It provides information and inspiration that clearly defines and outlines what is required in future for the organization. It also incorporates philosophy, goals, policies, rules and regulations (Fig. 2). The characteristics of mission include:

- It should be short, unambiguous and must have a clear meaning.
- It should be dynamic and should give a direction to frame philosophy, objectives and operational plans of the department.
- It delineates the organizational uniqueness.

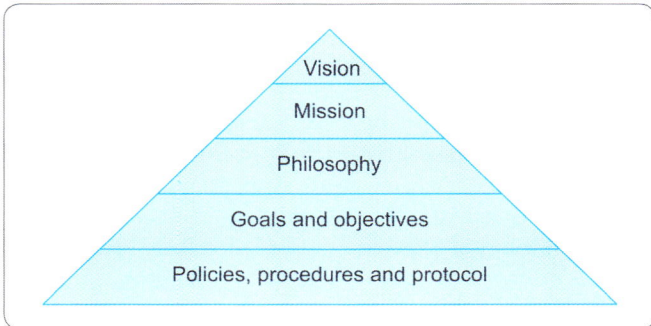

Figure 2: Planning hierarchy

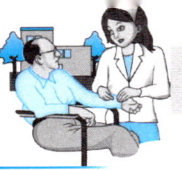

Uses of Vision and Mission

The vision and mission statements must be clear and precise. While formulating vision statements, the organization must have a look into the culture, values and strategies and have a view regarding the future. Vision and mission helps:
- To improve the efficiency and outcome of an organization
- Serves as a foundation for a broader strategic plan
- Motivates the employees to work together to achieve goals
- Acts as a guide for the employees in decision making
- Serves as a foundation for a strategic planning
- Inspires staff to achieve goals of the organization
- Serves as a tool for public relation
- Acts as a frame work for professional conduct and ethical behavior

Characteristics

- The statement of vision and mission statement are clear and simple.
- They must be broad and distinct.
- They should be motivating, unambiguous, powerful and dynamic.
- They should focus on desired outcome.
- They should be easy to communicate with all team members.

Table 2: Difference between vision and mission

Vision	Mission
Vision describes the future of an organization, its dreams and future plans.	Mission focuses on what the organization does to achieve the objectives. It shows what to do, how to do and the statements concentrating on present.
Vision communicates purposes and values and states what the organization wants to become	Mission communicates goals and primary objectives of the organization
The statements of vision are brief and guide functional level of planning	Statements are longer than vision and describe the present state of the organization

Examples of Vision and Mission Statement of a Hospital

Mission
As a center of excellence, the hospital provides comprehensive, high quality holistic health care to all patients who are seeking health care and their care givers with provision of learning facilities for students in medicine, nursing and other allied health sciences with special importance to evidenced based practice.

Vision of nursing educational institution
Establish college of nursing as a center of excellence in nursing practice, education and research imbibed with scientific culture and technology and service to the sick and needy people in the community through comprehensive, holistic health care.

Mission of Nursing education institution

Establish benchmark in the field of nursing by empowering nursing students who will be able to provide quality nursing service to all patients, caregivers and the people in the community based on advanced scientific technology and establish excellence in education, practice and research.

Philosophy

Philosophy is a statement of values and beliefs that directs an organization in its attempt to achieve its mission. When developing a philosophy, it is important to consider the historical background, education, theory, practice, research and nursing role in the overall organization.

It verbalizes the nurse manager and nurse practitioner's vision of what they believe nursing management practices are. Statements of philosophy are abstract and contain value statements about: human beings as clients or patients and as workers, about self care, about nursing as a profession, about education that brings competence among nursing workers, and about the setting or community in which nursing services are provided.

The philosophy of an organization is very often implicit and is not written down. Like mission statements, philosophy statements evolve from higher levels of management and practice.

For Example we believe that:
- We are dedicated to provide excellence in patient care, teaching and research in the field of healthcare practices. Everyone should be treated with dignity.

Organizational Philosophy

The organizational philosophy provides the basis for developing nursing philosophies at the unit level and for nursing service as a whole.

Nursing Service Philosophy

The nursing service philosophy may be described as an intentionally chosen set of values and purposes that is the basis for determining the means to accomplish nursing objectives, written in conjunction with the organizational philosophy. The nursing service philosophy should address fundamental beliefs about nursing and nursing care.

Unit Philosophy

The unit philosophy has been adapted from nursing service philosophy. It specifies how nursing care is provided in the unit, will correspond with nursing service and organizational goals. In developing this philosophy, the unit manager incorporates the unit's internal and external environments and an understanding of the unit's role in meeting organizational goals.

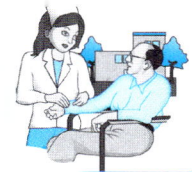

Societal Philosophies and Values

Societies and organizations have philosophies or sets of beliefs that guide their behavior. These beliefs which guide the behavior, are called values. MacPherson defines a value as "a quality having intrinsic worth for a society or an individual" and identifies individualism, the pursuit of self-interests, and competition as some of the most strongly held American values.

Individual Philosophies and Values

For the individual, personal philosophies and values are shaped by the socialization processes experienced by the individual. Therefore, the nurse leader must be self aware and provide subordinates with learning opportunities or experiences that foster increased self awareness.

McNally identified the following four characteristics that determine a true value. These are:
- It must be freely chosen from alternatives, only after due reflection.
- It must be prized and cherished.
- It must be consciously and consistently repeated.
- It is positively affirmed and enacted.

Hamilton and Kiefer identified seven steps to help determine and clarify values:
- Listen to your responses
- Differentiate internal sources from external sources
- Take time to experience full awareness of your internal responses.
- Act on your internal responses
- Evaluate your alternatives.
- Establish behavior patterns consistent with your values.
- Trust your beliefs, preferences, likes and dislikes.

Nursing managers must recognize that closely held values may be challenged by current social and economic constraints and that philosophy statements must be continually reviewed and revised to ensure on going accuracy of beliefs.

Goals and Objectives

Goals and objectives are the ends toward which the organization is working. All philosophies must be translated into specific goals and objectives if they are to result in action. Thus, goals and and objectives "operationalize" the philosophy.

Goal

Goal may be defined as the desired result towards which effort is directed. It is the aim of philosophy. Goals like philosophies and values change with time and they require periodic reevaluation and priorities. Goal should be measurable and ambitious.

Objective

Objectives are concrete and specific statements of the goals that nurse managers seek to accomplish. They are action commitments through which the mission will be achieved and the philosophy or beliefs will be sustained. They are used to establish priorities. They must be functional and useful.

Objectives must be selective rather than global and they must be multiple rather than single, so as to balance a wide range of needs and goals related to nursing services to clients or patients.

Objectives are the basis for work and assignments. They determine the organizational structure, the key activities, and the allocation of people to tasks. They give direction and make commitments that mobilize the resources and energies of nursing for the making of the future. They should be changed as necessary, particularly when there is a change of mission or when current objectives are no longer functional. For example, evaluation of patient care. To develop methods of measuring the quality of patient care can be an objective.

Goals and objectives are reflective of the mission statement. Goals relate to a desired outcome. From set goals, the objectives for achieving the mission and philosophy are developed. Goals are central to the entire management process. Objectives are specific statements that will be evident when the goal is accomplished.

ORGANIZING

Organizing is the basic function of management. It is a process of determining, grouping and assigning activities of an organization to achieve the goals.

Organizing provides the framework within which the managerial functions of planning, directing and controlling takes place for the successful functioning of an institution.

According to Fayol, to organize is to provide everything for the functioning - human resources, materials and capital.

Definition

Organization involves grouping of activities necessary to accomplish goals and plans, the assignment of activities to appropriate departments and the provision for authority delegation and coordination.
—*Koonts and O'Donnell*

Organizing may be defined as a group of individuals, large or small that is co-operating under the direction of executive leadership in accomplishment of certain common object.
—*Keith*

Organizing is the process of identifying and grouping the work to be performed, defining and delegating responsibility and authority and establishing relationship for the purpose of enabling people to work most effectively together in accomplishing objectives.
—*Louis A. Allen*

Organizing is the systematic arrangement of people brought together to accomplish some specific purpose.
—*Stephen P. Robison*

Organizing is the process of defining and grouping the activities of the enterprise and establishing the authority relationships among them.
—*Theo Haimann*

Organizing is a function by which the concern is able to

define the role positions, the job related and the coordination between authority and responsibility. —*Chester Bernard*

Importance/Significance of Organizing
- Organizing increases managerial efficiency
- Organization facilitates effective management by providing a conducive environment for the employees to work.
- It ensures growth and diversification of institution.
- Organization provides coordination between employees and it facilitates order and cohesiveness.
- Organizing stimulates creativity by motivating employees and providing innovative ways for doing things.
- It ensures better utilization of human resources through specialization.
- Organizing promotes awareness of responsibility and functions among members.
- It ensures stability of organization by ensuring delegation of authority, communication and leadership.
- Organization provides scope for training and development of employees.
- Organization promotes employee satisfaction so that effective administration can be possible.
- Organization reduces frequent turnover of employees.
- Organization helps for the growth and diversification of institution.
- Organization creates a structure of relationship within the institution.

A Sound Organization's Facilitates
- A sound organization is one which facilitates effective administration, promotes specialization, growth of institution and stimulates creativity and it can be achieved by active participation of all members of organization.

Characteristics of a sound organization are:
- Realization of objectives
- Reasonable span of control
- Unity of command
- Conducive working environment
- Stimulates creativity
- Increase employee satisfaction
- Motivate employees
- Proper utilization of resources
- Effective system of communication among members
- Provides facilities for development of employees
- Flexible
- Provision for development of the Institution

Nature of Organization
An organization is a group of people working together to achieve the objective. The nature of organization is given in Figure 3.

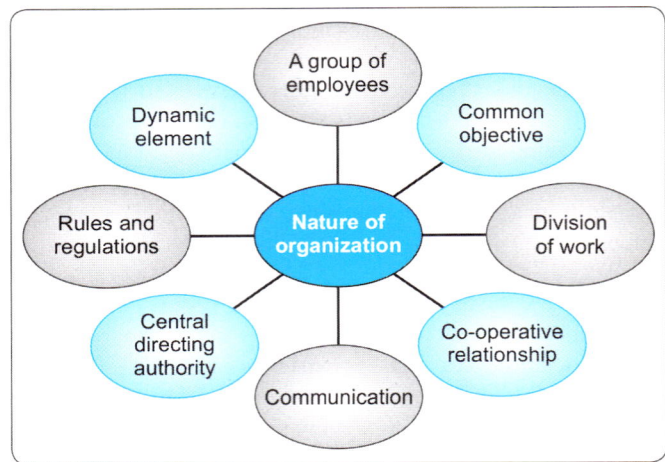

Figure 3: Nature of Organization

Principles of Organization
- **Principle of objective:** Every organization has some basic objective and a sound organization structure must focus on achievement of objectives. The principles of an organization must be clear to the employees and supervisors so as to work together.
- **Principle of specialization/division of work:** Precise division of work facilitates specialization and improves productivity and demands accountability from subordinates.
- **Principle of delegation:** Delegation involves assigning duties and delegating authority to subordinates. Delegation of authority to subordinates becomes necessary for the functioning of an organization. So there should be proper delegation of authority in an organization.
- **Authority and responsibility:** Along with delegation of authority to employees there is need for creating responsibility also. So that the individual workers are responsible for their respective job. Managers delegate authority and responsibility to his subordinates and encourages them to work effectively to achieve organizational objectives.
- **Principle of Coordination:** Coordination between employees in all departments are essential for the efficient functioning of an organization.
- **Unity of command:** The principle of unity of command means each and every employee must know who he or she is directed to.
- **The scalar chain:** Scalar chain means the hierarchy of authority or line of authority. There must be clear line of authority from top level management level to lower level of organization so that each employee may know his/her superior authority.
- **Principle of flexibility:** The organization structure should be flexible to accommodate the necessary modifications and technical or other changes in the environment of an organization. But at the same time it should be reasonably

stable to withstand changes and must facilitate growth of the organization.
- **Principle of span of control**: Span of control refers to the number of employees that a supervisor can effectively and efficiently control at a time. So every manager should have a limited number of subordinates to control.
- **Integration versus disintegration**: Integration means unification and disintegration means diversification. Line functions should be separated from the staff functions even when they are supplementary in character.

Process of Organization

Organizing involves developing structure and placing human resources to ensure achievement of goals. Organization structure enables human resources to work together. The steps involved in the process of organization are:

- **Reviewing plans and objectives:** The first step in the process of management is to review plans and determination of goals and objectives.
- **Identification of activities:** Determine tasks/activities and analyze the activities that are to be performed to achieve the objectives.
- **Classification of activities/tasks:** The tasks must be classified into manageable work units. These major categories of works are sub divided into smaller units to facilitate operations and supervision.
- **Appointing qualified employees for the job:** Human resources are the backbone of every organization to achieve objectives. Therefore, qualified employees who suit the need of job must be appointed.
- **Delegation of work and resources:** Delegation of work and resources is an important responsibility of manager to place right person in the right job which will help to avoid duplication of work and overlapping assignments of activities to subordinates. It creates responsibility among them and avoid duplication of work.
- **Developing relationship between authority and subordinates**.
- **Coordination of activities:** Coordination is essential to achieve harmony among individual efforts for the achievement of goals. Coordination creates relationship among positions and ensures cooperation among employees.
- **Evaluating the results:** Through evaluation, the effectiveness of performance of human resources can be analyzed and further modification can be recommended.

Theories of Organization

Theory is a set of interrelated concepts, statements, propositions and definitions which have been derived from philosophical beliefs of scientific data and from which questions or hypotheses can be deduced, tested and verified. There are several theories of management. It has attracted the attention of psychologists, sociologists, anthropologists, mathematicians, political scientists, economists and so on. They have given different theories based on management in later part of the 19th century and early 20th centuries.

Basic theories are
- Classical theory
- Neo-classical theory
- Behavioral science theory
- Modern theory

Classical Theory

- The term classical means something traditionally accepted or long-established.
- It does not mean that classical views are static and time bound that must be dispensed with.
- Some of the elements of classical theory are still with us, in one form or other.
  - **Inter-related functions:** Management consists of several inter-related and inter-dependent functions (planning, organizing, staffing, directing and controlling) which are exercised in a sequential form. This is repeated over and over again to bring order out of chaos.
  - **Guiding principles:** In order to increase the knowledge there are certain principles based on practical experience.
  - **Bureaucratic structure:** For maximum efficiency, this theory specified that the work must be logically divided into simple, routine and repetitive tasks. These tasks should then be grouped according to similar work characteristics and arranged in the form of departments. Work must be assigned to individuals based on job demands and the individual's ability to do the job. The organization has complex mechanisms, rules, regulations and procedures. The whole structure takes the shape of a pyramid. As the organization grows and develops—operation grows in size; communication becomes complex and more policies, procedures and further formalization is demanded. It would inevitably acquire a bureaucratic, pyramidal structure, as shown below in Figure 4.

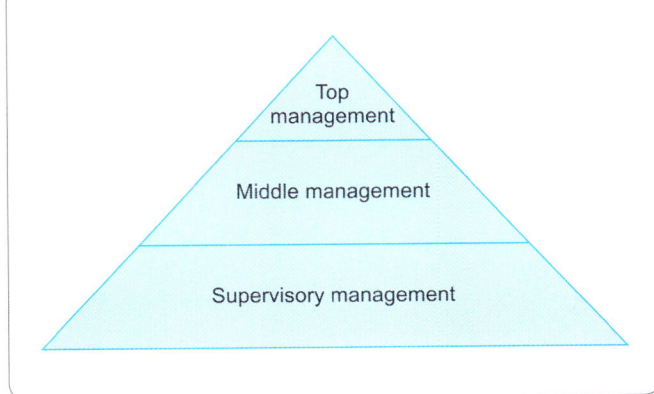

Figure 4: Pyramid structure of classical theory

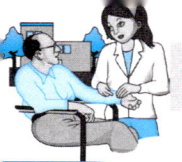

- **Reward punishment nexus:** Follow the rules, obey the orders, show the results and get the rewards. If you lag behind in the race, you will become a second-class citizen and not entitled to receive extra benefits. Great emphasis is put on efficient use of resources while producing results.

Branches of Classical Theory

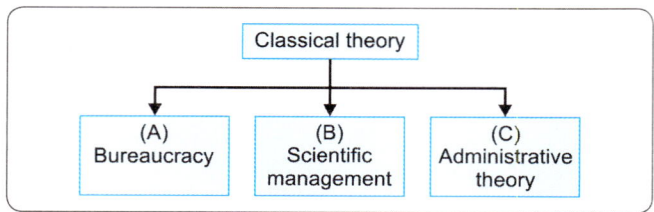

Bureaucracy

Classical organization especially as developed by FW Taylor. The word 'bureaucracy' implies an organization characterised by rules, procedures, impersonal relations and elaborate and fairly rigid hierarchy of authority—responsibility relationships. Persons with proper qualifications are selected so that the work is done efficiently.

Elements of bureaucracy

- **Hierarchy:** Hierarchy is a way of ranking various positions in descending order from top to bottom of an organization. Ultimately, no office is left uncontrolled in the organization.
- **Division of work:** The total work is divided into specialised jobs. Each person's job is broken down into simple, routine and well-defined tasks. Each employee knows his boundaries.
- **Rules, regulations and procedures:** The behavior of employees is regulated through a set of rules. Employees are expected to follow these rules strictly.
- **Records:** Proper records have to be kept for everything. Files have to be maintained to record the decisions and activities of the organization on a day to day basis for future use.
- **Impersonal relationships:** Everything should proceed according to rules. There is no room for personal involvement, emotions and sentiments. If an employee comes late, whether he is a manager or a peon, the rules must be same for all.
- **Administrative class:** Bureaucracies generally have administrative class responsible for coordinating the work. These officials are selected on the basis of their competence and skills. They are on paid salary, with increases according to age and experience and receive a pension when they retire. Promotion is based on seniority and achievement, decided by judgement of seniors.

Advantages of a bureaucratic structure

- **Specialization:** People can specialize in their respective fields and show improved performance.
- **Rationality:** Bureaucracy brings rationality to an organization. Judgements are made according to an objective and generally based upon criteria. Logical structuring of activities brings about orderly execution of assigned tasks.
- **Predictability:** The rules, regulations, training, specialization, structure and other elements of bureaucracy enable it to provide predictability and stability of an organization.
- **Democracy:** In bureaucratic organizations, decisions are arrived at according to an acceptable criteria. People are selected on the basis of merit. Patronage, favoritism are not given weightage. Because the opportunity to train, apply and be selected for a job is open to every citizen, a significant degree of democracy is achieved.

Disadvantages of bureaucratic structure

- **Rigidity:** Critics of bureaucracy claim that it is rigid, static and inflexible. Strict adherence to rules produces timidity, conservatism and technicism. In the name of following rules, people may even shirk away from their responsibilities.
- **Impersonality:** Bureaucracy emphasises on mechanical way of doing things. Rules and regulations are glorified in place of employee's needs and emotions.
- **Displacement of objectives:** Specialists e.g. may concentrate on their own finely toned goals and forget their goals area, mean for reaching the broader objectives of the organization.
- **Compartmentalization of activities:** Strict categorization of work restricts people from performing tasks that they are capable of doing.
- **Red tape:** Bureaucracies are paper mills. Everything is recorded on paper. Files move through endless official channels, resulting in inordinate delays.

Scientific management

Fredrick W. Taylor (1856-1915) has given the concept of scientific management. He is known as Father of Scientific Management. Scientific management is an approach that emphasizes the scientific study of work in order to improve worker's efficiency.

Basics of scientific management: It is based on four basic principles:

1. Each task must be scientifically designed so that it can replace the old.
2. Workers must be scientifically selected and trained so that they can be more productive on their jobs.
3. Bring the scientifically designed jobs and workers together so that there will be a match between them.
4. There must be division of labor and cooperation between management and workers.

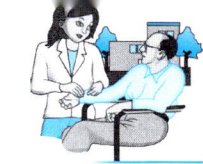

Knowledge

Taylor's Philosophy in a Nutshell
- Based on science, not rule of thumb
- Attained by harmony and not discard
- Can yield maximum output, in place of restricted output
- Maximum prosperity of employer, coupled with maximum prosperity of each employee

Limitations of scientific management

- **Exploitative device:** Emphasis on productivity rather than sharing the benefits with workers.
- **Depersonalized work:** Scientific management supplied standardized jobs to workers. They do the same job which leads to boredom and monotony, so workers do not like the ideas of becoming glorified machines.
- **Unpsychological:** Because there is no accurate information as to how the wages are to be given.
- **Undemocratic:** Because it overshadows the workers independence. It treats workers as unthinking animals.
- **Anti-social:** Because workers are treated as glorified economic tools only.
- **Unrealistic:** Only concentrated on physical and financial needs completely ignoring the social and ego needs of people.

Administrative theory

This theory was given by Henry Fayol (1841-1925).

An approach that focuses on principles that can be used by managers to coordinate the internal activities of an organization. His principles are as follows:

Fayol's six
- Technical (production)
- Commercial (buying and selling)
- Financial (use of capital)
- Security (protection of property)
- Accounting (keeping financial records)
- Managerial

Management functions
Forecasting and planning, organizing, commanding, coordination, controlling

Principles of management
- Division of work
- Authority and responsibilities
- Discipline
- Unity of command
- Unity of direction
- Subordination of individual interest to the common goal
- Remuneration of personnel
- Order
- Centralization
- Scalar chain
- Equity
- Stability of tenure
- Initiative
- Esprit de corps

Managerial skills
Fayol emphasized that managers should have certain skills in order to their work efficiently.
- Good Physical health
- Mental (ability to understand, learn, judgement)
- Moral (energy, initiative, loyalty, tact and dignity)
- Educational (acquaintance with matters)
- Technical (specialized knowledge relating to one's area of specialization)
- Experience (related to the work carried out)

Limitations of fayol's theory
- **Lack of empirical evidence:** e.g. the principle specialization does not tell us the way to divide the tasks.
- **Neglect of human factor:** Human attributes such as emotion, attitude, creativity have been totally ignored.
- **Pro-management bias:** It suffers from pro-management bias. It is more concerned with what managers should know and do rather than with a more general understanding of managerial behavior.

Neo-classical Theory

It is also known as Human Relations Theory. Neo-classical theory is the modification of classical theory including insights from behavioral sciences like psychology, sociology and anthropology. Human relations movement began with Hawthorne studies, which were conducted from 1924 to 1933 at Hawthorne Plant of Western Electric Company in Cicero by Elton Mayo and Chester Bernard.

"It is defined as movement in management thinking and practice that emphasized satisfaction of employees' basic needs as the key to increased worker productivity.

Characteristics of Neo-classical Theory

- Structure-organization is a social system.
- Behavior is a product of feelings, sentiments and attitudes.
- Primary focus is on small groups, on emotional and human qualities of employees.
- Emphasises personal, security and social needs of workers while achieving organizational goals.
- Democratic practices, participation of employees in decision making in order to improve morale and happiness of employees. It recognizes the importance of human dignity and values.
  - Happy employees try to produce more.

Behavioral Science Theory

It includes theories of leadership and motivation.

Theories of Leadership

Trait theory of leadership

Trait is defined as *a relatively enduring quality of an individual.* The trait approach seeks to determine 'what makes a successful

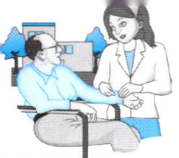

leader' from the leader's own personal characteristics. Research on leadership traits suggests that some factors differentiate leaders from non-leaders. The most important traits are a high level of personal drive, desire to lead, personal integrity, and self-confidence. Cognitive (analytical) ability, knowledge, charisma, creativity and flexibility are also desired. The various traits can be classified into innate and acquirable traits, on the basis of their source. These qualities are natural and often known as God-gifted. The individuals cannot acquire these qualities. Major innate qualities in a successful leader are:

- **Physical features:** Physical features of a man are determined by heredity factors. Heredity is the transmission of the qualities from ancestor to descendent. Physical characteristics and rate of maturation determine the personality formation which is an important factor in determining leadership success.
- **Intelligence:** For leadership, higher level of intelligence is required. Intelligence is generally expressed in terms of mental ability. Intelligence, to a very great extent, is a natural quality in the individuals because it is directly related to the brain.

Acquirable qualities of leadership are those which can be acquired and increased through various processes. Many of these traits can be increased through training programs. Following are the major qualities essential for leadership:

- **Emotional stability:** A leader should have high level of emotional stability. He should be free from bias, consistent in action, and refrain from anger. He is well adjusted, and believes that he can meet most situations successfully.
- **Human relations:** A successful leader should have adequate knowledge of human relations. An important part of a leader's job is to develop people and get their voluntary cooperation for achieving work. He should have intimate knowledge of how human beings behave and how they react to various situations.
- **Empathy:** Empathy relates to observing the things or situations from other's points of view. The ability to look at things objectively and understanding them from others' point of view is an important aspect of successful leadership. Empathy requires respect for the rights, beliefs, values and feelings of others.
- **Objectivity:** Objectivity implies that what a leader does should be based on relevant facts and information. He should make an objective diagnosis and implement the action required.
- **Motivating skills:** A leader should be self-motivated and have the requisite quality to motivate his followers. There is an inner drive in people for motivation to work. The leader can play an active role in stimulating the inner drives of his followers.
- **Technical skills:** The ability to plan, organizes, delegate, analyze, seek, advice, make decisions, control and win cooperation requires the use of important abilities which constitute technical competence of leadership.
- **Communicative skills:** *A* successful leader knows to communicate effectively. A leader uses communication skillfully for persuasive, informative and stimulating purposes.
- **Social skills:** *A* successful leader has social skills. He understands people and knows their strengths and weaknesses. He has ability to work with people so that he gains their confidence and loyalty.

Behavioral theory

According to this theory, a leader behaves according to the role expectations of the group. Strong leadership is the result of effective role behavior. To operate effectively, group needs someone to perform two major functions; a. Task related or problem solving functions and b. group maintenance or social functions.

Assumptions

- Leaders can be made, rather than are born.
- Successful leadership is based in definable, learnable behavior.

Behavioral theories of leadership do not seek inborn traits or capabilities. Rather, they look at what leaders actually *do*. This leadership theory focuses on the actions of leaders, not on mental qualities or internal states.

This theory failed to explain why a particular leadership behavior is effective in one situation, but fails in another situation. Thus, situational variables are not considered.

McGregor theory

Douglas McGregor categorized leadership style into two brand categories in his management theories, i.e. theory X and theory Y, having two different beliefs and assumptions about subordinates.

McGregor (1906-1964) postulated that managers tend to make two different assumptions about human nature.

> **Box: 1**
>
> **McGregor**
>
> **Theory X**
> - The average human being has an inherent dislike of work and will avoid it if he or she can.
> - Because of this human characteristic, most people must be coerced, controlled, directed, and threatened with punishment to get them to put forth adequate effort toward the achievement of organizational objectives.
> - The average human being prefers to be directed, wishes to avoid responsibility, has relatively little ambition, and wants security above all.
>
> **Theory Y**
> - The expenditure of physical and mental effort in work is as natural as play or rest.

Contd…

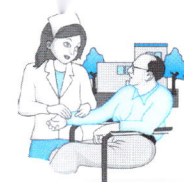

> **Box: 1**
> - External control and threat of punishment are not the only means for bringing about effort toward organizational objectives. People will exercise self-direction and self-control in the service of objectives to which they are committed.
> - Commitment to objectives is a function of the rewards associated with their achievement.
> - The average human being learns, under proper conditions, not only to accept responsibility but to seek it.
> - The capacity to exercise a relatively high degree of imagination. Ingenuity and creativity in the solution of organizational problems is widely, not narrowly, distributed in the population.
> - Under the conditions of modern industrial life, the intellectual potentialities of the average human being are only partially utilized.

Motivational Theories

Abraham maslow's need hierarchy theory

One of the most popular theories of motivation is the hierarchy of needs theory put forth by psychologist Abraham Maslow. Maslow saw human needs in the form of a hierarchy, ascending from the lowest to the highest, and he concluded that when one set of needs is satisfied, people will go for the next needs. He classified the human needs into five (Fig. 5).
- Physiological needs
- Safety needs
- Social needs
- Esteem needs
- Self actualization needs

Maslow later refined his model to include a level between esteem needs and self-actualization: The need for knowledge and aesthetics.

Implications for management

Maslow's theory has some important implications for management. This model helps the managers to understand and deal with issues of employee motivation at work place. Managers who understand the need patterns of their staff can help the employees the kinds of work activities and some of the implications are to meet,
- **Physiological needs:** Provide lunch periods, rest breaks, and wages that are sufficient to purchase the essentials of life.
- **Safety needs:** Provide a safe working environment, retirement benefits, and job security.
- **Social needs:** Create a sense of community via team-based projects and social events.
- **Esteem needs:** Recognize achievements to make employees feel appreciated and valued. Offer job titles that convey the importance of the position.
- **Self-actualization:** Provide employees a challenge and the opportunity to reach their full career potential.

Frederick herzberg's motivation-hygiene theory or herzberg's two factor theory (Fig. 6)

Herzberg stated that there are certain satisfiers and dissatisfiers for employees at work. They are intrinsic factors related to job satisfaction and extrinsic factors associated with dissatisfaction. Removing dissatisfying characteristics from a job does not necessarily make the job satisfying.

The two factors identified by him are:
- **Hygiene factors** → Which can demotivate when not present, e.g. security, status, relationship with subordinates, personal life, salary, work conditions, relationship with supervisor and administration.
- **Motivational factors** → Which will motivate when present, e.g. growth prospects, job advancement, responsibility, challenges, recognition and achievements.

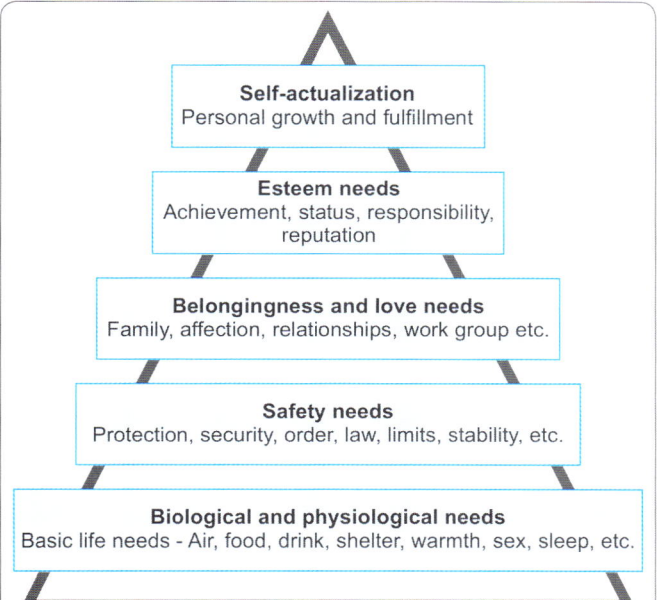

Figure 5: Maslow's Hierarchy of Needs

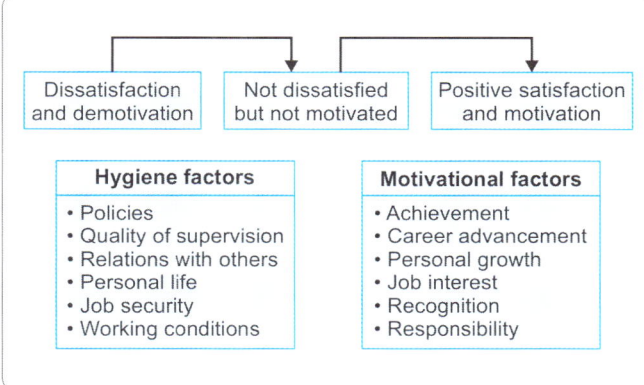

Figure 6: Herzberg's two-factor theory

Herzberg states that presence of certain factors like security, status, relationship with subordinates, personal life, salary, work conditions, relationship with supervisor and administration in the organization does not lead to motivation. However, their absence leads to dissatisfaction. These are called hygiene factors (or) dissatisfiers.

Similarly the absence of certain factors like growth prospectus, job advancement, responsibility, challenges, recognition and achievement causes no dissatisfaction, but their presence has motivational impact. These are called motivational factors or satisfiers.

Implications

In order to motivate employees, the manager must ensure to provide the hygiene factors and then motivating the motivating factors. So if we want to motivate employees on their jobs, it is suggested to give much importance on those job content factors such as opportunities for personal growth, recognition, responsibility and achievement. These are the factors of intrinsic motivation.

Herzberg model sensitizes that managers should utilize the skills, abilities and talents of workers.

Modern Approach

In this, modern management thought (MMT) combines the valuable concepts of classical theory with the social and natural sciences. The source of inspiration of MMT is the system analysis.

Characteristics of MMT

- **Open system view:** It treats the organization as an open system. Because it interacts with the environment continually, in order to survive and flourish. It receives input from the environment, processes them into meaningful services and offers to the environment
- **Dynamic and adaptive:** Modern theory is dynamic. Changes according to change in outer environment.
- **Multilevel and multidimensional:** MMT is both micro and macro. It is macro when considered with respect to the entire nation or industry; it is micro with respect to internal parts of the organization.
- **Multimotivated and multidisciplinary:** MMT recognizes that the behavior is the product of multifarious factors. As worker can be motivated with salaries and extra wages and benefits. Similarly, multidisciplinary as embraces the economics, sociology, engineering, psychology, etc.

This applies system theory and contingency theory.

System Theory (Fig. 7)

It tries to solve problems by diagnosing them within the framework of input, transformations processes, output and feedback.

Relevance and usefulness of system's theory:

- In a system, a manager operates with a view to complete all tasks which give relevant results to the organization.

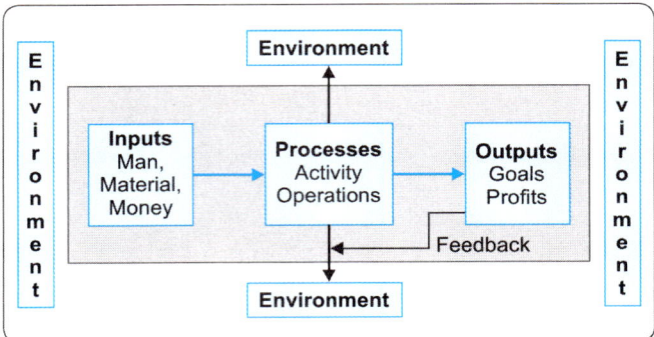

Figure 7: System theory

- They think before they act, evaluate their works after implementation.
- It makes a good balance between various parts of the organization and goals.

Contingency Theory

(Situational approach): It argues that appropriate managerial action depends on the particular parameters of the situation.

Important elements in contingency theory:

- According to it, effective management varies with the organization and its environment.
- Spells out the relationship of organization to its environment clearly.
- Each organization is unique.
- More pragmatic and action-oriented
- Tries to identify nature of inter-dependence between various parts of an organization and their impact on various things.

Organizational Structure

A good organizational structure is needed so that each employee in the organization is assigned a role and responsibility and necessary authority. Organizational structure includes arrangement of organizational activities and assignment of resources in those activities to achieve goals of organization. It is the way in which the activities of each department in the organization are coordinated and integrated to achieve organizational objectives. In a good organizational structure each employee is assigned a responsibility and the activities of employees in each department are coordinated and integrated to achieve goals.

Steps in Organizational Structuring

The organization needs to be structured in such a manner that human and physical resources are brought to action to achieve the goals and objectives. The following are some of the steps to build organizational structure.

- **Determination, identification and enumeration of activities:** After setting vision, mission, goals and objectives identify the activities required to achieve these objectives. These activities are again divided in to sub activities so

that each employee knows his role, responsibilities and relationship with the others.
- **Grouping and assigning of activities:** All similar activities are grouped together and the activities are further divided into sub activities as purchasing, budgeting etc. These groups of activities are assigned to various divisions or departments. The departmental heads delegate and distribute the job to their subordinates.
- **Delegation of authority:** The persons who are assigned the particular activity of job are responsible for performing their work in an optimal manner. So they must be given corresponding authority also. Responsibility is actually the accountability of authority.

Benefits of Good Organizational Structure

- **Achievement of objectives:** A good organizational structure facilitates attainment of objectives.
- **Minimum conflicts:** Conflicts between employees are found to be less in good organizational structure as each employee is assigned a particular job to perform.
- **Reduction in duplication of work:** Since a good organizational structure requires that the duties be clearly defined and assigned, duplication of work is less.
- **Interpersonal relations and communication:** A good organizational structure facilitates effective communication at all levels of organizational hierarchy and maintains good interpersonal relations.
- **Effective planning:** A well organized organizational structure provides a sound basis for effective planning. Since the goals are clearly established and resources are clearly identified, planning becomes more focused and realistic.
- **Increase in cooperation and proper coordination:** A good organizational structure results in increased cooperation and a sense of pride among members of the organization. Also, because of clear cut accountability and recognition of skill, the employees develop their own initiative and a spirit of motivation and creativity.

Forms of Organizational Structures

The types of organization structure based on the authority and responsibility are:

Line Organization

Line Organizational Structure is the oldest and simplest form of organization. In line organizational structure, the authority flows vertically from top to bottom and each employee knows to whom they areanswerable. The line of authority is vertical and workers at the same level perform the same function. The direction flows from top, transmitted through the managers to the supervisors and then to the workers and staff.

Advantages of line organization

- It is simple to establish and easily understood by employees.
- There is a clear unity command and all employees are directly involved in achieving the objectives.
- It facilitates prompt decision making.
- It is economically effective.
- It ensures better discipline and there is unified control.
- It provides opportunity for the development of managers as every manager has to perform a variety of functions.

Disadvantages

- It cannot be used for large organization.
- It is rigid.
- There is lack of expertise to give advice. Managers are responsible for both planning and execution of work.
- All decisions come from top level.
- There is inadequate communication from bottom to top level.

Line and Staff Organization

- In line and staff organization, there are staff specialists who give expert advice to line managers to perform their duties. The staff specialists have the right to recommend but have no authority. This type of organizational structure is most commonly seen in large organization. The combination of line organization with expert staff constitute the lines and staff organization.

Advantages of line and staff organizational structure

- There is possibility to receive specialized advice from experts.
- The work load is reduced and managers can utilize enough time for creative thinking.
- The line and staff organizational structure is highly flexible because new activities may be introduced without disturbing line authority.
- There is a chance for better decision making process.
- The principle of unity of command is followed in line and staff organizational structure.

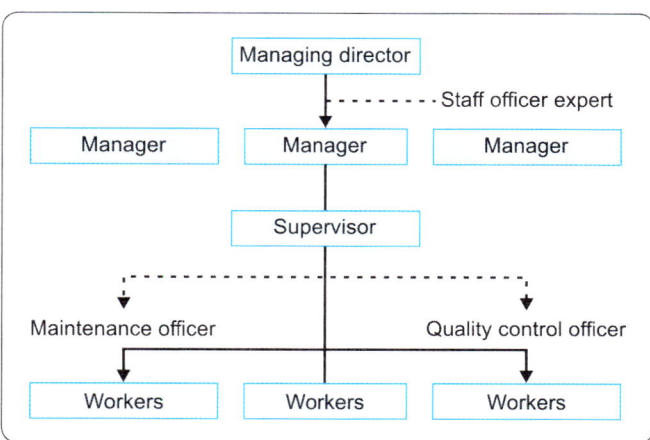

Figure 8: Line and staff organization

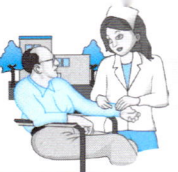

Disadvantages

- There is possibility for conflicts between line managers and staff specialists.
- Line managers sometimes depend too much on staff experts.
- Staff specialists have no authority.
- There are chances of role confusion among staff and line officers.

Functional Organization

In functional organizational structure, the organization is divided in to a number of functional areas, i.e., organization is grouped according to its purpose. The whole activities of organization are divided into various functions and each functional area is put under the charge of a functional manager. In hospitals, the functional areas may be classified into nursing care services area, laboratory services, pharmacy service etc.

Advantages

- **High specialization:** Every functional head is an expert in his area and all employees get the benefit of his expertise.
- **Better control** and coordination.
- Duplication of work can be kept minimum and there is clarity in functioning.
- Helps to improve efficiency of employees.
- Facilitates adequate supervision

Disadvantages

- **Complex relationship:** Each employee is accountable to several superiors which results in conflicts between workers and specialists.
- As there are many cross relationships, an employee may receive conflicting orders.
- **Slow decision making:** As several specialists may involve in decision making process, there is delay in decision making.

Project Organization

In project organizational structure each project is organized under a semi autonomous project division. A project team consists of specialists in different areas. The activities of the project team members are coordinated by a project manager. Once a particular project is completed, the project division undertakes a new project.

Advantages

- It facilitates more attention to completion of complex projects.
- It permits maximum use of knowledge, skill and experience of employees.
- It provides better coordination of organization resources.

Disadvantages

- Project manager has to deal with specialties from a number of diverse fields. The specialists have different approaches and interests. It delays the decision making process.
- The job of project manager becomes difficult due to lack of clarity defined, responsibility and lack of clear communication.

Matrix Organization

Matrix organization is an organizational form in which there are multiple lines of authority and is used in large multinational organization. It is a combination of functional and project organization and it is otherwise called grid organization.

There are several departments under matrix organization. The available resources of the organization can be used by each department along with the coordination of other departments in an organization.

A matrix organizational structure is any organization that employs a multiple command system, that includes not only the multiple command structure, but also related mechanisms and there are associated organizational structures and behavior patterns.

—*SM Davis and PR Lawrence*

Under matrix organizational structure, the project teams are formed using personnel from permanent functional structure. Different project managers share resources and authority with functional head. The employees are subjected to dual line of command from the project manager and functional head. When one project is over, the resources are diverted to new projects.

Advantages

- Better utilization of resources in the organization
- The matrix structure offers operational freedom and flexibility.
- In matrix organizational structure employees learn new skills which helps in their development.
- It helps to maintain professional identity.
- Under matrix structure, the motivation and morale of employees are lightened.

Disadvantages

- **Double line of commands:** In matrix organizational structure, working relationships become complex and there is great confusion among employees due to double line command. As the employees get command and from different superiors like, functional or department manager and project manager, unity of command is violated.
- **Problem of adjustment:** In Matrix organizational structure, after completion of one project, people are assigned to some new project and employees face problems of adjustment.
- **Delayed decisions:** There are chances for delay in taking decisions.

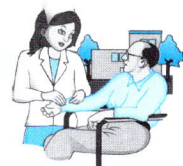

CENTRALIZATION AND DECENTRALIZATION

Centralization is the process of transfer of administrative authority from a lower level to a higher level of organization.
—*LD White.*

In a centralized organizational structure, most of the power and critical decision making responsibilities are concentrated within a few administrators. The authority for most decisions is concentrated at the top of managerial hierarchy.

In decentralization, the authority is dispersed by extension and delegation through all levels of management. Decentralization refers to systematic efforts to delegate to the lowest levels of authority except that which can only be exercised at central points or decentralization is the process of systematically delegating power and authority throughout the organization to middle and lower level managers. No organization is ever completely decentralized or completely centralized.

Some of the variables as being primary in determining the need for a centralized or decentralized structure isolated by research studies are size and complexity of the organization, competency of top management, competency of subordinates, desirably of creativity in the organization, adequacy of communication system, etc.

Advantages of Centralization

- The quality of decision is expected to be higher since the top management who makes decisions are more experienced and knowledgeable.
- It is a means for adopting and enforcing uniform policies and it achieves coordination since all decisions are made at one point.
- Centralization results in optimum utilization of human and physical resources.
- Centralization provides prestige and power and is highly motivating for executives.
- Centralization makes it easier to achieve balance among the activities of different departments and areas.

Demerits of Centralization

- As decisions are taken by the top level management, the role of subordinates in executive functions are less.
- There is less involvement by specialists as all decisions are taken by top level managers.

Advantages of Decentralization

- It provides foundations for the development of future executives.
- It helps to reduce the work load of top executives.
- Decentralization is highly motivational for subordinates and provides a feeling of status and recognition to subordinates.
- There may be possibility for prompt action and quick decisions at lower level itself.
- Decentralization results in effective control over operations and processes.
- Decentralization creates delegation of authority which provides effective supervision and control.

Disadvantages of Decentralization

- **Lack of coordination:** In decentralization each department has autonomy. Hence coordination becomes difficult.
- As large number of managers and supervisors are required in decentralization, which leads to substantial increase in cost of operation.
- As different departments work independently, there will be difficulty in control.

ORGANIZATIONAL CHARTS

Organizational charts and manuals are prepared for the purpose of describing the organization structure. These are used as tools of management control. They give full information on a particular organization. An executive finds out his exact place in the organization structure from the charts and manuals.

It shows the responsibility and authority of an executive. He knows his superior for whom he is responsible and his subordinates whom he has to supervise.

Definition

"An organization chart is a diagrammatic representation of the framework or structure of an organization". —*J.Batty*

"An organization chart is a diagrammatical form which shows the *important aspects* of an organization including the major *functions* and their respective *relationship*, the channels of supervision and the relative *authority* of each employee who is in charge of each respective function".
—*Terry*

Contents of Organizational Charts

- Basic organization structure and flow of authority
- Authority and responsibilities of various executives
- The relationship between the line and staff officers
- Names of components of organization
- Positions of various office personnel
- Number of persons working in the organization
- The present and proposed organization structure
- Ways of promotion
- The requirements of management development
- Salary particulars

Principles of Organizational Chart

- **Observation of lines of authority by top executives:** The executives should never by pass the lines of authority. The

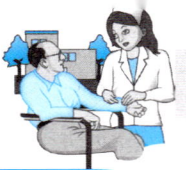

executives should give orders or obtain information by following the lines of authority.
- **Observation of lines of authority** by subordinates
- **Defining lines of position:** The position of each individual in an organization should be clearly stated. The staff should be assured that there would not be overlapping and two persons would not be appointed for the same position when their authorities and responsibilities are different.
- **Non-assignment of same duty twice:** An individual should not be compelled to work under two masters for the same work performance.
- **Avoid unique concentration of duty:** All work or maximum work should not be concentrated in a single point. The work should be divided according to the duties and responsibilities of each worker and the administrative relationship with others.
- **Organizational charts should be above personalities:** A position should not be assigned to a person since he is the son or relative of any one of the top executives of the organization. Prime importance should be given to an organization than to an individual.
- **Simple and flexible:** understandable. Size and nature of the organization may be changed in course of time. Need may arise for periodical modification in the organization chart. Then the existing organization chart should permit these modifications.

Example of an organization chart has been illustrated in Figure 9.

Types of Organizational Chart

All use a spatial relationship (i.e., a distance between) to illustrate differences in rank, authority or status.

Basic (Vertical chart)

The basic relationship is that between superior and subordinate and usually this is shown vertically. The lines of command flows from the top level to the bottom in vertical lines. This vertical chart is in the form of a graph. This type is followed in companies.

Superior-supervisor, etc   A
Subordinate-operator, clerk, etc   B

This fig shows superior/subordinate relationship.

Horizontal Chart

The lines of command flows horizontally. In this, the supervisor is on the left side of the chart and the subordinate on the right side or vice versa. This is not followed in any organization.

Advantages of Organizational Charts

- They give a clear picture of the organization in a simple way.
- They show the levels of authority and relationship prevailing among employees at a glance.
- Dual reporting relationships and overlapping positions come to light in the preparation of organization chart.
- Instructing work is simplified.
- Newly hired personnel can understand their role in the organization and behave accordingly.
- Strengths and weaknesses of an organization are evaluated.
- It acts as authoritative source of information.
- The lines of authority shown are definite and formal.
- The lines of promotion can be understood.
- Organization charts help planning and improve communication both inward and outward.
- Correct methods of checks and balances in the organization are provided.
- The degree of contribution to organization and achievements can be identified.
- The obstacles to the efficient functioning of the management can be found while drawing the organization's chart.
- The outsiders can have a quick understanding of each department and original disputes can be solved in the organization.

Limitations of Organizational Charts

- The organization charts create more rigidity of relationship prevailing among the employees of the organization.
- It is very difficult to maintain and ensure that the organization charts up-to-date. The employees of the organization are very reluctant to put up with the organization changes.
- The organizational charts don't show the informal relationship existing among the organization's staff members.
- If the charts are not correctly prepared, they will lead to misleading inference. A false picture may be developed by following the over simplified structure of organization.
- There is no differentiation between line officers and staff officers in an organization chart.
- The organization charts produce a psychological complex such as superiors, inferiors etc., in the minds of the employees.
- The relationship shown in an organization's chart does not actually prevail among the employees.
- The words and lines used in an organizational chart gives different meanings to different people.

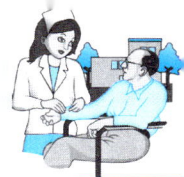

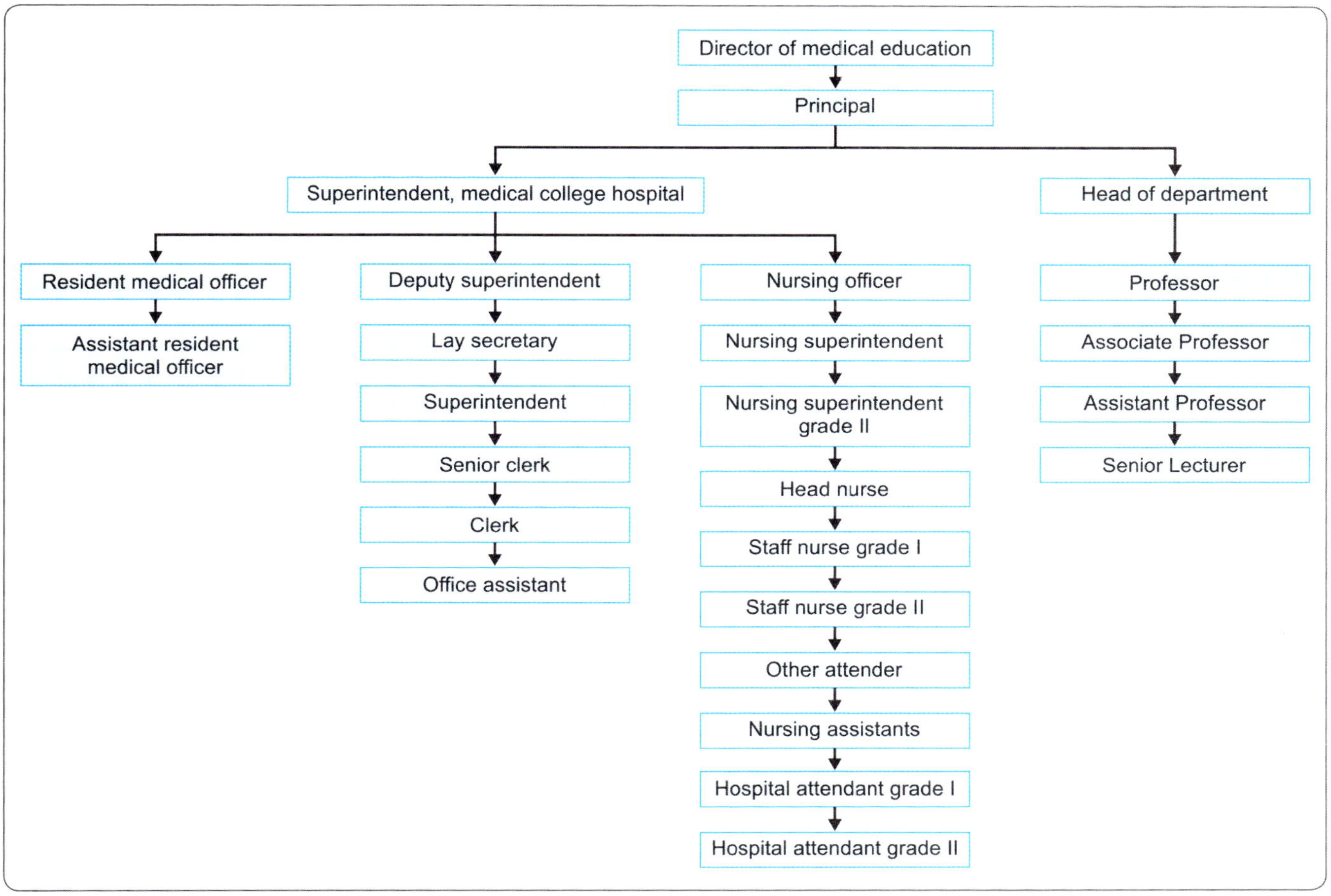

```
                        Director of medical education
                                    ↓
                               Principal
                    ┌───────────────┴───────────────┐
                    ↓                               ↓
         Superintendent, medical college hospital        Head of department
    ┌───────────┬───────────┬───────────┐                ↓
    ↓           ↓           ↓                         Professor
Resident    Deputy      Nursing officer                  ↓
medical    superintendent    ↓                    Associate Professor
officer        ↓        Nursing superintendent           ↓
    ↓       Lay secretary    ↓                    Assistant Professor
Assistant      ↓        Nursing superintendent           ↓
resident   Superintendent  grade II                Senior Lecturer
medical        ↓              ↓
officer    Senior clerk   Head nurse
               ↓              ↓
             Clerk       Staff nurse grade I
               ↓              ↓
         Office assistant Staff nurse grade II
                              ↓
                         Other attender
                              ↓
                        Nursing assistants
                              ↓
                    Hospital attendant grade I
                              ↓
                    Hospital attendant grade II
```

Figure 9: Example of an organization chart

STAFFING

Staffing is a constant challenge for health care facilities. Staffing is the most crucial function of management to have a competent person for job to achieve high quality service in an organization. Proper staffing helps to ensure optimum utilization of human resources. Before the selection of the employees, one has to analyse about the requirements of a particular job, which are required by an organization.

Definitions

Staffing is selection, training, motivating and retaining of a personnel in the organization.

Staffing is the systematic approach to the problems of selecting, training, motivating and retaining professional and non-professional personnel in any organization. It involves manpower planning to have the right person in the right place.

Philosophy of Staffing in Nursing

Nurse administrators of a hospital nursing department must adopt the following staffing philosophy:

- Nurse administrators believe that the needs of critically ill patients should be met by professional nurses, as the condition of certain patients may be more complex in nature.
- Nurse administrators believe that patient's assessment, work quantification and job analysis should be used to determine the number of personnel in each category to be assigned in care for patients of a particular disease condition.
- Nurse administrators believe that a master staffing plans, policies and protocols in all units should be prepared centrally by the nursing department heads of nursing service.
- Nurse administrator believes that the staffing plan should be administered at the unit level by the head nurse, so that selected plan details, such as shift start time, number of staff assigned to go on holidays, and number of employees assigned to each shift could be modified to accommodate the unit's workload and workflow.

Objectives of Staffing in Nursing

- Provide sufficient staff to permit 1:1 nurse-patient ratio for each shift in every critical care unit.

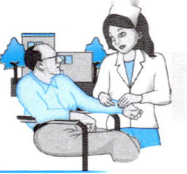

- Staffing the unit by following hospital policy
- Head of nursing services should be involved in designing master staffing program.
- Head nurses should be held responsible for planning schedules in their wards.
- Empowering the head nurse to adjust work schedules for unit nursing personnel to get rid of problems associated with any staff excess or deficiency which may be caused by census fluctuation or employees absence. Also consider staff on special vacation or holidays.
- Reward employees for long-term services like, special time requests to individauls, on the basis of seniority. .

Norms of staffing (S I U- Staff Inspection Unit)

Norms

Norms are standards that guide, control and regulate individuals and communities. For planning nursing manpower in a hospital we have to follow some norms. The nursing norms are recommended by various committees, such as; the 'Nursing Man Power Committee, The High-power Committee, Dr. Bajaj Committee, The Staff Inspection Committee, TNAI and INC'. The norms have been recommended taking into account the workload projected in the wards and the other areas of the hospital.

All the above committees and the staff inspection unit recommend the norms for optimum nurse-patient ratio, such as: **1:3** for non teaching hospital and 1:5 for the teaching hospital.

Staff Inspection Unit

The Staff Inspection Unit (SIU) is the unit which has recommended the nursing norms in the year 1991-92. As per this SIU norms the present nurse-patient ratio is based and practiced in all central government hospitals.

Recommendations by SIU

- The norms for providing staff nurses and nursing sisters in government hospital is given in this report. The norms have been recommended taking into account the workload projected in the wards and the other areas of the hospital.
- The posts of nursing sisters and staff nurses have been clubbed together for calculating the staff entitled for performing nursing care work. The work that is assigned to the nursing staff will be continued even after he/she has been promoted to the existing scale of nursing sister from the post of staff nurse.
- Out of the entitlement worked out on the basis of the norms, 30% posts may be sanctioned as nursing sister. This would further improve the existing ratio of 1 nursing sister to 3.6 that is the ratio of staff nurses fixed by the government, in settlement with the Delhi Nurse Union in may 1990.
- The assistant nursing superintendents are recommended in the ratio of 1 ANS to every 4.5 nursing sisters. The ANS will perform the duty presently performed by nursing sisters and perform duty in shift also.
- The posts of Deputy Nursing Superintendent may continue at the level of 1 DNS per every 7.5 ANS.
- There will be a post of Nursing Superintendent for every hospital having 250 or more beds.
- There will be a post of 1 Chief Nursing Officer for every hospital having 500 or more beds.
- It is recommended that 45% posts added for the area of 365 days working including 10% leave reserve (maternity leave, earned leave and days off as nurses are entitled for 8 days off per month and 3 national holidays per year when doing 3 shift duties).

Most of the hospitals today are following the S.I.U. norms. In this the post of the nursing sisters and the staff nurses has been clubbed together and the work of the ward sister remains same as staff nurse even after promotion. The 'Assistant Nursing Superintendent' and the 'Deputy Nursing Superintendent' have to do the duty of one category below their rank.

HUMAN RESOURCE MANAGEMENT

Human beings are the most important resources of an organization and management. Human resources are a challenge for the administrator to manage. Human resource management (HRM) is the function within an organization that focuses on recruitment, management and providing direction for the people who work in the organization.

Definition

Human resource management is the function performed in organizations that facilitates the most effective use of people to achieve organizational and individual goals.
—*Ivancevich and Gluck*

Human resource management is defined as a process of acquiring, training, appraising and compensating employees and attending to their labor relation, health safety and fairness concerns.
—*Dassler.*

Human resource management is planning, organizing, directing and controlling of the procurement, development, compensation, integration, maintenance and separation of human resources to the end that individual organizational and social objectives are accomplished. —*Edwin B Flippo*

Human resource management is a strategic and comprehensive approach for managing people and the work culture and environment.

Human resource management ensures effective utilization and maximum development of human resources and to develop and maintain a quality of work life. Sound HRM helps to maintain high morale and job satisfaction among employees.

Human resource planning for health is the process of estimating the required health work force to meet future health service requirements and the development of strategies to meet those requirements.

Human health resource planning is defines as the process of ensuring that the right health workers are in right place at the right time with the right skills. —*Gavel, 2004*

Importance of Human Resource Management

Human resource management is important in organizations for achieving the goals and objectives. HRM helps for the replacement of employees–those who have retired from services or died or became disabled.

- HRM helps in attracting and retaining employees in an organization.
- It helps in effective utilization of human resources.
- HRM helps to create team spirit among employees.
- HRM helps to meet the challenges occurring in the field of health due to expanding needs of human resources.
- HRM creates a positive working environment for workers.
- HRM provides opportunity for effective utilization of individual employees and their talents.
- HRM provides opportunity for development of employees and facilitates professional growth.
- HRM provides opportunity to manage and identify future requirements of human resources and provides the basis for recruitment and selection.
- HRM helps for the effective utilization of nursing personnel.
- It helps to create a balance in a situation where there is a mandate to cope with the changing technology and rising needs as well as demands.
- HRM also facilitates for preparation of appropriate human resource budget for each department.
- HRM helps to improve quality of patient care services.

So through sound HRM, the managers are able to place the right number of employees with right skill at the right place and thereby provide quality health care services to public. Effective HRM enables human resources to contribute in productivity to attain the goals of an organization. Human resource management includes the following:

- Conducting job analysis
- Planning personnel needs and recruitment
- Selecting the right people for the job
- Facilities for orientation and continuing education
- Determining and managing wages and salaries
- Providing benefits and incentives
- Appraising performance
- Communicating with employees at all levels.

Human Resource–Philosophy

The philosophy of human resource should be based on the following beliefs:

- Human beings are the most important assets in the organization.
- Human beings can be developed to a great extent as they have creative energy which is utilized only partially.
- Human beings feel committed to their work in the organization if they develop belongingness with it.
- Human beings are likely to develop a feeling of belongingness if the organization takes care of them and their needs of satisfaction.
- Human beings contribute to the maximum if they get an opportunity to discover their full potential and to use it.
- It is the responsibility of the organization to create healthy and motivating week climate characterized by openness, enthusiasm, trust and collaboration.

Human Resource Philosophy Cardinal Beliefs

- **Self managing resource:** Human being is a fundamentally different and unique resource in that employee is a source and a resource at the same time and lies at the end of all economic and social activities.
- **Potential:** Believe in the inherent potential of people. There are different kinds and degrees of potentials which can be developed and utilized in the context of task challenges, responsibility and commitment.
- **Limitations:** Any apparent limitations in people are the results of a variety of situations and factors and can be overcome with support.
- **Quality of work life:** The institution can provide high quality of work life for all its members through opportunities for a meaningful carrier, job satisfaction and professional achievements.
- **Meritocracy:** Believe that people accept meritocracy as a just and equitable system and contribute best under condition of open opportunities and challenges.
- **Actualization:** Believes that update of human resource management system is able to enrich the skills and creation of good environment and it is ongoing process. The philosophy of HRM is to develop people/employees as per their aspirations and individual goals and motivate them to help in achieving organizational goals.

STAFFING PROCESS

- Recruitment
- Selection
- Placement and indoctrination
- Training
- Development
- Appraisal and remuneration

Recruitment

Recruitment is an important function of health manpower management, which determines whether the required output will be available at the work spot, when a job is actually undertaken. Recruitment procedures include the process and the methods by which vaccancies are notified, posts are advertised, applications are handled and screened, interviews

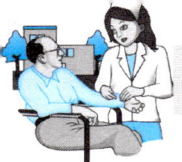

are conducted and appointments are made. Recruitment of nurses are a major concern in healthcare settings. It is a process of searching for prospective employees and stimulating them to apply for job in an organization.

In a simple term, recruitment is understood as the process of searching for and obtaining applicants for job and from these the right people is selected.

Recruitment refers to the process of attracting, screening, and selecting qualified people for a job at an organization or firm. Recruitment is a process of securing applicants to fill vacant positions. It covers both, the filling of new and replacement of previously established posts which fall vacant. Recruitment is defined as the process of searching for prospective employees and stimulating them to apply for job in the organization. —*B Flippo*

Recruitment is a process to discover the sources of manpower to meet the requirements of the staffing schedule and to employ effective measures for attracting the manpower in adequate numbers to facilitate effective selection of an efficient working force. —*Yoder*

Recruitment is the development and maintenance of adequate manpower resources. It involves the creation of pool of available labor upon whom the organization can draw when it needs additional employees. —*Dale S Beach*

Factors Affecting Recruitment Policy

- Organizational objectives
- Personnel policies of the organization and its competitors.
- Government policies on reservations
- Preferred sources of recruitment
- Need of the organization
- Recruitment costs and financial implications
- Size of the organization
- Employment conditions in the community

In the field of nursing, in addition to the above mentioned factors, some of the additional factors must be considered. They are—nurse patient ratio, increasing number of hospital departments, bed occupancy, foreign job opportunity etc.

Planning for Recruitment

The shortage of nurses highlighted the need for health agencies to actively market nursing positions to available applicants. Marketing is a planned approach to promote an exchange relationship with a desired candidate.

Marketing encompasses four concepts i.e. product, place, promotion and price.

To market employment to professional nurses, the recruiter should *describe the product* as a nursing position with opportunity for personal adventure, professional enrichment and social expansion that can be shaped to satisfy an incumbent's needs and showcase her or his abilities.

In addressing place, the agency and the nursing unit should be described as settings for high-quality care of selected types of patient and enriching professional experience for nurses of the applicants' description.

In planning promotion of the job to applicants, the recruiter must decide who can most persuasively convey the facts about the job and when and how this information should be transmitted to attract the highest quality candidates.

In marketing job, *the price factor* should include present salary, insurance benefits, in-service educational opportunities, pension or retirement provisions and promotional opportunities.

Sources of Recruitment

Internal Sources

These sources include the employees already on the payroll i.e. present work force. Whenever any new vacancy arises, people from within the organization will be upgraded, promoted and transferred. The process of filling job openings by selecting from among the pool of present work force can be implemented by the following methods:

- Reviewing the personnel records
- Job posting and job bidding
- Inside moonlighting and employee's friends

Internal Recruitment

It is done when the business looks to fill the vacancy from within its existing workforce. They can be:

- Present permanent employees (based on programs of career development)
- Present temporary/casual employees
- Retired employees
- Dependents of deceased, disabled, retired and present employees

Advantages of internal recruitment

- Motivation to the employees
- Helps to develop a sense of security
- Performance of employees may improve
- Increase morale of workers
- Reduce staff turnover
- More experienced employees can be recruited

Disadvantages

Talented persons may lose the opportunities

External Recruitment

Recruitment is called external recruitment
Is when the business looks to fill the vacancy from any suitable applicant outside the business.

External Sources

External sources lie outside an organization. Here the organization can have the services of:

- Employees working in other organizations
- Job aspirants registered with employment exchanges
- Students from reputed educational institutions

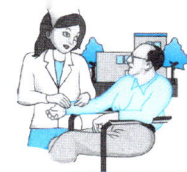

- Candidates referred by unions, friends, relatives and existing employees
- Candidates forwarded by search firms and contractors
- Candidates responding to the advertisements, issued by the organization
- Unsolicited applications/walk-ins.

	Advantages	Disadvantages
Internal Recruitment	Cheaper and quicker to recruit	Limits the number of potential applicants
	People already familiar with the business and how it operates	No new ideas can be introduced from outside the business
	Provides opportunities for promotion within the business – can be motivating	May cause resentment amongst candidates not appointed
	Business already knows the strengths and weaknesses of candidates	Creates another vacancy which needs to be filled
External Recruitment	Outside people bring in new ideas	Longer process
	Larger pool of workers from which to find the best candidate	More expensive process due to advertisements and interviews required
	People have a wider range of experience	Selection process may not be effective enough to reveal the best candidate

The numbers given in the Figure 10 above are:
1. Identify vacancy or job requirement
2. Prepare job description and person specification
3. Deciding the source of recruitment and selection methods
4. Advertising the vacancy
5. Managing the response
6. Short-listing of the candidates
7. Conducting interview and select and appoint successful candidates

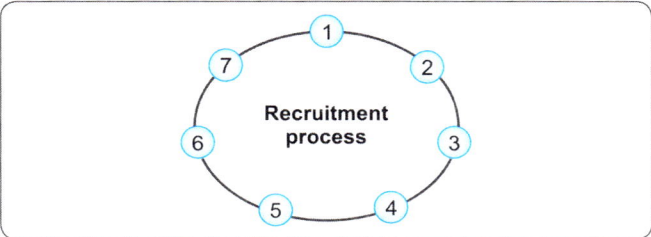

Figure 10: Recruitment process

The **recruitment process** is immediately followed by the selection process i.e. the final interviews and the decision making, conveying the decision and the appointment formalities.

Recruitment Methods

Recruitment can be done by different methods as,
- **Recruitment by campus method**
- **Recruitment by job centers:** They usually provide a shortlist of candidates based on the people registered with the agency. They also supply temporary or interim employees.
- **Recruitment by advertisements:** They can be found in many places such as:
  - Newspaper
  - Job posting on job sites
  - Ads on websites related to positions recruited.
- **Database search on job sites:** Company can buy data from job websites for a week or a month to search candidates.
- **Contract staffing**
- **Word-of-mouth recruitment/personal recommendation:** Often referred to as 'word of mouth' and can be a recommendation from a colleague at work. A full assessment of the candidate is still needed however but potentially it saves advertising cost.
- **Free online ads:** You can post your recruitment ads at free websites such as social forums, blogs, etc...
- **Career-day programs:** In some places nursing schools and colleges hold, annual career-day programs during which recruiting officers from local health agencies inform senior students about employment opportunities in respective organizations.
- **Open house:** It is a showcase of the opening of a new service or educational program. If health agency is well organized, and their settings attract idealistic, service-oriented nurses then the candidates apply for job. Invitation to an open house may be sent to individual nurses, groups of specialty nurses, professional organizations, final year student nurses and alumni of schools/colleges to attend open house for recruitment.
- **Promotions and transfers:** This is a method of filling vacancies from within through transfers and promotions. A transfer is a lateral movement within the same grade, from one job to another. It may lead to changes in duties and responsibilities, working conditions, etc but not necessarily salary. Promotion on the other hand, involves movement of employee from a lower level position to a higher level position accompanied by (usually) changes in duties, responsibilities, status and vision.
- **Employment exchanges:** As a statutory requirement, companies are also expected to notify their vacancies

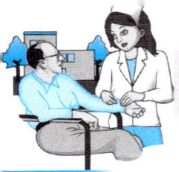

through the respective employment exchanges, existing all over India for helping unemployed youth, displaced persons, ex-military personnel, physically handicapped, etc.
- **Gate hiring and contractors:** Gate hiring is for job seekers, generally blue collar employees, who present themselves at the factory gate and offer their services on a daily basis.
- **Unsolicited applicants/walk-ins:** Companies generally receive unsolicited applicants from job seekers at various points of time.
- **e-hiring:** The first step in e-hiring is to get a URL (Universal Resource Location) that people can conveniently use and thus they do not have to use a search engine. There is no point in being a famous company if people cannot find you without trouble on the net.

Selection

Selection is the process of choosing the right candidate. It is the process of picking individuals who have relevant qualifications to fill jobs in an organization. The basic purpose is to choose the individual who can most successfully perform the job from a pool of similarly qualified candidates.

The purpose of selection is to pick up the most suitable candidate who would meet the requirements of the job and the organization best and to find out which job applicant will be successful, if hired. To meet this goal, the company obtains and assesses information about the applications in terms of age, qualifications, skills, experience, etc. The steps which constitute the employee selection process are the following:

Screening and receiving the application
- Conducting preliminary interview .Interview by personnel department
- Pre-employment tests
- Interview by department head
- Decision of Administrator to accept or reject
- Medical Examination
- Check for references
- Issue of appointment order

Interviewing

It is the main method of appraising an applicant's suitability for a post. The objectives of interview are:
- Decide suitability for post
- To give candidate complete picture of post and organization
- To obtain additional information

Pre-employment tests
- For certain category of posts there is a need for testing professional competence of candidates for assessing certain characteristics that can't be properly assessed otherwise. These tests include:
  - Tests in general ability
  - Tests in specific ability
  - Tests for achievement
  - Personality tests
  - Intelligence tests
  - Aptitude test

Role of Nurse Manager
- Ensure fairness in selection process.
- Accept that our perceptions to understand others can't be accurate every time and it can act as a stumbling block.
- Create an environment of minimal pressure to elicit maximal performance.
- Advocate the use of reliable and valid tools for selection.

Placement

Placement refers to the allocation of people to jobs. Placement is defined as the appointment of right employees at the right place that arouse the will to work in the mind of the operators. Placement is a decisive step and should consist of matching job requirements and offers.

Advantages of Appropriate Placement
- Increases intensity and duration of human efforts.
- Lessens labor turnover and absenteeism
- **Improves work performance**

Staff Training and Development

Discussed in detail in unit 6

Appraisal and Remuneration Promotion

Promotion refers to a change for better prospects from one job to another job by the employee. The factors implying promotion are:
- Increase in salary
- Increase in job prestige
- Upliftment in hierarchy of jobs
- Additional supervisory ability
- A better future

Unions generally favor promotions on the basis of seniority and managements usually favor promotion on the basis of merits. However, it is an ideal to have following factors which must be the basis of promotion.
- Outstanding services in terms of quality as well as quantity
- Above average achievement in patient care
- Experience
- Seniority
- Initiative
- Leadership qualities
- Particular knowledge and experience necessary for a vacancy
- Record of loyalty and cooperation

RETENTION

The loss of nurses is unsustainable in a workplace environment as nurses' shortage continues to increase. High increase in number of nurses turnover can impact negatively on an organization's capacity to meet patient needs and provide quality care. **Nurse turnover** is a recurring problem for health

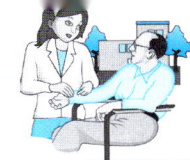

care organizations. Nurse retention focuses on preventing nurse turnover and keeping nurses in an organizations employment. At the nursing unit level, high turnover affects the morale of nurses and the productivity of those who remain to provide care while new staff members are hired and orientated.

Nurse Turnover Determinants

Job Satisfaction

- Job satisfaction factors include extrinsic rewards, scheduling, family/work balance, co-workers, interaction, professional opportunities, praise/recognition and control/responsibility. Job dissatisfaction has been frequently identified as the reason why nurses leave their jobs. Low job satisfaction was concentrated in young, newly qualified and highly educated nurses, and is associated with administration, promotional prospects, employment security and amount of time for clinical duties.
- **Moderators of nurse turnover:** Some studies suggest that certain moderators apart from external, personal and work-related variables also influence job satisfaction like, turnover intention and turnover behavior. Poor management and communication, burnout etc. add to these factors.
- **Stress, workload and burnout:** Heavy workload increases stress which results in burnout and lowering morale and thus increases likelihood of turnover.
- **Management style:** Good management style is needed for retention. It may be facilitative communication, flexible working hours, decentralized organizational structure etc, resulting in higher levels of job satisfaction and lower nurse turnover. .
- **Empowerment and autonomy:** Empowerment is associated with nurse retention. Structural empowerment is the perception of the presence or absence of empowering conditions in the workplace, psychological empowerment is the employees' psychological interpretation or reaction to these conditions.
- **Promotional opportunities**
  Career development and life-long learning activities in nursing promotes retention of nurses and enable continued provision of high-quality care. Dissatisfaction with promotion and training opportunities has been shown to have a strong impact on nurse turnover.
- **Work schedules:** To promote balance between work and home, potential benefits of self-scheduling strategies have been documented, especially for nurses who have home responsibilities such as young children; long shifts, overtime, weekend duties, night dutiess, overtime on holidays and weekends were found to be predictors of anticipated turnover.
- **Individual factors and turnover:** Certain socio-demographic characteristics of nurses predispose to turnover. An inverse relationship between age and turnover has been demonstrated. It is suggested that mature nurses have greater job satisfaction, productivity and organizational commitment. Highly educated individuals are more likely to quit in order to seek career advancement, especially if there are limited opportunities in their current organization.
- **Economic factors and nurse turnover:** Studies that include remuneration as one component of job satisfaction are inconsistent in their findings. For example, pay does not have as strong an impact as work environment.

Consequences of Nurse Turnover

There is overall consensus that undesirable nurse turnover is costly as well as detrimental to nurse and patient outcomes. Patients do suffer more physically and emotionally in health care environments experiencing high nurse turnover.

Direct costs are those incurred during the hiring process, such as advertising, recruiting agency for hiring of nurses. Indirect costs are due to orientation and training and decreased productivity. Indirect costs of nursing turnover could be significant because of the decreased initial productivity of new employees and the decrease in staff morale and group productivity that imposes nursing turnover.

Role of Nurse Manager

- **Passion**—Show your involvement and commitment to the organization at all levels, as well as during participation in community activities.
- **Due diligence**—Hire right person, the first time itself.
- **Orientation**—Use a program to provide an excellent orientation in a safe work environment.
- **Staying power**—Give employees a reason to stay.
- **Put the staff first**—To create a patient-centered environment and actualize the mission of the organization, it is important to put the staff first who would then put the patient first. It includes caring about them as people, meeting their needs, treating them with respect and high regard, using appreciation and recognition liberally; listening and responding to them and providing support.
- **Forge authentic connections**—It includes taking time to connect with employees. Each employee needs to have a personal, individual connection with the manager.
- **Coach for and expect competence**—Focusing on the growth and development, both personal and professional on the people with whom they worked. Setting high standards and clarifying expectations, coaching and supporting development, modeling the behavior they expected from staff and managing the performance of people within the department help to accomplish this goal.
- **Partner with the staff**—Adopt a leadership style based on a partnership relationship of which visibility and accessibility are key aspects.

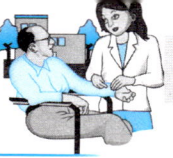

SEPARATION

Separation occurs when an employee leaves the organization.

Types of Separation
- Voluntary separation
- Involuntary separation

Voluntary Separation

Voluntary separation occurs when the employee decides to terminate his or her relationship with the organization.
- **Quits:** An employee decides to quit when his or her level of dissatisfaction with the present job is high or a more attractive alternative job is awaiting the individual.
- **Retirements:** Retirements occur when the employee reach the end of their career.

Involuntary Separation

Employers resort to termination for the below mentioned reasons:
- Organization is passing through lean period and is unable to maintain existing labor
- Initial faulty hiring
- Employee exhibiting deviant behavior vitiating the environment
- **Discharges:** Discharge or termination takes place when the employer discovers that it is undesirable to keep an employee. Termination needs to be viewed as a last resort.
- **Resignation:** It refers to the termination of employment at the insistence of employee.

Role of Nurse Managers
- Facilitate the process of separation
- Make provision for the replacement of vacant places
- Support employee during the transition
- Do as needed to maintain reputation of organization.

DIRECTING

Directing is one of the most important function of management. While managing an enterprise, managers have to get things done through people. In order to be able to do so, they have to undertake many activities, like guide the people who work under them, inspire and lead them to achieve common objectives. Direction helps the managers in ensuring quality performance of jobs by the employees and achievement of organizational goals.

According to Koontz and O'Donnel Directing is a complex function that include all those activities which are designed to encourage subordinates to work effectively and efficiently in both the short and long run.

Directing involves determining the course, giving order and instruction and providing dynamic leadership (Marshall).

Direction consists of the process and techniques utilizing in issuing instruction and making certain that operations are carried out as planned.

Directing is concerned with instructing, guiding, supervising and inspiring people in an organization to achieve its objectives. It is the process of telling people what to do and seeing that they do it in the best possible manner. The directing function thus, involves:
- Telling people what is to be done and explaining to them how to do it.
- Issuing instructions and orders to subordinates to carry out their assignments as scheduled.
- Supervising their activities.
- Inspiring them to meet the mangers expectation and contribute towards the achievement of organizational objectives.
- Providing leadership.

Features of Direction
- Direction is an important managerial function. Through direction, management initiates actions in an organization.
- Direction is performed at every level of management. It is performed in the context of superior-subordinate relationship and every manager in the organization performs his duties both as superior and as subordinate.
- Direction is a continuous process. Every manager needs to direct his subordinates on a continual basis.
- Direction initiates at the top level in the organization and follows to bottom through the hierarchy. It emphasizes that a subordinate is to be directed by his superiors only.
- Direction has dual objectives. It aims at getting things done by subordinates and also provides opportunities to superiors for doing some more important works which their subordinates cannot do.

Importance of Direction
- **Direction initiates action:** It guides and helps the subordinates to complete the given task properly and as per schedule.
- **Direction integrates employee's effort:** Each individual's performance affects the performance of others in the organization. Hence individual efforts need to be integrated so that organization achieves its objectives in the most efficient manner.
- **Direction attempts to get maximum out of the individual:** It provides the necessary motivation to subordinates to complete the work satisfactorily and strive to do their best.
- **Direction facilitates changes in the organization:** Organization exists in society and any change in the society changes organizational process. To incorporate and implement these changes, management should motivate individuals affected by these changes, which is an essential part of direction.

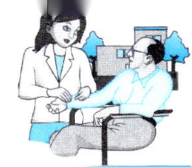

- **Direction provides stability and balance in the organization:** Effective leadership, communication and motivation provide stability in the organization and maintain balance in different parts of the organization.

Elements or Techniques of Direction

Communication, supervision, motivation and leadership are the four essential elements of directing.

Motivation

"Motivation is the complex force starting and keeping a person at work in an organization. Motivation is something that moves the person to action, and continues to keep him in the course of action already initiated."

Both monetary and non-monetary incentives are given to employees for motivation.

Motivation is one of the important elements of directing. It may be in the form of incentives like financial (such as bonus, commission etc.) or non-financial (such as appreciation, growth etc.), or it could be positive or negative. Basically, motivation is directed towards goals and prompt people to act.

Roles and Functions of Motivation in Directing

- Recognize each worker as unique individual who is motivated by different things.
- Identify the individual and collective value system of a unit, and implement a reward system that is consistent with those values.
- Encourage workers to stretch themselves in an effort to promote self-growth and self-actualization.
- Maintain a positive and enthusiastic image as a role model to subordinates in the clinical settings.
- Encourage monitoring and coaching with subordinates
- Devote time and energy to create an environment that is supportive and encouraging to the discouraged individuals
- Develop a unit philosophy that recognizes the unique worth of each employee and promotes reward system

Leadership

"Leadership is the process of influencing and supporting others to work enthusiastically towards achieving objectives."
—*Bamard Keys and thomas case*

Leadership plays an important role in directing. The objectives of any organization can only be fulfilled if its employees are working towards accomplishment of set objectives. To make people work in the desired manner, proper instructions and guidance are necessary. And this direction process becomes effective when the persons who give such direction have leadership qualities. Leadership is essential in functioning of any organization. Its importance and benefits are varied.

Roles and Functions of Leadership in Directing

- To lay down goals and policies to persuade the subordinates to work with zeal and confidence.
- To shape the organization on scientific lines with the view to make its various components operate sensitively and reliably.
- The leader should be capable of taking pioneering decisions on all vital aspects of administration.
- The leader should consult the group in framing the policies and lines of action and in initiating any radical change in them.
- He should exercise authority whenever necessary to implement the general policies in the interest of the group.
- He should keep the employees well informed of their duties and obligations and adopt motivational exercises to stimulate them for the performance of task.

Communication

"Communication is defined as the process by which people seek to share meaning via the transmission of symbolic messages".
—*FEX Dance*

Communication is a basic organizational function, which refers to the process by which a person (known as sender) transmits information or messages to another person (known as receiver). The purpose of communication in organizations is to convey orders, instructions or information so as to bring desired changes in the performance and/or the attitude of employees. Proper communication results in clarity and securing the cooperation of subordinates. Faulty communication may create problems due to misunderstanding between the superior and subordinates.

Roles and Functions of Communication in Directing

- **Information function:** Information is vital for the functioning of any organization. The technology of communication has greatly enhanced man's information generating capabilities.
- **Command and instructive function:** Those who are hierarchically superior often initiate communication not only for the purpose of informing their subordinates, but also for the purpose of telling them what to do, directing them or commanding their behavior in some way.
- **Influence and persuasive function:** In management, influence and persuasion together represent one of the several functions. Managers can influence others either through coercively or communicatively. Since influence through coercion has its limitation in organizational settings, managers can influence others through effective communication.
- **Integrative function:** Communication performs the integrative function by relating various components of the organization and maintaining equilibrium among them. The integrational aspects include all behavioral operations which serve to keep the system in operation.
- **Other functions:**
  - Communication helps employees to understand their role clearly and perform effectively.

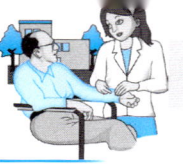

- It helps in achieving coordination and mutual understanding which in turn, leads to industrial harmony and increased productivity.
- Communication improves managerial efficiency and ensures cooperation of the staff.
- Effective communication helps in molding attitudes and building up employees' morale.
- Communication is the means through which delegation and decentralization of authority is successfully accomplished in an organization.

Supervision

"Supervision is defined as the authoritative direction of the work of one's subordinates."

Supervision means overseeing the employees at work. The effectiveness of the workers depends largely on the supervision they reserve. In other words, quality of work is directly related to the degree of supervision. Managers play the role of supervisors and ensure that the work is done as per the instructions and the plans. Supervisors clarify all instructions and guide employees to work as a team in cooperation with others. Supervisors are expected to maintain the best and friendly relations with their seniors as well as with the workers and enjoy the trust and confidence of both management and operatives

Roles and Functions of Supervision in Directing

- **Orientation of newly posted staff:** All newcomers should be informed about their functions, the method that they should use, the personnel whom should they work with, etc. All these things need orientation.
- **Assessment of the workload of individuals and groups:** It must be ensured that the work load is within the physical and mental competence of a worker. Otherwise job should not be assigned to them.
- **Arranging for the flow of materials:** A supervisor must find out the need for supplies and equipment and arrange for their supply in good time.
- **Coordination of the efforts:** A supervisor coordinates the work of his/her workers and agencies and promotes team work.
- **Promotion of effectiveness of workers:** This may be done through performance evaluation and introducing concept of staff development.
- **Promotion of social contact within the work team:** Social contacts help to bring the staff together and increase group cohesiveness.
- **Helping the individuals to cope with their personal problems:** A sympathetic understanding of the individual's personal problems improves the employee's morale.
- **Facilitating the flow of communication:** A free flow of communication among members is necessary for team work. Supervisor should encourage free communication among the employee.
- **Raising the level of motivation:** All good works should be given due recognition. Supervisor must provide opportunities for growth and achievements.
- **Establishment of control:** A supervisor should know what work is being done and with what effectiveness. Techniques such as observation and review of recordscan be used for this purpose.
- **Development of confidence**: Supervisors should know the background of workers and try to develop mutual confidence.
- **Record keeping:** They should maintain good record system for many purposes like.

CONTROL IN MANAGEMENT/CONTROLLING

Control is one of the most important functions of management. Control is concerned with securing good individual performance and organizational performance. The function of control includes the activities that are undertaken to ensure that the events do not deviate from pre-arranged plans.

Control is an executive process. It involves three elements – standards, evaluation and corrective action. Individual and organizational performances are measured and evaluated against standards to ensure actual results against expected results.

Definition

Controlling is determining what is being accomplished, that is evaluating the performance and if necessary applying corrected measures so that performance takes place according to plan.
—*Terry*

Management control is systematic effort to set performance standards with planning objectives to design information feedback systems, to compare actual performance with the pre-determined standards to determine whether there are any deviations and to measure their significance and to take any action required to assure that all resources are being used in the most effective and efficient possible way to achieve objectives.
—*Robert J. Mockler*

Importance of Control

Control is a fundamental managerial function. The importance of control includes:

- **Insurance of value of control:** The basic function of control includes regulating activities in such a way as to ensure achievements of pre-determined objectives.
- Control is the basis of future action.
- **Control facilitates coordination:** Coordination is facilitated by control functions of management.
- Control methods can be used to standardize quality of performance in the organization.
- Control helps to conserve assets of the organization.

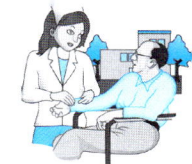

- Control is used to evaluate the performance of employees in an organization through internal audit, budgeting, etc.
- Control helps top level management for keeping plans and programs in balance through policy making, preparation of master budget, etc.
- Control ensures organizational efficiency and effectiveness.
- Control methods can be used to motivate the employees through recognition for achievement, promotions and other methods of recognition.

Characteristics/Features of Control

- Control is an ongoing activity and it is exercised by all managements.
- Unity is an integral part of control.
- There should be flexibility in management system.
- Control must be forward looking or futuristic.
- Control process must be work focused.
- Control is a continuous process.
- Control is a coordinated and integrated system.
- Pervasiveness

Requirements for Effective Controlling

Control is necessary in every organization to ensure that every action is going properly. So every organization should have an effective control system.

- Control system should reflect the organizational needs.
- **Accuracy:** Accurate data is necessary for effective control.
- **Flexibility in control:** An effective control system is one that can be changed quickly as and when need arises.
- Control must be simple and balanced.
- **Acceptable:** Control measures should be acceptable to employees.
- Control must be forward looking and motivating.
- **Integration:** When control becomes an integrated part of organizational environment and it becomes effective.
- **Economic feasibility:** Control system must be economically feasible and reasonable to operate.
- **Strategic control points:** For maintaining balance and economy in all control systems, control is exercised on strategic points.

Steps in the Control Process

The steps in control process are:

- **Establishment of control standards:** Standards are established in every organization which are criteria against which actual results are measured. For effective control of care services to patients, establish standards of performance against which activities can be verified and compared. Standards established must be specific and clear and understood by all employees. Standards are formulated to assess the expenditure involved in the function of an organization to assess the level of quality of patient care services and level of performance of employees in the institution.
- **Measurement of performance:** The second step in the controlling process is to monitor and measure the actual performance by using standards of performance set. Assessment of performance must be a continuous activity and involves collection of data that represents the actual performance. Measurements can be performed to assess whether resources are adequate in meeting the needs, to assess effectiveness of patient care achievement of planned goals, the efficiency of employees and the effectiveness of institution. The performance is qualitative and intangible such as human relations, employee morale etc. It can be measured by psychological tests and opinions surveys.
  According to Peter Drucker, for measuring tangible and intangible performance, measurements must be clear, simple and having rationale, relevant, reliable, self-announcing and understandable.
- **Evaluating performances:** The third step is the comparison of actual performance and standard performance. For that first identify the extent of deviations and then find out the cause of deviations. This information should be informed to the employee and his immediate supervisors so that improvement in performance can be ensured. Evaluation of the work progress is reviewed so that management can make necessary adjustments for improving final outcome.
- **Taking corrective actions:** After measurement and evaluation of performance, corrective actions must be made. The action should be taken to maintain the desired degree of control system or operation. Such control actions may be taken to,
  - Review plans and goals and change therein on the basis of such reviews.
  - Change in the assignment of tasks.
  - Change in existing technique of direction.
  - Change in organization structure, provision of new facilities, etc.

Control Areas

Controls are needed in every area, in the process of management. Peter Drucker has identified eight key areas where objectives should be set and controls should be exercised. These are: market standing, innovation, productivity, physical and financial resources, profitability, managerial performance and attitude development, work performance and public responsibility. The following are some of the areas where control can be established.

- **Controls over policies:** Policies are formulated to govern the behavior and actions of personnel in the organization and are prepared by top management.
- **Control over organization:** Organization charts and manuals are used to keep control over organization structure.
- **Control over employees:** The manager may keep control over personnel in the organization.
- Control over wages and salaries

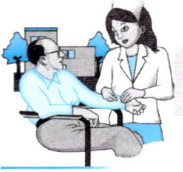

- **Control over costs:** Cost control is exercised by making comparison between standard cost and actual cost. Cost control can also be ensured by budgetary control system
- **Control over methods and manpower:** This helps to ensure that the individual is working properly. So periodic analysis of activities is needed. The methods adopted and time consumed must be controlled.
- **Control over capital expenditure:** The budget must be prepared and evaluated.
- **Control over research and development:** As research and development are highly technical activities therefore they must also be controlled indirectly.
- Control over public relation
- **Overall control:** Control over each segment of organization contribute to overall control.

PLANNING METHODS

For planning and scheduling of programs or projects there are Mainly 3 major methods. They are Gantt Chart, Program Evaluation and Review Technique (PERT) and Critical Pathway Method (CPM).

Gantt Chart

Gantt chart was initiated by Henry L. Gantt to measure tasks in a project. It is one of the most popular methods of showing activities (tasks and events) displayed against time. Gantt chart is most commonly used for tracking project schedules. It helps to visualize and plan project tasks and helps in monitoring project progress. Gantt chart is graphical illustration of a schedule that helps to plan and coordinate specific task in a project. Gantt chart shows various activities, the beginning and ending of each activity, the period schedule for each activity and whether activities overlap or not.

A Gantt Chart is formulated with a vertical axis representing the task that makeup the project and horizontal axis representing time span of the project broken down into days, weeks or months. Each task is represented by a bar and the bar shows the start, duration and end date of each activity.

Steps of Construction of Gantt Charts

- The first step in preparing a Gantt Chart is to identify the task involved in completing a project.
- In the next step, calculate the expected time required for each task.
- Organize the sequence of each of the activities identified.
- Draw a horizontal time axis, along the top or bottom of the page. Mark it in an appropriate scale for the length of tasks (days/weeks).
- On the left side of the page, write each task and milestones of the project in order. For the activities that occur over a period of time, draw a bar that represents appropriate items on the timeline. Align the left end of the bar with the time when the activity begins and align the right end with time when the activity concludes.

Table 4: Calculations of ET for Gantt chart

Task	O	M	P	TE
I	1 month	2 months	5 months	2.33
II	2 months	4 months	6 months	4
III	3 months	4 months	7 months	4.33
IV	5 months	6 months	8 months	6.1
V	2 months	6 months	4 months	4

For example, if there are 6 tasks in a project labelled from I to V. Calculate the time estimate for these 6 tasks and the three time estimates are,

O – Optimistic time
M – Most likely
P – Pessimistic time
We can calculate expected time (ET) by using formula
$TE = (O + 4M + P) \div 6$

Characteristics of Gantt Chart

- The bar in each row indicates the corresponding tasks (Fig. 5)
- The horizontal position of the bar indicates start and end times of the task.
- The bar length represents the duration of the task.
- Task duration of one can be compared easily with another.
- Precedence relationships can be represented using arrows.

Advantages

- Simple to create
- Used for planning and scheduling projects
- Provides easy graphical representation of progression of activities
- It allows both planning, monitoring and control.
- Gantt chart represents a clear order of work.

Limitations

- Gantt chart clearly indicates details regarding the progress of activities.
- Gantt chart does not indicate relationship between separate activities.
- It does not explain the reason behind the duration of each activity.
- It does not explain the course of project or the resources being utilized in the project.

Program Evaluation and Review Technique (PERT)

PERT is a mathematical and schematic network technique developed in 1958 by Boos, Allen and Hamilton. In the 1950s, Project Evaluation Review Technique was developed by the US Navy to manage the Polaris submarine missile program of their Special Projects Office. The Program Evaluation and Review Technique is a traditional project management tools that is used to schedule, organize and coordinate tasks within

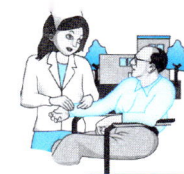

Task	Duration ET	February	March	April	May	June	July	August	September
I	2.33	██████████							
II	4	████████████████████						
III	4.33		████████████████████				
IV	6.1			██████████████████████████████			
V	4				████████████████████		

Figure 5: Gantt Chart

a project. It is a sophisticated version of the network technique comprising a number of events and activities. It is a complex, task oriented technique of activities.

Program Evaluation and Review Technique provides a visual depiction of major activities and sequence in which they are computed. Program Evaluation and Review Technique uses statistical method for estimating time required for each activity (Fig. 6).

According to Harold Kerzner, Program Evaluation and Review Technique is basically a management planning and control tool. It can be considered as a road map for particular program or project in which all major events have been completely identified together with their corresponding interactions.

Program Evaluation and Review Technique shows a list of activities within a project, their duration and relationship between them. PERT is a technique used for problems that occur once or for a few times and that has a definite starting point and finishing (completion) point.

Two paths can be identified here. One traced by the events ABCEGH and the other ABDFGH. The question before the manager is: Which is the critical path that determines the earliest possible completion date of the project under consideration. The critical path is the path in the project network that takes the longest time to complete. It is the sequence of various activities in a project that the management is most anxious to determine, monitor and shorten, since a delay in any of these activities will cause corresponding delay in the entire project.

Steps of PERT
PERT Involves the following Steps
- **Identify the specific activities and milestones:** The first step in formulation of PERT is to identify the activities or tasks that are required to complete the project. The milestones are the events marking the beginning and the end of one or more activities.

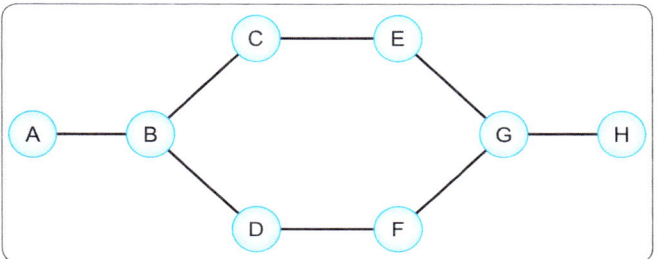

Figure 6: A hypothetical construct of PERT

- **Determine the sequence of activities:** In this step, the manager has to organize the activities in a sequence so that it become easy to chart PERT network.
- **Create a network diagram:** Using these sequences of activities, a network diagram can be drawn in which they can be represented by using arrow lines and the sequence by circles.
- **Estimate the time required:** The weeks or months are commonly used to estimate the time required for each activity. For each activity, the model usually includes the three time estimates, the optimistic time, realistic time and the pessimistic time. Estimate the time using the calculations mentioned below. Shift the green highlighted text here
- **Determine the critical path**: The critical path is determined by adding the times of each activities in each sequence and determining the longest path in the project. If activities outside the critical path speed up or slows down, the total project time does not change. The amount of time that a non-critical pathway activity can be delayed without the project is referred to as slack time.
- **Update PERT chart** as the project progresses.

In Program Evaluation and Review Technique, the time required for activity is based on the assumption that activity's duration follows a probability distribution instead of being a single value and three time estimates are required to compute the parameters of an activity, duration and distribution. These are the optimistic time, realistic time and expected time.

Optimistic time: The least time or the minimum possible time required to complete an activity (O).

Realistic time: Most likely time of an activity (M) ie, how much time is required to complete the activity under normal circumstances.

Pessimistic time: The maximum time of activity (P)

In order to calculate the time estimate of an activity

$$\text{Expected time} = \frac{O + 4M + 9}{6}$$

For example, to compute a project in public health,

If, O = 12 days
M = 18 days
P = 60 days

$$\text{Expected time} = \frac{12 + 4(8) + 60}{6} = 24 \text{ days}$$

Structure of PERT chart: The Program Evaluation and Review Technique chart consists of arrows and nodes or circles. The arrows represent the activities and the nodes represent the sequence of activities from starting point to finishing point of diagram which is called as path (Fig. 7).

e.g.: PERT for conducting a community health project with 11 tasks ranging from Task A to Task K. At first, the manager has to list down the tasks/activities and milestones and find out the expected time. If the expected time are as follows:

S. No.	Task	Expected time
1	A	12
2	B	8
3	C	5
4	D	10
5	E	18
6	F	10
7	G	10
8	H	20
P	I	4
10	J	10
11	K	9

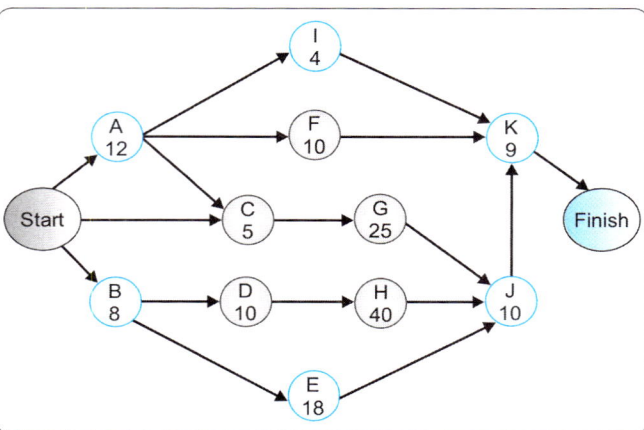

Fig. 7: PERT

In preparation of Program Evaluation and Review Technique chart, first the manager has to develop a relationship among the activities. Next is assigning of time and/or cost estimate to each activity and then computing the critical path. Use the network to help to plan schedule, monitor and control a project.

Uses of PERT
- Useful for organizing task and establishing time frames.
- It helps to plan, analyze and co-ordinate tasks within the project.
- It results in efficient utilization of resources and facilities.

Advantages
- Gives special emphasis to each activity
- Enables managers to make advanced planning for activity
- Allows identification of critical path and the minimum time needed to complete the total project.

Limitation
- Over emphasis on critical path
- Specified precedence relationship
- It is difficult to update or change project plan.

Critical Path Method (CPM)

Critical path method is a project modelling technique developed in the late 1950 by Morgan R Walker and James E. Kelly.

Critical path method is a step by step project management technique for process planning that defines critical and non-critical tasks with the goal of preventing time frame problems. It is an effective tool for project management. In Critical Pathway Method calculate the longest path of planned activities to the end of the project and the earliest and latest that each activity can start and finish without making the project longer. This process determines which activities are critical and which activity can be delayed without making the project longer.

Steps in Critical Pathway Method
- Identify each activity or task involved in the project.
- Determine the sequence of activities – A complete and thorough understanding of sequence of activities are needed to prepare Critical Pathway Method.
- Draw the critical path analysis chart or network diagram. The network diagram is a visual representation of the order of activities based on sequence (Figs 8A and B).
- Estimate activity completion time. We can use a 3 – point estimation method.
  a—the best case estimate
  m—the most likely estimate
  b—the worst case estimate
  E—(a+4m+b)/6
- Identify the critical path
- Update the critical path diagram to show progress

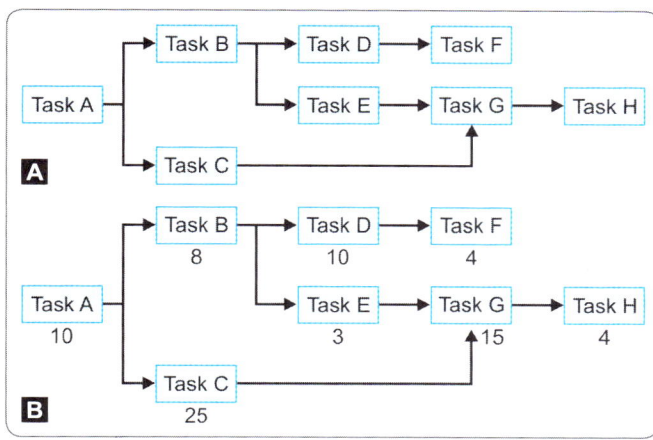

Figures 8A and B: A. Critical pathway method; B. Critical pathway after estimation of completion time

BENCH MARKING

Benchmarking is a process of comparison and measurement of a health care organization's performance against other health care organizations.

Benchmarking is a measurement tool for monitoring the impact of governance, management, clinical and logical functions. 　　　　　　　　　　　　　　*—Braillon 2008*

Bench marking in health care is a process of comparative evaluation and identification of under lying causes leading to high level of performance. 　　　　　　　*—Ellis 2006*

American Society for Quality (ASQ) defines benchmarking as a technique in which an organization measures its accomplishments against performance of the best organizations and according to ASQ subjects that can be bench marked include strategies, operations and processes.

Many health care organizations are using benchmarking as a tool for identifying desired standards of organizational performance as through benchmarking we are measuring products, practices and services against best performing organizations.

For example: Clinical benchmarking in hospital includes the area of hospital acquired infection, catheter associated urinary infection etc. The process involves the comparison and sharing of practices regarding management of catheter associated infection with best practices of another institutions.

Importance of Benchmarking

- Benchmarking improves current practices in an organization
- Benchmarking ensures sharing of evidence based practices between health care organizations at national level.
- It helps to improve customer's satisfaction and enables quality improvement.
- Benchmarking establishes high standards of excellence in health care facilities by comparing best health practice services from other organizations.

The Steps in Bench Marking

The process of benchmarking according to Pitarell and Monrier (2002)
- Select activity of bench marking
- Identify reference points
- Collect and organize data
- Identify the competitive data gap by comparing against external data
- Set future performance objectives
- Communicate the bench marking results
- Develop action plans
- Take concrete action
- Monitor progress

The different steps in benchmarking process include:
- Identify the area of practice–Identify the area to be bench marked, for example material management, human resource management etc.
- Comparing hospital performance
- Develop action plans
- Implement plans and monitor progress. Periodically assess and report the progress.
- Compare revised performance to bench marks of past.

Types of Bench Marking

Some specific types of benchmarking are:
- **Internal benchmarking:** This type of benchmarking means benchmarking process between departments in the same organization. In internal bench marking, standardized data is readily available and less time and resources are needed for the same.
- **External benchmarking:** External bench marking is comparison of performance against the best practices of another organization and this method takes significant time and uses resources to ensure the comparability of data and information.
- **International benchmarking:** In this types of benchmarking, best practitioners are identified and analyzed elsewhere in the world. Globalization and advances in health care information system are increasing opportunities for this.
- **Competitive benchmarking:** It is a process of comparing practices and performances with that of its most successful competitors.
- **Functional benchmarking:** Functional benchmarking includes comparing performance against best businesses operating in the similar field which perform similar activities.

Advantages of Benchmarking

- Enables sharing of best practices between health care facilities.
- Helps to maintain quality in service.
- Benchmarking improves current practices in the organization.

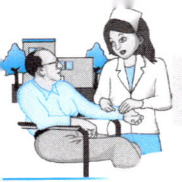

- It is a cost effective way of establishing innovative changes and brings improvement in quality and productivity.
- Provides opportunity to understand strengths and weaknesses in performance of the organization.

Benchmarking efforts may fail due to incompetent leadership, lack of adequate resources and facilities, lack of commitment on the part of management and workers. For effective benchmarking, the administrators must be competent with leadership abilities. The organization must allot resources for implementation of the process. Staff members from top level to bottom level must be educated and informed about their goals because staff of the institution plays a major role in implementation of bench marking.

BUDGET

A budget is a document that translates plans into money - money that is required to be spent to fulfil planned activities (expenditure) and money that will be generated to cover the costs of getting the work done (income). It is an estimate, or informed guess, about what you will need in monetary terms when you do your work.

Meaning of Budget

The word Budget is derived from the old English word "budgettee" means a sack or pouch which the chancellor used to keep his papers before presenting them in the Parliament for sharing financial schemes in the Government for the current year.

Now the term "budget" refers to the financial papers, certainly not to the sack. —*Definition of Budget*

"Budget" is a concrete precise picture of the total operation of an enterprise in monetary terms. —*HM Donovan*

It is financial blueprint or action plan for an organization. It translates the strategic plans into measurable expenditures and anticipated returns over a certain period of time.

"Budget" is an operational plan, for a definite period usually a year and is expressed in financial terms and is based on expected income and expenditure.

Purposes of Budget

- To assist in assessing the financial requirement of an agency.
- To indicate the lines on which the money raised or received will be spent.
- To provide participation of staff members in the preparation of budget.
- To guide the staff of a college in spending money allocated on various schemes.
- To provide adequate reporting system.
- To facilitate comparison of actual performance with targets and thereby to help controlling function.

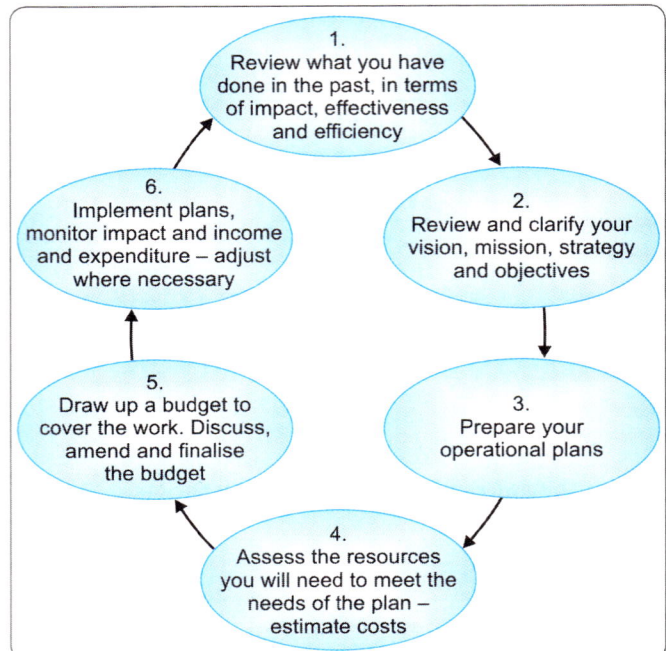

Figure 9: Budget planning

Budget Planning

Budget planning entails identifying the sources of income and taking into account all current and future expenses, with an aim to meet an individual's financial goals. The primary aim of a budget planner is to ensure savings after the allocation money for spending (Fig. 9).

How is Budget Planning Done?

By following good budgeting strategies, one can ensure the successful management of his or her expenditure and the recording of savings so that investments may be made for securing one's future.

Guidelines for Preparation of Budget

- The budget estimates should be prepared on realistic basis under relevant heads.
- The provision to be included in respect of each item should be based on what is expected to be or spent during the year including areas of previous year.
- Obsolete items should be omitted. The estimates for the current year must never be adopted blindly as a basis for framing those of the following year.
- Lump sum provisions to be avoided. As a rule details should be worked out for any item of expenditure included in the budget estimates.
- The number of posts budgeted in the current year and those for which provision is in the next year, should be clearly indicated, both for permanent and temporary posts.
- The minimum and maximum of scales of pay should also be indicated and provision should be made on the actual pay drawn by each individual.

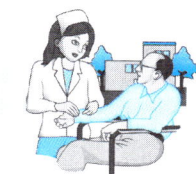

Essential Requisitions for Budget Preparation

- **Forecasting:** Sound forecasting may be related for making decisions on purchases, expansion, advertising, services, working capital needs etc.
- **Accounting:** Good accounting system must be needed to compare the budget information with actual accomplishments. The cost information tells us tabout how much it will cost to produce or give service.
- **Lines of authority:** Budget preparation, operation and supervision require clearly defined lines of authority.
- **Budget committee:** Budget preparation needs budget committee in an organization.
  - To receive and approve all forecasts, departmental budgets and periodic reports showing comparison of actual and budgeted income and expenditure.
  - To request for special studies of deviations from the budget and consider revision of budget to meet changed conditions.
- **Business policies:** Clearly defined business policies serve as basis for budget preparation.
- **Statistical information:** It is provided in the form of figures, i.e. estimates regarding the budget terms and this is essential for budget.
- **Top level management support** is essential to ensure successful installation of budget program.
- **Period of budget:** Length of budget period (usually a year) should be specified.

Factors Influencing Budget Planning

Any alteration in one or more factor/factors from the below mentioned factors require reviewing, modifying or even changing the budget. These factors are:
- Internal and external economic environment, as well as financial means.
- Changing demands of the clients and/or providers.
- Availability of human resources.
- Capacity of the organization (as opening a new, or closing a working unit).
- Service costs/market price.
- Organizational goals and strategic directions.
- Plans and objectives of one or more department.

Steps of Budget Planning

First Step–Assessment

- Assess what needs to be covered in the budget.
- Review the budget in the past, in terms of impactness, effectiveness and efficiency.
- Unit managers develop goals, objectives and budgetary estimates with input from colleagues and subordinates.

Second Step-Planning

How Planning is done?
- Selecting the optimal time frame for the budgeting.
- A budgeting cycle that is set for 12 months is called fiscal year budget, which may or may not coincide with the calendar year is then usually broken down in to quarters or subdivided into monthly, quarterly or semi-annual periods.
- Most budgets are developed for one year but a perpetual budget may be done on a continuous basis each month, so that 12 months of future data is always available.

Third Step- Implementation

- In this step, ongoing monitoring and analysis occurs to avoid inadequate or excess funds at the end of the fiscal year.
- In most of the health care institutions, monthly computerized statements outline each department's projected budget and any deviation from the budget.
- Each manager is accountable for budget deviation in his or her unit.

Fourth Step: Evaluation

- The budget must be reviewed periodically and modified as needed through the fiscal year.
- With each successive year of budgeting, managers can more accurately predict their unit's budgeting requirements.

Budget for College of Nursing

Budget for college of nursing is designed to support the college staff and students to carry out various activities and to protect money from being misused or wasted.

Preparation of Budget

Budget required for the nursing college is a cooperative activity of the principal and her associates as department heads, including the faculty members. It is prepared under the direction and supervision of the administrator or finance officer. The administrator supplies special forms for the budget. Budget request may be broken down to different units e.g. salaries, equipment and other purchase goods. The principal of college of nursing has certain specific functions in the preparation of budget request for programmed planning, estimating the cost, justification of request and for administration of budget in the college.

Generally the items which have to be included in the budget for college of nursing are following:
- Salaries for professional, clinical and domestic staff
- Stipends for student
- New equipment and repair
- Linen and other household supplies
- Office supplies, including stationary and postage
- Maintenance of transport and cost of conveyance
- Maintenance of library and purchase of books and journals
- Funds for educational tours, professional activities.

Types of Budget

- **Incremental budget:** It is based on estimated changes in present operation, plus a percentage increase for inflation. All of which is added to previous year's budget.

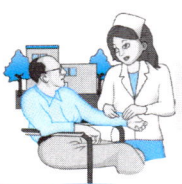

- **Open ended budget:** It is a financial plan in which each operating manager presents a single cost estimate for each program in the unit, without indicating how the budget should be scaled down if less funding is available.
- **Fixed ceiling budget:** It is a financial plan in which the upper most spending limit is set by top executive before the unit and divisional managers develop budget proposals for their areas of responsibility.
- **Flexible budget:** It is based on the fact that operating conditions rarely confirm the expectations.
- **Roll over budget:** It is a budget that forecasts programmed revenues for a period greater than a year.
- **Performance budget:** For example direct nursing care, in service education, quality improvement, nursing research.
- **Programmed budget:** It is a budget in which costs are computed for a total program i.e. grouping total costs or budget of each service being programmed e.g. MCH, FP and UIP etc. These base budgets require the nurse manager to examine and justify each cost of every programmed budget, both old and new in every annual budget preparation.
- **Sunset budget:** It is designed to "self destruct" within a prescribed time period to ensure the cessation of spend in by a predetermined date. In a public policy, a sunset provision or clause is a measure within a budget which provides that certain clause shall cease to have effect after a specific date, unless further legal action is taken to extend the clause.
- **Sales budget:** It is an estimate of sales for a upcoming financial period. It is used to set department goals, estimate earnings and forecast requirements of production. Sales budget are compiled in terms of quality as well as of values. The sales budget affects both: other operating budgets and the overall master budget of a company.
- **Production budget:** It is the budget that aims at securing the economical manufacture of products and maximizing the utilization of production facilities.

It is expressed in financial terms and takes the nature of a preformed income statement for the future. It may be prepared in a detailed form or as an abstract statement showing the items of profit and loss under classified headings.

Classification of Budget

Since budget expresses plans and an organization may have different types of plans, there may be different types of budgets. The budget may be classified on the basis of:
- **Coverage of functions:** Master budget and functional budget.
- **Nature and activity covered:** Capital and revenue budget.
- **Period of budget:** Long term and short term budgets.
- **Flexibility adopted:** Fixed and flexible budget

Master and Functional Budget

It is prepared for the entire organization incorporating the budget of different functions. For example, when we refer to the annual budget of Govt. of India, it incorporates the budget outlays of different ministries.

A functional budget is prepared by incorporating a major function and its sub functions. Since an organization may have a number of functions, numerous functional budgets are prepared. For example, production budget, cash budget etc.

Capital and Revenue Budget

An organization's activity involves creating facilities for carrying out activities and actual performance activities. These include capital expenditure and whole returns accrued over a number of years. For such activities, capital budget is prepared which is essentially a list of what management believes to be worthwhile or projects for acquisition of new assets together with the estimated cost of each project.

Capital budget is prepared by following step by step process by an organization to determine the merits of an investment project. For example, a business house may approve a social or charitable project not for return but more on the desire to foster goodwill and to contribute back to its community.

Revenue budget involves the formation of target for a year or so in respect of various organizational activities such as production, marketing, finance, etc. Thus a revenue budget includes expenditure and earning for a specific period, like one year.

Long Term and Short Term Budget

A budget with a term usually longer than one year is called **long term budget**. It involves more uncertainty as compared with short-term budget because, market movements and the business cycles can be more easily predicted in the short term budget. Many organization integrate their yearly budgets with long term projection of business activities along with yearly budget. They prepare budgets for a longer period of 2–3 years. The budgets may be prepared for the next year and subsequent 2–3 years.

The **short term budget** is for a year and is divided into a number of periods for effective implementation. For example, cash budgets are prepared on yearly basis as well as on monthly or quarterly basis to facilitate better cash management.

Fixed and Flexible Budgets

Fixed budget is a budget that doesn't change due to any change in activity level or output level in an organization. Generally, organizations prepare budgets which pertain to only certain projected fixed volume of operations for a year or so such budget are known as fixed or static budgets. When an organization's volume of business can be predicted with fair amount of precision, the fixed budget is satisfactory.

A budget which is designed to change in accordance with the activities of the organization is known as **flexible budget**. It considers several levels of activities and assures that labor, material or facilities used in production and hence cost varies with a known relationship to the actual volume of activity.

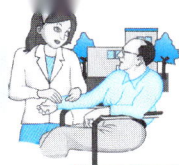

Functions of Budget in Nursing

- Identifies the importance of and develops short and long range fiscal plans that reflects unit's needs.
- Articulates and documents units' needs effectively to higher administrative levels.
- Assesses the internal and external environment of the organization in forecasting to identify driving forces and barriers of fiscal planning.
- Demonstrates knowledge of budgeting and uses appropriate technique.
- Provides opportunities for subordinates to participate in relevant fiscal planning.
- Co-ordinates unit level fiscal planning to be congruent with organizational goals and objective.
- Accurately assesses personal needs using predetermined standards or an established patient classification system.
- Co-ordinates the monitoring aspects of budget control.
- Ensures that documentation of client's need for services is clear and complete.

Table 5: Budgeting for college of nursing 40 students intake

Description		Account No.	Previous year 2017	Current year 2018	Future estimation 2019
Income					
Capital Items	Funds		50000.00	56000.00	
	Grants		100,000.00	1,50,000.00	
	Scrap sale		20,000.00	15,000.00	
Recurrent items	Bed charges		1,50,000.00	2,00,000.00	
	Lab investigation		75,000.00	85,000.00	
	Diagnostic tests		36,000.00	50,000.00	15,00,000.00
	Consultations		30,000.00	35,00000	
	Nursing services		50,000.00	75,000.00	
	Registrations		35,000.00	45,000.00	
	Pharmacy		50,000.00	75,000.00	
	Canteen and diet		35,000.00	40,000.00	
	Others		1,40,000.00	1,76,000.00	
			7,71,000.00	10,02,000.00	
Income (A) = 10,02,000.00					
Expenses					
Capital items	Equipment		20,000.00	40,000.00	
	Tax		10,000.00	12,000.00	
Recurrent items	Salaries		2,50,000.00	3,00,000.00	
	Maintenance and repairs		50,000.00	65,000.00	
	Electricity and water		25,000.00	30,000.00	10,00,000/-
	Supplies		40,000.00	55,000.00	
	Pharmacy		70,000.00	85,000.00	
	Diet		30,000.00	45,000.00	
	Transport		6,000.00	10,000.00	
	Miscellaneous		20,000.00	25,000.00	
			5,21,000.00	6,67,000.00	

Expenses (B) = 6,67,000.00

$$
\begin{aligned}
\text{Income (A)} &= 10{,}02{,}000.00 \\
\text{Expenses (B)} &= 6{,}67{,}000.00 \\
\text{Contingency (C)} &= \frac{667000 \times 10}{100} = 66{,}700 \ (10\% \text{ of expense}) \\
\text{Profit} &= A-(B+C) \\
&= 10{,}02{,}000.00 - 7{,}33{,}700.00 \\
&= \mathbf{2{,}68{,}300.00}
\end{aligned}
$$

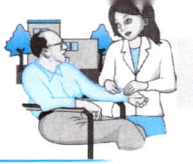

Table 6: Budgeting for 40 students intake BSc (N)-con

Description		Account No.	Previous year 2017	Current year 2018	Future estimation 2019
Income					
Capital Items	Student fees		30,00,000.00	40,00,000.00	
	Grants/funds			1,00,000.00	
Recurrent items	University sanctioned			5,00,000.00	50,00,000.00
	Exam fee			40,000.00	
	Miscellaneous			5,000.00	
				46,45,000.00	
Income (A) = 46,45,000.00					
Expenses					
Capital items	Salary			12,00,000.00	
	LCD projector			60,000.00	
	Furniture			1,00,000.00	
	OHP			30,000.00	28,00,000.00
Recurrent	OHP marker, transparencies			5,000.00	
	Transport			10,00,000.00	
	Miscellaneous			10,0000.00	
				24,95,000.00	

Expenses (B) = 24,85,000.00

Present year budget is excess income over expenditure

Future year budget (2019) is estimated approximately at Rs. 15,00,000.00 (income) and Rs. 10,00,000.00 (expense)

Signature of Finance Officer

Contingency (C) = $\frac{2495000 \times 10}{100}$ = 249500.00

Profit = A-(B + C)
  = 46,45,000 - 27,44,500
  = **19,00,500.00**

Signature of finance officer

Role of the Nurse administrator in Budgeting

Budget required for the nursing department is a cooperative activity of the nursing superintendent and his/her associates including the supervisors. It is prepared under the direction and supervision of the financial officer. The officer supplies special forms to guide the budget. The budget request may be broken down to different units, e.g. salaries, supplies, equipment and other purchase requirements.

The responsibilities of nursing administration in budget include the following:
- Participation in planning budget.
- Consult and take assistance of his/her subordinates in determining the needs of the unit for ensuring year, on the basis of information received.
- Request sufficient funds to suggest a sound financial management such as to provide for developing program provision, expansion of program to attract and to hold qualified staff, to provide for expansion of physical facilities, supplies, equipment, aids for improving teaching instructions and also to carry out adequate functions of the institution.
- Submit budget is alloted and. The administrator should support the budget. He/she should interpret the subordinates any change that may affect instruction services for the adopted budget. Once the budget is adapted, it is the responsibility of the administrator to see that expenditure should not exceed the appropriate limits.
- Since the nurse administrator also is responsible for budget, she/he should cover the routine budget control.

Roles

He/she:
- Is visionary in identifying or forecasting short and long term unit needs, thus inspiring proactive rather than reactive fiscal planning.
- Demonstrate flexibility in fiscal goals setting in a rapidly changing system.
- Anticipates, recognizes and creatively solves problem constraints.
- Influences and inspires group members to become active in short and long range fiscal planning.
- Recognizes when fiscal constraints have resulted in an inability to meet organizational or unit goals and communicates this insight effectively.

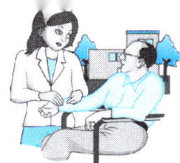

Suggested Reading

- Swansburg RC–Management and Leadership for Nurse Managers, Jones and Bartlett Publishers, Pp. 46–53.
- Marquis BL, Huston CJ- Leadership Roles and Management Functions in Nursing Theory and Application, 2nd edition, Lippincott Company, Pp. 57–65.
- Avasthi, Maheshwari – Public Adminstration, 153–157.
- Chatterjee SS – Management: Its Principles and techniques, 2nd edition, 1–23.
- Budget. From Wikipedia the free encyclopedia.
- Chatterjee Satya Saran. An Introduction to Management Its Principles and Techniques. 3rd ed; 1963:241-248.
- Heinz Weihrich, Mark V Cannice, Harold Koontz. Management A Global and Entrepreneurial Perspective. 12th edn. Tata McGraw – Hill Publishing Company Ltd.
- Usha Malik. Management and Leadership for Nurse Administrators. KPH Nursing Books.

Assess Yourself

LONG ANSWERS

1. Define planning. Explain the mission and philosophy of planning. Enlist the characteristics of good planning.
2. Define planning. Describe the elements and principles of planning. Explain in detail about types of planning.
3. Explain the scope of personal management/human resource management. Describe the principles of personal management.
4. Define recruitment. Explain in detail about the sources of recruitment with merits and demerits. Describe the methods and techniques of recruitment.
5. Define selection. Write down the stages of selection procedure in detail.
6. Define training. Explain the importance of training and discuss various types of training.
7. Define budgeting. Enlist the types of budgeting. Explain the steps in preparing budgetary statement in nursing services.
8. Define staffing. Describe the methods of assigning nursing personnel and the role and functions of manager in staffing.
9. Define organization and explain the principles of organization. Prepare an organization chart of school of nursing.
10. Plan a budget proposal for a college of nursing with 40 students annual intake.

SHORT NOTES

1. Retirement and promotion
2. Bench marking
3. Directing
4. Planning
5. Budgeting
6. PERT
7. Types of budget
8. Principles of organization
9. Organization chart

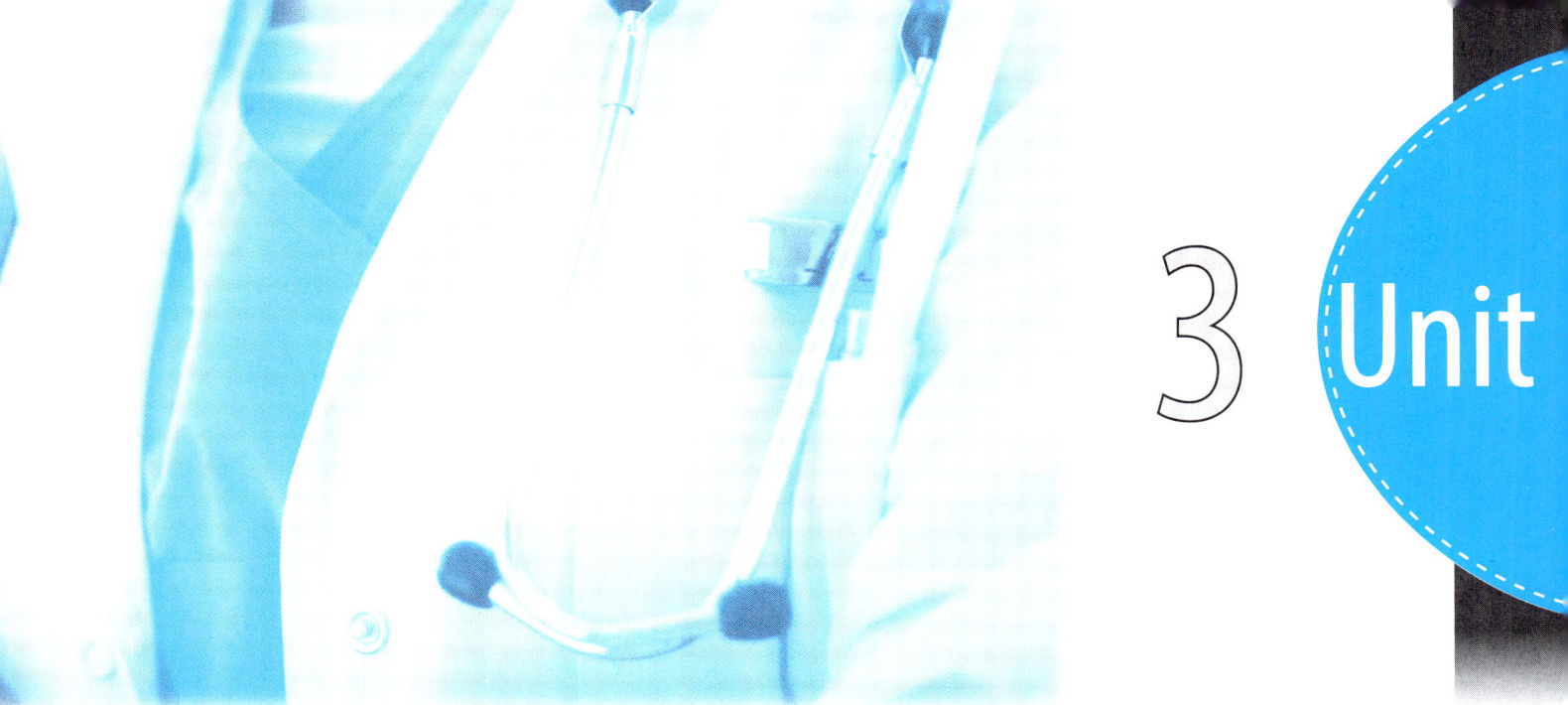

Unit 3

Management of Nursing Services in the Hospital and Community

Unit Outline

- Nursing Service Administration
- Organization of a Hospital
- Hospital Planning
- Elements/Divisions of a Hospital
- Hospital Departments
- Hospital Ward
- Patient Classification Systems
- Progressive Patient Care
- Factors Influencing the Quality Patient Care
- Duty Roster
- Job Analysis
- Job Responsibilities of Different Categories of Nursing Personnel
- Steps in Budgetary Process
- Material Management
- Inventory Control
- Delegation
- Supervision
- Standards in Nursing
- Nursing Manuals
- Role of Head Nurse in Clinical Teaching
- Nursing Rounds
- Bedside Clinic
- Nursing Care Conference
- Ward Management Role of Head Nurse
- Accountability
- Quality Assurance
- Continuous Quality Improvement
- Total Quality Management
- Patient Record System/Documentation
- Documentation
- Records and Reports of the CNO Office
- Telemedicine/Tele Health
- Telenursing
- Electronic Medical Records
- Performance Appraisal
- Nursing Audit
- Conclusion
- Disaster Management
- Phases of Disaster
- Disaster Nursing: Role of Nurse Administrator

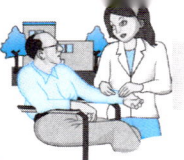

NURSING SERVICE ADMINISTRATION

Nursing profession is an art and service, the aim of nursing service department is to provide quality nursing service which is cost–effective, competitive and based on newer technology. Nursing service department administers services like preventive, curative and rehabilitative etc. to patients, families and community. Nurse manager has a critical role in organizing nursing service department to satisfy nursing needs of the community.

WHO expert committee on nursing defines nursing services as part of total health organization which aims to satisfy the major objectives of nursing services, prevention of disease and promotion of health.

Philosophy of Nursing Service Department

The nursing service department of hospitals functions to uphold the values of nursing personnel and promoting the nursing services. The philosophy of nursing service department is:

- Believes that the primary objective of nursing service department is to provide high quality and cost effective nursing care.
- Believes that each individual is unique, so it provides services to all patients with dignity and compassion without any discrimination to age, sex, color, caste, nationality and socio-economic status.
- Believes in multidisciplinary team approach for providing comprehensive nursing services to patients.
- Believes in maintaining a therapeutic environment for comfort of patients and to promote quality care.
- Believes that family is an extension of patient and family members must be involved in patient's progress.
- Teaching and education are integral part of nursing service.
- Believes in evidence-based approach. Encourages applications of research evidences during nursing intervention.
- Believes that human resources are the greatest assets of an organization. The nursing service department ensures professional growth and development of employees in the department through performance appraisal, in-service education, participation in professional organization and research.
- Believes that when job of nursing personnel is designed, employee's autonomy will be encouraged and improved patient satisfaction will be provided.
- Believes that continuous monitoring and evaluation of nursing practice is important for quality care.

Objectives

- To provide high quality nursing care services as preventive, curative and rehabilitative services to patients in coordination with other departments
- To maintain therapeutic environment for patient care services
- To establish adequate staffing pattern
- To participate in preparation of hospital budget
- To promote team work and co-operation with related departments
- To develop and implement good communication system
- To ensure adequate supplies, equipment and good inventory control
- To develop sound constructive program of leadership in nursing
- To develop and initiate supervision and periodic evaluation system
- To maintain proper documentation system
- To promote career development of each employee
- To initiate orientation program for new staff
- To delegate responsibilities without confusion and plan patient's assignments carefully
- To create conducive environment to give proper learning experience to students
- To encourage and participate in research activities and to continue nursing education
- To evaluate performance of nursing staff in the unit.

Characteristics Essentials of Good Nursing Services

- Clear and specific goals and objectives of nursing service in accordance with hospital philosophy
- Organization chart
- There should be well organized plan of organization
- Nursing procedure manual and protocol must be included in it
- Adequate infrastructure and equipment must be provided
- Clearly formulated hospital policies and administrative manuals
- Well planned nursing service budget
- Master staffing pattern which is the number and composition of nursing personnel assigned to work in hospital in different departments and units in a hospital which serves as guide for planning daily, weekly and monthly schedule
- Clearly written job description and job specification
- Therapeutic environment conducive to good nursing care
- Staff health and welfare services
- Well maintained documentation system
- Good communication system and referral services
- Regular conduct of nursing service administrative meetings for planning, organization and evaluation of nursing services
- System for infection control and biomedical waste management
- Proper evaluation and periodic appraisal system

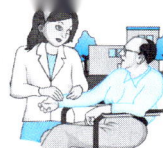

Planning of Nursing Service

The following are the elements of sound organizational planning of hospital nursing service.

- **Aims and objectives:** Set objectives according to the philosophy of hospital. Objectives should be specific, clear and measurable and is formulated by considering newer trends and issues in the field of health in consultation with experts and reviewers.
- **Policies and administrative manuals:** Policies and procedure manuals are required for proper organization and maintenance of hospital nursing service. It should be reviewed and revised regularly based on changing concepts.
- **Nursing service budget:** Properly planned budgets are necessary for proper functioning of nursing service department. Preparation of budget include analysis of previous year budget and anticipate future revenues and expenses.
- **Job description and job specification:** It is the responsibility of the administrator to ensure that job description and job specification are available to each category of employees. It will help to reduce conflict, frustration and act as guide for evaluation and appraisal.
- **Supplies and equipment:** Supplies and equipment are important contributing factors for proper functioning of ward and patient care for providing comprehensive nursing care. Adequate resources must be available for the department.
- **Registers and records:** Records are legal and scientific documents and it should be clear, concise, neat and legible. The administrator should ensure proper documentation and keep confidentiality.
- **Master plan for staffing pattern:** It is the plan that indicates the number and composition of nursing personnel assigned to work in different departments or wards in a given period of time. It includes daily plan, weekly, monthly and yearly schedules.
- **Regular conduct of staff meeting:** Staff meeting provide opportunity for planning, organizing and evaluation of nursing service. Nursing care problems and issues can be discussed freely in these meetings.
- Staff development programs and welfare services should be organized for the professional growth of employees.
- Nursing service appraisal and evaluation helps to improve quality of service and job competencies.
- Formulation of an advisory committee with experts who give necessary direction and advice for issues and matters related to nursing service.

Steps in Planning Nursing Service Unit

- **Formulation of Goals:** The goals and objective are formulated based on philosophy. Formulate goals that are specific, clear and informative to employees of the nursing service department. Some examples of the activities concerned with the management of the ward are assignment as duties and responsibilities as a nurse, distribution of supplies and equipment, purchase and inventory, periodic checkup, evaluation, activities concerned with cleaning of wards as fumigation, dusting, disposal of biohazard waste materials etc.
- **Assessment of resources:** It is the duty of nurse manager to assess resources available for achievement of objectives. The administrator estimates demands in terms of nursing personnel and materials required for efficient functioning. While planning manager must consider the facts like, total number of hospital beds, availability and experience of staff, total number of patients, patient assignment methods, number of available non nursing staff, physical facilities etc.
- **Establishment of planning premises:** Premises refers to the factors in the environment that affect the achievement of goals. They are assumptions about future or understanding the expected situation, e.g. emergency management
- **Securing participation:** The plans formulated by the nurse administrator must be communicated to subordinates properly for increasing their awareness regarding proposed action and to get their co-operation. The plans and programs should be informed to first and middle level managers by top level authority. The first and middle level managers are the person organize work at unit or department level.
- **Write up the formulated plan:** Writing or formulating monthly or weekly duty plan, maintenance of stock register, formulation of protocol.
- **Programming and implementation:** It is the key step in planning process. Implement a well–organized nursing service unit based on formulated goals and objectives.
- **Evaluation and feedback:** Follow-up and evaluation can be made by regular supervision, feedback, use of records and registers etc.

Role and Functions of Nurse Manager/Administrator

Nursing service department is responsible for providing quality nursing service to all patients in collaboration with other departments. Some of the responsibilities of nurse manager are given below.

- **Administration**
  - Develop mission, vision and goals of nursing service department
  - Formulating nursing care delivery model in accordance with philosophy and objectives
  - Formulate policies and procedure manual
  - Plan and organize nursing service plans and activities
  - Formulate nursing service budget
  - Recruit and select qualified nursing professional and supporting staff

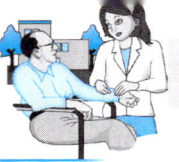

- Co-ordinate all activities in the department
- Establish general pattern of delegation, responsibilities and assignments
- Recruit and select qualified nursing professionals
- Co-ordinate the activities of other departments
- Evaluate performance of nursing staff
- Ensure infection control practices and biomedical waste management
- **Organization and implementation**
  - Ensure to start each day's duty on time and take measures to avoid interruptions as possible.
  - Assign duties and responsibilities to various categories of staff.
  - Ensure standard discipline of staff at all time.
  - Supervise and evaluate performance of employees
  - Promote and maintain effective relationship with various administrative department of hospital and community
  - Promote team work by coordinating different departments of the hospital.
  - Establish a general pattern of delegation of responsibility and authority.
  - Co-ordinate the activities of all nursing departments
  - Maintain good order and discipline
  - Promote teamwork and establish trust
  - Promote and maintain effective relationship with other departments
  - Evaluate periodically effectiveness of work of staff
  - Utilize opportunities for development of staff through regular conduct of ward rounds, nursing care conference etc.
  - Conduct periodic staff meeting in each nursing unit. Organize in-service training program for all categories of nursing staff
  - Report to higher authority all matters concerning neglect of duty or malpractice
  - Ensure that welfare services of employees are properly implemented.
- **Education and Research**
  - Conduct update/refresher courses based on needs/changing trends in health care.
  - Responsible for organizing and conducting staff meeting
  - Organize orientation programs for newly joined staffs and in-service education programs
  - Encourage employees to participate in continuing nursing education programs
  - Encourage scientific research in nursing care to support changes in health system
  - Conducting nursing care conferences regularly to discuss nursing care issues and problems
- **Records and reports:** Maintain a well-established documentation system as patient records and registers as they are legal documents. Maintain daily weekly, monthly and yearly duty plan leave account, stock register etc.
- **Public relation:** Promote and maintain relationship with various departments of hospital and other related community health agency and maintain cordial relationship with patients and their relatives attending hospital.

ORGANIZATION OF A HOSPITAL

Hospital is an integral part of a social and medical organization, the function of which is to provide complete health care to people, both curative and preventive and outpatient services to reach out to the family and its home environment. The hospital is also a center for the training of health workers and biosocial research.
—*WHO*

Hospital is a social organization and logical combination of activities of a number of persons with different levels of knowledge and skill for achieving a common goal of patient care through a hierarchy of authority and responsibility.

A hospital is a multi faceted organization that requires highly trained employees, efficient systems and control, necessary supplies, adequate equipment and facilities.

A hospital system is an organization that mobilizes the skills and efforts of divergent group of professionals and non-professionals so as to provide services to individual patients.

A modern hospital is an institution which possesses adequate accommodation and well qualified and experienced personnel to provide curative, restorative and preventive character of highest quality possible to all people regardless of race, color or creed economic status. Hospital also conducts educational and training programs for students particularly required for efficacious medical care and hospital services and it conducts research, assisting the advancement of medical service and hospital services.

Objectives of the Hospital

- Provide curative, preventive and rehabilitative services to all people who seek health care
- Training of professionals who are involved in health care
- Facilitate biomedical research
- Render high quality health care services to public

Functions of the Hospital/Hospital Services

- **Essential services**
  - Outpatient department services
  - In patient department service
  - Emergency department service
  - Intensive care services
  - Operation theater services
  - Nursing services
- **Supportive services**
  - Radiological services
  - Laboratory services
  - Pharmacy services
  - Central sterile supply services

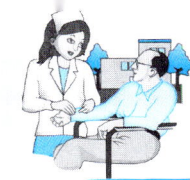

- Blood bank
- Rehabilitation services
- Medical records
- **Utility Services**
  - Dietary services
  - Hospital engineering services
  - Laundry services
  - Public relation and communication
  - Fire and safety
  - Canteen services
  - Mortuary
  - Stores and purchase
  - Hospital security services
- **Administration services**
  - Personal management
  - Financial management
  - Material management
  - House-keeping management
  - General/community services
- **Biomedical research**
  - Training of health professionals
  - Health education
  - Integration with other health care institutions supporting community needs and
  - outreach service
  - Medical camps/mobile clinics
- **Educative function**
  - Medical, dental and nursing education
  - Paramedical education

Classification of Hospitals

- **According to ownership and control**
  - Public hospital/Govt. Hospital
    - Central Govt. hospital
    - State Govt. hospital
    - Corporation/local bodies
  - Semi Govt./autonomous bodies
  - Voluntary agencies hospital
  - Private hospital
  - Corporate hospitals
  - Charitable hospitals
- **According to regional basis**
  - General Hospitals, e.g. District Hospital, Taluk Hospital
  - Rural Health Centers
  - Teaching cum Research Centers
  - Specialized Hospitals
- **According to speciality**
  - General Hospital
  - Specialist Hospitals e.g. Maternal Hospital, Paediatric Hospital
  - Superspecialty Hospitals e.g. Cardiothoracic Hospital, Neuro hospital
- **According to size of hospital**
  - Teaching Hospital 500 (bed to be increased according to number of students)
  - District Hospital 200 (may be raised up to 300 depending on population)
  - Taluk Hospital 50 bedded (may be increased depending upon population to be served)
  - PHC 6 beds (may be increased up to 10 depending upon needs
- **According to systems of medicine**
  - Allopathic Hospitals
  - Ayurvedic Hospitals
  - Homeopathic Hospitals
  - Unani Hospital
  - Siddha Hospital
- **According levels of health care**
  - Primary level Health Care Centers e.g. Primary Health Center
  - Secondary level Health Care Centers e.g. General hospital
  - Tertiary level Health Care Centers e.g. Medical College Hospital
- **According to teaching facilities**
  - Teaching Hospital
  - Non-teaching Hospital

Organizational Functions of Hospital

Patient Care Services

- Organization of structure
- Formulation of policies, rules and regulations
- Developing patient care services
- Arrangement of physical facilities
- House-keeping and biomedical waste management

Staff Management

- Manpower planning
- Recruitment and selection
- Wages and salary
- Training and development
- Rewards and promotion
- Finance and budgeting
- Budget planning
- Recurring capital
- Accounting

Material Management

- Material planning
- Procurement and storage
- Inventory control
- Disposal and condemnation

Hospital Information System

- Medical record keeping
- Control function
- Patient feedback system
- Public relation
- Communication

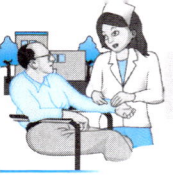

Quality Management
- Medical and nursing audit
- Quality assurance
- Evaluation and performance appraisal

Legal and Statutory Function
- Constitutional rules and acts
- Notification of birth and death

Ethics and Code of Conduct
- Code of conduct for patient, family and staff
- For research issues

HOSPITAL PLANNING

The concept of health care delivery centers are changing. Epidemiologic and geographical changes, advances in medical science and technology, enhanced standards of care etc. are the challenges in health care. In the last few decades we can see spectacular development and changes in the field of health. Hospital consciousness of the Indian public is changing now a days. The essential health care services needed for the community can be met economically only through proper planning, designing, construction and administration of health care services and the hospital must be designed to serve people.

Aims of Hospital planning
- To render high quality patient care services including preventive, promotive, curative and rehabilitative services to patients and community
- To increase utilization of hospital facilities
- To improve productivity of the hospital
- To improve efficiency of services provided by the hospital

Principles in Hospital Planning
- Patient care of high quality
- Effective community orientation
- Economic viability
- Orderly planning
- Sound architectural plan

Stage of Hospital Planning

The various stages of hospital planning are:
- **Conceptualization of hospital:** This is the first stage where the administrator formulates a conceptual idea of the hospital and compares his idea with existing hospitals and formulate a small organization with chairman and other members with specific aims of the project and finding out resource for completion of the project.
- **Market survey/feasibility survey:** Market survey help to determine the viability of the project. So conduct a feasibility study of the area selected for the construction of hospital. Market surveys are conducted for assessing the character, need and possibilities of organizing hospital in that particular area. Assess the geographic area, educational status of people, cultural habits, beliefs and customs. During survey assess the character need and possibility, type and size of hospital and financial condition of the community. Collect details of demographic profile as population, age and sex structure of population, economic status, health status of people as data regarding morbidity and mortality. Collect details regarding environmental statistics as sources of water supply, basic sanitation facility etc.

  It is important to collect data regarding availability and types of **hospitals** in **that area. Other** facilities as bank, transportation facilities, communication network and availability of medical manpower, health needs and changing trends in health care, etc. must be arranged.
- **Preplanning work schedule:** Prepare preplanning work schedule. For that we can depend on management techniques as PERT or critical pathway method. This helps to explain the different tasks for completing the project within time limit and the administrators can assess the progress of work.
- **Organization of governing board or planning the team:** Hospital administration can be made effective by constituting the governing board of the hospital or planning the team under the chairman of Board of Directors. The team members include, hospital consultants, medical administrators, financial expert, legal advisor, specialists from all clinical departments, nursing administrators, engineers from different specialty, architects and representatives from local bodies.

  All members plan, organize and function as a team to make the dream effective. The responsibilities of hospital consultant are to develop and prepare master plan based on findings of feasibility survey and assess the financial feasibility.
- **Financial planning:** Financial planning is the assessment and planning of financial resources as estimating cost of construction, source of income and the funding agencies/stake holders. Preplanning is necessary to identify source of money required for constructing, equipping, staffing hospital, revenue generation process as patient fee, bed charges, treatment charges based on ownership of hospital as whether it is public or private. Also plan the sources for operating fund including salaries, other maintenance expenses.
- **Selection of site:** After organization has been constituted the next step is selection of site for construction of hospital. The site should be wide enough for future expansion and development and there must be accessibility for transport with adequate parking facility for vehicles. Avoid low lying areas and nearby places as possible. The area should be free

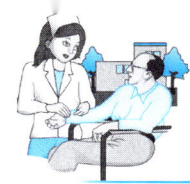

from undue noise, smoke, dust, flood and it is ideal to be away from railroads and industrial areas. The area should get adequate supply of portable water 24 hours a day and electricity and there should be public sewerage system. Also take measures to select areas free from air pollution, insects and vectors of diseases, noise pollution etc.

All departments need to be linked by internal traffic routes for use of patients and staff. The space selected should be of adequate size according to type of hospital and bed strength. Availability of fresh air and facilities for biomedical waste disposal are to be considered.

Determine the scope of future expansion and planning various departments with experts.

- **Planning the team:** The responsibilities of senior architect are site selection, orientation, adapting building design etc. And he has to transform his dream into reality in consultation with engineers from various department as public work or civil engineer, mechanical engineer, electrical engineer, electronic engineer and biomedical engineer.
- **Equipment planning:** Equipment are necessary for the proper functioning of the hospital. Administrators in consultation with heads of each department and experts equip each department with necessary equipment for the smooth functioning of the hospital. Room by room/departmental equipment lists are formulated by experts from each department and should be reviewed and verified by the administrator.

Categorization of Hospital and Space Requirements (Table 1)

According to minimum standards for allopathic hospitals under Clinical Establishment Act, 2010, the different levels of hospital include:

- **Hospital Level 1(A):** General medical services with indoor admission facility provided by recognized allopathic medical graduate(s)
  Example: PHC, Government and Private Hospitals.
- **Hospital Level 1(B):** This level of hospital shall include all the general medical services provided at level 1(A) and specialist medical services provided by doctors from one or more basic specialties namely General Medicine, General Surgery, Pediatrics, Obstetrics and Gynecology and Dentistry, providing indoor and OPD services.
  Level 1(A) and Level 1(B) Hospitals shall also include support systems required for the respective services like Pharmacy, Laboratory, etc.
  Example: General Hospital, Single/multiple basic medical specialties provided at Community Health Center, Sub Divisional Hospital, Private Hospital of similar scope. Nursing Home, Civil/District Hospital in few places etc.
- **Hospital Level 2 (Non-Teaching):** This level may include all the services provided at level 1(A) and 1(B) and services through other medical specialties given in addition to basic medical specialty given under 1(B) like;
  - Orthopaedics
  - ENT
  - Ophthalmology
  - Dental
  - Emergency with or without ICU
  - Anesthesia
  - Psychiatry
  - Skin
  - Pulmonary Medicine
  - Rehabilitation etc.

  Example: District hospital, corporate hospitals, referral hospital, regional/state hospital, nursing home and private hospital of similar scope, etc.
- **Hospital Level 3 (non-teaching) super-specialty services:** This level may include all the services provided at level 1(A), 1(B) and 2 and services of one or more of the super specialty with distinct departments and/or also Dentistry if available. It will have other support systems required for services like Pharmacy, Laboratory, and Imaging Facility, Operation Theater etc.
  Example: Corporate Hospitals, Referral Hospital, Regional/State Hospital, Nursing Home and Private Hospital of similar scope etc.
- **Hospital Level 4 (Teaching):** This level will include all the services provided at level 2 and may also have Level 3 facilities. It will however have the distinction of being teaching/training institution and it may or may not have super specialties.

Table 1: The minimum space requirements proposed by Clinical Establishment Act 2010–XXX

Hospital	Level I	Level II	Level III
• Wards, ward bed and surrounding space	6 m²/bed	6 m²/bed	6 m²/bed
• Minor operation theater procedure room	10.5 m²/table	10.5 m²/table	10.5 m²/table
• Labor room, labor room table and surrounding area	10.5 m²/table	10.5 m²/table	10.5 m²/table
• 4. Other areas, Nurses station, doctor's duty room, store, clean and dirty utility circulating area, toilets	10.5 m² for clean utility and store. 7 m² for dirt utility, 3.5 m² for toilet.	10.5 m² for clean utility and store, 7 m² for dirt utility, 3.5 m² for toilet.	10.5 sqm for clean utility and store, 7 m² for dirt utility. 3.5 m² for toilet.

Contd…

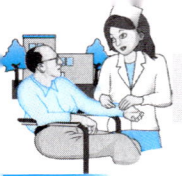

Hospital	Level I	Level II	Level III
• Biomedical waste	10.5 m²	5 m² for <50 beds, 10 m² for 50-100 beds 20 m² for >100 beds	5 m² for <50 beds, 10 m² for 50-100 beds 20 m² for >100 beds
• ICU, ICU, CCU, • Neuro ICU, Trauma, ICU etc.		10.5 m² bed	10.5 m² bed
• Operation Room area		24.5 m² operating room	30.5 m² operating room
• Emergency and casualty		10.5 m²/bed	10.5 m²/bed
• Pharmacy		0.8 m² per patient	5% of total clinical visit to OPD at the rate of 0.8 m/patient

Wards

- The ward shall also have designated areas for nursing station, doctors' duty room, store, clean and dirty utility, janitor room.
- For a general ward of 12 beds, a minimum of 2 hand wash basin shall be provided
- Distance between beds shall be 1.0 meters
- Space at the head end of bed shall be 0.25 meters
- Door width shall be 1.2 meters and corridor width 2.5 meters

Intensive Care Unit

- The unit is to be situated in close proximity of operation theater, acute care medical and surgical ward units
- Suction, oxygen supply and compressed air is to be provided for each bed
- Adequate lighting and uninterrupted power supply shall be provided
- Adequate multi-sockets with 5 ampere and 15 ampere sockets and/or as per requirement to be provided for each bed
- Nurse call system for each bed
- ICU shall have designated area for nursing station, doctors' duty room, store, clean and dirty utility, circulating area for movement of staff, trolley, toilet, shoe change, trolley bay, janitor closet etc

Labor Room

- The obstetrical unit shall provide privacy, prevent unrelated traffic through the unit and provide reasonable protection of mothers from infection and from cross-infection
- Measures shall be in place to ensure safety and security of neonates
- Resuscitation facilities for neonates shall be provided within the obstetrical unit and convenient to the delivery room
- The labor room shall contain facilities for medication, hand washing, charting, and storage for supplies and equipment
    - The labor room shall be equipped with oxygen and suction.

Operation Theater

- The operation theater complex shall have appropriate zoning.
- The operation theater complex shall provide appropriate space for other areas—nursing station, doctors' duty room, scrub station, sterile store, clean and dirty utility, dress change room and toilets.
    - Sterile area consists of operating room sterile store and anesthesia room
    - Clean zone consists of equipment/medical store, scrub area, pre and/or postoperative area and linen bay
    - Protective zone consists of change room, doctors room and toilets
    - Dirty area
    - Due considerations are to be given to achieve highest degree of asepsis to provide appropriate environment for staff and patients.
- Doors of pre-operative and recovery room are to be 1.5 m clear widths.
- Air conditioning to be provided in all areas. Window AC and split units should preferably be avoided as they become a source of infection.
- Appropriate arrangements for air filtration to be made.
- Temperature and humidity in the OT shall be monitored.
- Oxygen, nitrous oxide, suction and compressed air supply should be provided in all OTs.
- All necessary equipment such as shadow-less light and Boyle's apparatus shall be available and must be in working condition.
- Uninterrupted power supply

Note: For Eye Hospitals, only where procedures are done in local and or regional anesthesia, minor OT criteria may be applicable.

Emergency Room

- Emergency bed and surrounding space shall have minimum 10.5 m²/ bed area.
- There shall be designated space for nurse station, doctor duty room store, clean and dirty utility, dressing area, toilet etc.

Clinical Laboratory

The laboratory area shall be appropriate for activities including test analysis, washing, biomedical waste storage and ancillary services like storage of records, reagents, consumables, stationary and eating area for staff.

- The department shall be located at a place which is easily accessible to both OPD and wards and also to emergency and operation theater
- As the department deals with the high voltage, presence of moisture in the area shall be avoided
- The size of the department shall depend upon the type of equipment installed.
- The department/room shall have a sub-waiting area preferably with toilet facility and a change room facility, if required.

Central Sterilization and Supply Department (CSSD)

- Sterilization, being one of the most essential services in a hospital, requires the utmost consideration in planning.
- Centralization increases efficiency, results in economy in the use of equipment and ensures better supervision and control.
- The materials and equipment dealt in CSSD shall fall under three categories:
  - Those related to the operation theater department
  - Common to operating and other departments
  - Pertaining to other departments alone.

Other Departments

Other departments shall have appropriate infrastructure commensurate to the scope of service of the hospital.

Hospital Design

An architect who is specialized in hospital construction can prepare a hospital plan and get approval by local authorities. While planning, all major departments need to be connected by internal routes for use of patients and their relatives, and staff and for the delivery of supply areas to their point of use. Plan departments carefully with the aim to provide best quality service to public. Those departments which are closely linked with community should be planned nearby places to entrance and be accessible area, for example, outpatient departments, casualty etc. Support services like X-ray and laboratory services need to be located near OPD.

During construction of ward, ICU, other allied departments, maintenance of a therapeutic environment should be given first consideration. Hospital hygiene is a critical element in designing a hospital and take precautions to minimize risk of cross infection.

While planning, the circulation routes of hospital site and within building must be given due consideration. The two types of circulation in the hospital include internal circulation i.e. the space involves corridors, stairways, lifts and corridors with less than 8 feet width. Protection corners heading is also a necessity in hospital corridors. While planning external circulation, it is desirable that the entrance and exit points should be wide enough to take two lines of traffic.

The distances must be minimized for all movements of patients and relatives and hospital staff. Separate space should be there for parking of vehicles of employees and public. Landscaping and garden gives very good visual effect if space is available.

Bed Distribution

The number of beds in a hospital is a yardstick that is applied when referring to the size of hospital. Bed distribution among various specialties may vary according to following range.
- Medical : 30-40%
- Surgical : 25-30%
- Obstetrical : 15-18%
- Psychiatric : 10-12%
- Miscellaneous : 10-15%

Land Requirement (Table 2)

Table 2: **Land requirements for different hospitals**

No. of beds	LAND area	Storey of building
50 beds	10 acres	Single storey
100 beds	15–20 acres	Double storey
200 beds	20–25 acres	Double storey
500 beds	55–70 acres	3–5 storey
700 beds	80–90 acres	4–6 storey
1000 beds	90–100 acres	6–9 storey

Bed Planning

$$\text{Population} = \frac{A \times S \times 100}{365 \times PO}$$

A - Number of patients admission/1000 population/year
S - Average length of stay
PO - Percentage of occupancy

Hospital Building

While construction of hospital, the following needs consideration—therapeutic environment, screened windows, entrance and exit points, traffic flow corridors, fine escape routes and safety, short traffic roots and fire safety is very important while planning a building.

Hospital Commissioning

When hospital building is ready, equipment has been procured, staffs have been recruited, the hospital is ready for commissioning. The hospital building, the staff and equipment are all brought together to a state of operational readiness. During this period good publicity should be given through mass media, to project the right image of the hospital in the minds of the people. (Fig. 1).

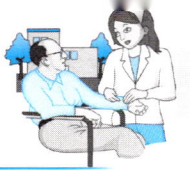

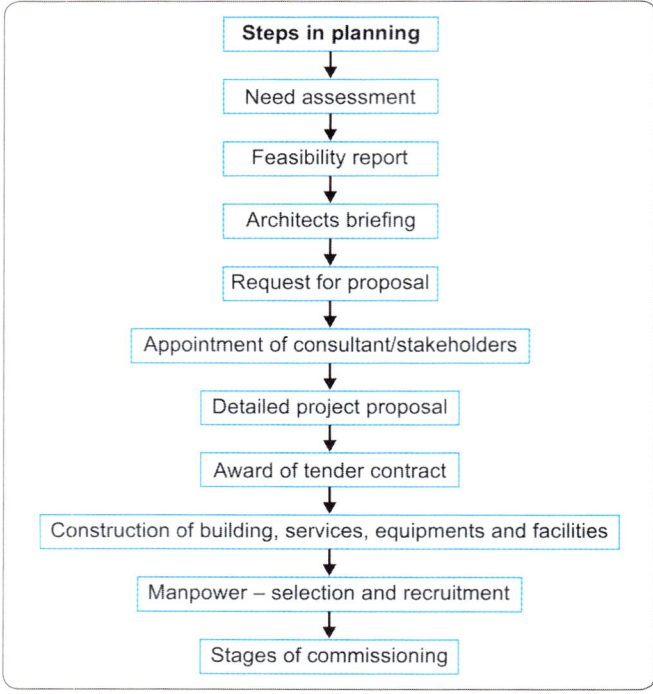

Figure 1: Stages of hospital commissioning

ELEMENTS/DIVISIONS OF A HOSPITAL

- Administrative division
- Outpatient division
  - Outpatient clinic
  - Pharmacy
  - Emergency department/casualty
- Diagnostic service division
  - Laboratories
  - Radiology department
- Therapeutic services
  - Physiotherapy
  - Radiology
- Internal medicine treatment division
  - Operation theater
  - Intensive care units
  - Maternal and child health section
  - Central sterilization department
- Inpatient division
  - Patient's ward
  - Inpatient services
- General service division
  - Kitchen
  - Laundry
  - Storages
  - Workshops
  - Mechanical services
  - Mortuary
- Security
- Parking
- Landscaping, etc.

HOSPITAL DEPARTMENTS

- **Outpatient department:** Outpatient department is an important area in the hospital which should be easily accessible to public. It is better to have direct approach to outpatient department from the road. The size of outpatient department depends upon the volume of patients attending the hospital. Outpatient department shall function 6 days on a week from 8 am–5 pm. The space requirement is usually 0.66 – 1 sq ft area/annual outpatient attendance. Generally in OPD there should be a large hall to function as waiting area with adequate furniture so that patients can wait comfortably. There should be a separate area for reception and enquiry and separate area for registration. In the OPD there should be area for medico – social worker, insurance services, cash counters, OPD, pharmacy, treatment/procedure room, clinical lab, imaging section, area for public relations office and staff zone. Signboards or display boards should be there to direct patients without confusion. OPD is manned by doctors, nurses and paramedical staff.
- **Medical department:** All hospitals have medical departments headed by Professor and Head and there are professors and lecturers. The department provides direct patient care by diagnosis and appropriate treatment. The department of medicine is further divided into various sub specialties as cardiology, endocrinology, gastroenterology, nephrology etc. where doctors are specialized in each specialty provide needed services.
- **Surgery department:** Surgery department deals with surgical management of patient. In surgery department also there are surgeons, specialized in various sub specialties. The sub specialties of surgery department include general surgery, orthopedic, urology, neurology, depending upon the level of health care centers.
- **Obstetrics and gynaecology department:** The department of obstetrics and gynaecology mainly provides prenatal care, care during delivery, care of mother after delivery, neonatal and newborn care. The number of labor rooms and other facilities depends on the annual number of delivery and level of health care institution.
- **Pediatric department:** Children are grouped by age than by diagnosis and attention is to be given to the emotional development of child. Pediatric department deals with medical care of infants, children and adolescents. In the pediatric department there should be a unit for care of premature infants. In newborn nursery, glass walled cubicles are desirable for each infant and each cubicle should be equipped with devices to control temperature and humidity and other emergency equipment. Strict aseptic technique must be observed in these units.

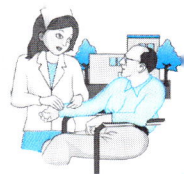

- **Operation theater:** It is preferable that operation theater should be close to surgical wards or intensive care units. At the entrance of operation theater, there must be waiting area, premedication room, changing room for various categories of staff followed by sterile zone with scrub room, anesthesia room and there should be disposal rooms and janitors. Operation theater is staffed by surgeon, anesthesiologist, nurses, technicians, cleaning staff etc. There should be policy guidelines for infection control in operation theater.
- **Intensive care unit:** Intensive Care unit provides highly skilled care to critically ill patients at the acute stage of their illness. It is good if intensive care units are situated near operation theater or recovery room in concerned departments attached to wards. A minimum of 15 sq ft of clean floor area and minimum head wall width of 1.2 ft/bed and 8 feet between beds is recommended for Intensive Care Unit. There should be movable partition between beds and a hand sanitizer besides each bed. The nurses' station should be located in center to have complete visualization control of all beds. Each bed should be well illuminated and lighting of non–reflecting type for the patient. Maximum permissible noise level is 50 db with a humidity of 50-60%. All emergency drugs should be kept ready for use. Staff in intensive care units include medical and nursing staff specialized in critical care medicines, junior consultants with a nurses' ratio 1:1. Adequate monitoring equipment and ventilators in good working condition must be available in intensive care unit.
- **Emergency department:** In emergency department patient arriving at hospital in need of immediate care are cared for. It must be on the ground floor of the hospital and is easily accessible to all those who seek acute care. It works 24 hours per day with easy access to vehicles and ambulances. In casualty there should be triage, resuscitation room, major trauma intensive care unit, patient waiting area, minor procedure room, emergency operation theater, 24 hour pharmacy, nurses station, emergency care room, doctor's room etc. There should be a well organized triage area for emergency care and a well–planned disaster plan in emergency department. Staff working in emergency department include physicians, surgeons, anesthetist, resident medical officer, nurses; technicians like lab technician, ECG technician, radiographers, nursing assistants, cleaning staff etc. All medico-legal cases should be reported to proper authority.
- **Nursing service department:** The primary responsibility of nursing service department is to restore and maintain the health of patients. Further explanation of nursing service department will be explained in this unit.
- **X-ray department:** Department of imaging provides services to inpatients and outpatients and medical imaging technology is used for diagnosis and treatment of disease. Medical imaging department is ideal to be situated in the ground floor near OPD/emergency department. The main areas in X-ray department are reception, film processing and distribution area, film drying area, darkroom located between two X-ray room, administrative area, dressing room, toilet etc. Other areas are CT scan area, MRT area, mammography, nuclear imaging, PET scan area etc. There should be adequate area for free movement of patient's caregivers and staff. X-ray department is manned by radiologist technicians, nurses, other staff etc. Well-organized policies and procedures regarding handling of radio nuclide, protection to staff and patients, distance between radiation source and staff, use of personal protective equipment etc. should be there.
- **Dietary serviced:** The dietary department provides catering of therapeutic diet to patients, canteen facilities for relatives of patients and staff, diet counseling and health education. It is good if dietary department is situated on the ground floor. The recommended space requirement is 15 sq ft per bed. The various divisions of the department include cooking area, preparation area, cold rooms, dish wash area, storage area, offices of staff etc. and there should be LPG stove and refrigeration facilities. The menu should be planned to meet patient's needs by dietitians. There should be food safety control system with specific guidelines and policies.
- **Laundry services:** The image of the hospital depends on the clean and neat appearance of wards which can be rendered by a well functioning laundry department. The laundry can be either attached to hospital or nearby to hospital and should have separate entry and exit. It is recommended to have a mechanized laundry in the basement with proper drainage system. The department is managed by supervisors and semi–skilled and unskilled workers. This department provides clean, safe, adequate and timely supply of linen to different areas as wards special room, ICU's, operation theaters etc. linen from operation theater needs to be washed and sterilized separately.
- **Laboratory services:** Laboratories in hospitals help to confirm diagnosis, assist in the treatment and follow up of patients. The different laboratories attached to hospitals are clinical pathology lab, biochemistry lab, histopathology, cytology, microbiology lab etc. It is preferable to have laboratories in the ground floor or first floor. The size and type of labs varies according to the level of hospital. The different areas of lab include receptions, sample collection area, specimen toilet, glass washing and sterilizing unit, areas for utility services, issue of reports, storage area etc. Staff in lab include doctors qualified in pathology, biochemistry etc. Scientific officers, Laboratory technicians etc. There should be specific policies and standard operating policies for all services, collection of sampling, disposal of waste, policy for blood born infections etc. **Quality Control of laboratories:** National Accreditation Board of laboratory (NABL) accreditates to laboratories as a quality indicator.

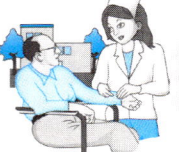

- **Human resource department:** Human resource department in health care institutions are essential to enable delivery of efficient medical services and to provide quality patient care.
- **Central sterile supply department:** This department is an important supportive service and this department is responsible for processing, issuing and control of sterile supply to different units of hospital. The supplies include sterile linen, OT packs, sterile articles and other surgical supplies. The recommended area is 1.64 m²/bed for up to 400 bedded hospitals and for more than 400 beds an area of 1 m²/bed. Staff working in CSSD area include supervisors, technicians, cleaning staff etc.
- **Medical records department:** Medical records are the legal document relating to patient care in hospital. Medical record is a scientific data for assessing the medical and nursing services. Medical records department is responsible for processing of medical records, coding, indexing and storage of medical records, filing and retrieval system. The department secures all electronic and written medical records in a health facility. The Medical Records Department officer is incharge of the department.
- **Public relations department:** Public relations department deals with media coverage of the activities of the hospital including visits, meetings, conferences etc. This department also prepare booklets and posters with the aim of educating people regarding various aspects of health.
- **Medical maintenance and engineering department:** The function of this department is repair and maintenance of hospital equipments, security and safety system. This department is responsible for the daily operations and proper maintenance of hospital equipments. It includes workshops for electrical equipments, air conditioning etc. Bio medical engineering division is responsible for condemnation and disposal of hospital equipment. The department is manned by biomedical engineers, technicians, helpers, etc.

HOSPITAL WARD

Hospital ward is a division of a hospital shared by patients need similar kind of call.

Ward is that area of hospital where all amenities – physical, social and especially medical care are made available to facilitate patient treatment.

Hospital Inpatient Service

The objectives of hospital inpatient services are:
- To render nursing care to all patients
- To provide equipment, essential drugs and other requirements in an organized manner
- To provide opportunity for training to medical, nursing and paramedical students including research work

Factors Affecting Ward Design
- Type of ward
- Category of patients
- Movement space
- Number of beds
- Bed spacing
- Ancillary and auxiliary services
- Nursing station
- Toilet and other facilities

Types of Ward
- General ward
- Specialty wards, e.g. maternity, pediatric, psychiatry etc.

The different types of ward according to ward design are:
- **Nightingale ward:** It is a type of ward designed in 1770 by Frenchman and later it was adopted by Florence Nightingale and is known by her name. Nightingale ward is rectangular in shape containing 25-30 beds located in two long rows. Nurse's station, Doctor's room etc. are at one end of the ward. There may be side rooms attached with ward in which patients who need isolation can be admitted. Toilets and other facilities are attached to the other end of ward.

  The advantages of Nightingale ward are that there is possibility of nurses to have a view on all patients and facilities for good ventilation. This type of ward is found to be economic. The main disadvantages are that there is no privacy for patients and there are increased risk of infections.
- **Modified nightingale ward:** In modified Nightingale ward nurse's station is designed in the center of the ward. The advantage is that it is time saving for nurses and supervision of patient is more improved in this type of ward.
- **Rigg's ward:** It is designed in Rigg Hospital in 1990 in Copenhagen. Here the ward is divided into small cubicles for 1-4 patients. The beds are arranged parallel to the longitudinal wall.

The advantages of Rigg's ward are:
- Privacy can be maintained
- Neat and tidy appearance

The disadvantages of Rigg's ward are:
- Difficulty in communication between nurses and patients.
- More number of staff nurses are required to provide care
- Construction and maintenance are expensive.

Components of Ward Unit
- Patient's bed/patient's rooms
- Nurse's station
- Ancillary services as dietary services, physiotherapy area, utility room, ward pantry, stores.
- Auxiliary facilities as housekeeping section/store, lecture hall or seminar hall, doctor's and nurse's resting room, visitor's room, ward lab, etc.

- Sanitary facilities as bathroom, toilet, sluice room, washing area etc.

Head Nurses' Responsibility for Effective Functioning of Ward

The head nurse or ward in charge is the key person to control the day to day activities in the ward. She is responsible to ensure high quality nursing care services to patients. For that ward in charge is responsible:

- To endorse patients and give attention to patient's comfort and safety
- Delegate/assign duties to nurses and other ancillary nursing personnel
- Ensure that the supplies and equipment are adequate, clean and in good working condition
- Create a safe and comfortable environment for patients
- Guide and provide nursing care to patients with cooperation from other members of health team
- Supervise and evaluate the job performance of nursing staff and other ancillary nursing personnel. Assess the efficiency of patient care services and identify nursing care service problems and assist to find out solutions
- Take active steps in procurement storage, inventory, distribution and disposition of hospital supplies, materials and equipment
- Ensure infection control practices are following properly by staff working in the unit.
- Maintain properly the electrical, mechanical, communication equipment and allied facilities
- Determine and make recommendations regarding ward facilities

Factors Affecting Good Ward Management

The head nurse is the first line nurse manager of each ward/unit. The nurse in charge of the unit or wards is responsible to provide quality nursing care to patients. Quality nursing service can be provided only if the wards are well organized, adequately equipped and properly arranged. The factors involved in good ward management are:

- **Standards and policies:** Policies and procedures should be prepared based on the aims and objectives of the hospital. Policies and standards in relation to organizing, staffing, evaluation etc. will influence the functioning of the ward. Nursing standards and ward policies greatly influence good ward management and the head nurse can plan activities of the ward based on that.
- **Plan each day's program:** For that the head nurse must have adequate knowledge regarding hospital policies, ward policies and procedures, methods of patient assignments, hospital routines rules and regulations etc. Plan each day's duties and assignments in advance with special attention to special days as admission day, discharge day etc. The daily, weekly and monthly assignment should be prepared in advance.
- **Start the day on time:** Good ward management is facilitated by starting the day's program in time and each and every staff should be in the ward on the assigned hours. Punctuality of the staff and students will influence functioning of ward.
- **Orientation of new staff members:** In order to acquaint new staff with ward policies and routines, arrange orientation program to newly joined staff. During orientation program introduce the new staff to ward routines, ward policies and procedures, equipment and supplies, patient assignment methods, various departments of the hospital, line of responsibility etc.
- **Adequate equipment and supplies:** Supplies and equipment are important contributing factor for quality care. Continuous supply of materials is essential for managing the ward. Good material management and inventory control ensures materials required for patient care in right quantity and quality at the right time to the right cost.
- **Proper maintenance of records and reports:** Patient clinical records are the documents which have legal, scientific and educational value. So it should be accurate, neat and legible and should be signed by the health care workers. Proper maintenance of records and well organized reporting system help to ensure good ward management.
- **Delegation:** Delegation enables managers to distribute their work to subordinates. Delegation helps to enhance confidence, job satisfaction, motivation and morale of subordinates and thereby improve quality of nursing care services.
- **Good supervision and evaluation:** Evaluation and supervision are administrative techniques through which patient care can be safeguarded and staff can be helped to improve their quality of care. A good performance appraisal system is essential for maintaining good quality patient care.
- **Maintain good working relationship and morale:** Good communication and interpersonal relations among health team members in the ward are essential to create a therapeutic environment thereby good ward management. Work performance is always better when morale is good.
- **Staff development programs:** Conducting regular staff development program will help to update knowledge and skill of staff which will also be a contributing factor for quality care to patients.
- **The methods of assignment:** The patient care assignment can be planned according to the hospital policy, patient care area, and type of patients, members of nursing staff available etc. Effective methods of patient assignment will be a contributing factor for good ward management.
- **Time management and time planning:** Proper time management and management of duty time of staff in the ward will ensure effective ward management.

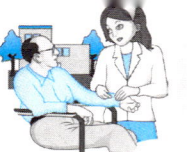

PATIENT CLASSIFICATION SYSTEMS

The patient classification systems (PCS) is a method of categorizing patients according to severity of their illness and amount and complexity of their nursing care requirements. PCS is an indicator for measuring quality of medical care service in a hospital. PCS helps to improve patient satisfaction by providing quality patient care.

Purpose of PCS

- PCS helps the nurse manager to differentiate the intensity of care needed by individual patients and thereby delegate responsibilities
- PCS provides opportunity for tracking changes in patient care needs
- PCS helps to plan, schedule and control nursing services
- PCS can be used to measure patients' needs
- It helps to determine work load of staff
- PCS helps to determining nursing hours needed to provide quality nursing care based on standards of care
- PCS also helps to assess the level of support services needed

Types/Styles of PCS

The different types of PCS widely used are,

Prototype Evaluation System

In prototype evaluation system, the symptoms of patient typical of each care category are listed and patients are categorized on the basis of severity of categories of patients in prototype evaluation system:

Category I

In self-care categories patients no longer require intensive or moderate care. Self-care category patients require nursing services 1-2 hours/day. Patients with acute, chronic, episodic disease, who will return to their pre-illness level of functioning and for them the goal of nursing is complete elimination of present condition.

Category II

This category includes patients who need minimal care requiring 3-4 hours nursing care per day. For example, patients who are recovering from a severe illness or surgery. The goal of care is management of chronic health problem with treatment without ongoing nursing service.

Category III

This category patients require intermediate care, nursing service 5-6 hours per day. For them the care goal is rehabilitation to a maximum level through continuous nursing care.

Category IV

Patients who are sick or acutely or severely ill and who have high level of dependency, come under this category. They need close supervision. For example, patients who are admitted in intensive care units or patients in unstable condition requiring close supervision.

Category V

This category includes patients with end stage of illness and for them the goal of nursing care is assurance and comfort throughout the terminal stage of illness.

Factors Evaluation System

In factor evaluation system a number of critical care descriptors are identified, and patient's care needs are scored according to patients' dependency level.

Measurement of Patient Classification System

$$\text{NCH/PPD} = \frac{\text{Nursing care hours worked}}{\text{Patient census}}$$

Patient Assignment

Objectives of Assignment Planning

- To provide the patient with the best possible nursing care.
- To plan assignments which are interesting to nurses and stimulating to their professional growth.
- To provide a well-rounded educational experience for student nurses.

Principles of Assignment Planning

Principles that should be kept in mind by the nurse manager when planning assignment

- Activities are better performed when each is made the responsibility of a single person.
- Assignment of patients and duties should not be changed frequently
- The care required by all patients in the group assigned to one nurse must be considered when making assignments
- Assignment planning is closely related to time planning
- The best use will be made of the nurse's time if the patients assigned to one nurse are geographically close together

Methods of Assignment

The different methods of patient assignment are:

Patient Method/Case Method

Total patient care delivery is the oldest method of patient assignment. In this method one professional nurse is responsible for providing comprehensive care for one or more patients. The nurses are responsible for planning, organizing and performing all care, including medicine and injection administration, emotional support, health education, attending hygiene needs required by the assigned patients during the assigned duty hours.

This method is best used in intensive care units and in teaching nursing students. As the nurses assume total responsibility for meeting all the needs of assigned patients, each and every patient receives holistic and unfragmented care.

Advantages
- Quality of patient care is high
- Higher degree of autonomy and responsibility for nurses
- Continuity of care can be facilitated
- Patient satisfaction is high

Disadvantages
- Each registered nurse have a different approach to care
- Not cost effective
- High cost
- There may be lack of adequate nurses.

Functional Method

The functional method of delivering nursing care evolved as a result of World War II. Because nurses were in great demand oversee and at how many ancillary personnel were used to assist patient care. It is an organizational mode of assigning nursing personnel that is task and activity oriented using auxiliary health workers trained in different skills. In this method, the unskilled workers were trained to do simple tasks and they gain skill by repetition.

Work assignments are divided in to tasks and assigned to nursing and ancillary personnel. It is a task focused method. A charge nurse makes the assignment and coordinates the care of all patients in the unit.

All responsibilities of the unit are assigned to selected people in accordance with their expertise (Fig. 2).

Advantages
- Economic and cost effective
- Minimum number of nurses are required
- Nurses completes tasks quickly
- Useful in emergency situations
- A nurse can become particularly skilled in performing assigned job tasks
- It is easy to organize the work of the unit and staff

Disadvantages
- Patient care may become fragmented
- There is neglect of individual needs of patients
- Patient may get confused with many care givers
- Less satisfaction for both nurses and patients
- There is less opportunity for staff development

Team Method of Assignment

Team nursing developed in 1950's is based on the philosophy in which a group of professional and non-professional personnel work together to identify, plan, implement and evaluate comprehensive client oriented care. Team leader is responsible for providing a cooperative environment and maintaining clear communication

In this method, a group of health care workers with different skills and training works together towards a common goal providing qualitative comprehensive nursing care. The entire ward may be organized in to teams or there may be one team for a group of patients. The main feature of team method of assignment is the team conference, where the members of the team discuss the progress and problems of patients and discuss future plan of care (Fig. 3).

Advantages
- High quality comprehensive care can be provided
- Each member of the team is able to participate in decision making and problem solving
- Continuity of care is facilitated
- Patients receive high quality care
- High work satisfaction for nurses
- Development of leadership skills.

Disadvantages
- Unstable staffing pattern make team nursing difficult
- Time is needed for conducting team conferences
- Establishing team for care takes time and effort.

Team nursing is an effective, efficient method of patient assignment. Team leader must have strong clinical skills, good communication skill, delegation ability and decision making ability.

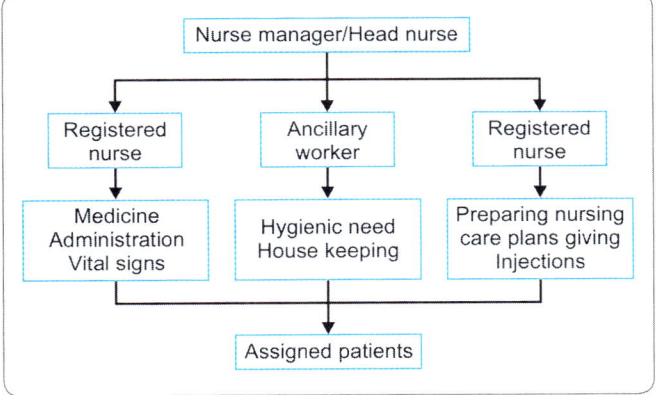

Figure 2: Functional methods of work assignment

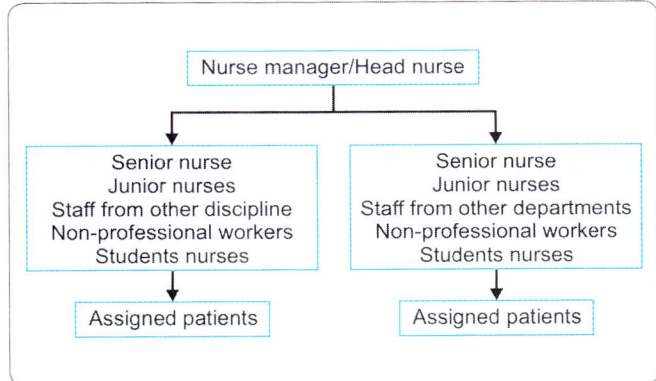

Figure 3: Team method of work assignment

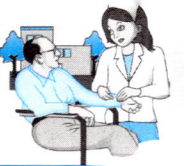

Modular Nursing

Modular nursing is a modification of team nursing and focuses on geographic location for staff assignment. The goal of modular nursing is to increase the involvement of nurses in planning and coordinating care. The concept of modular nursing calls for a small group of staff providing care for a smaller group of patients.

The patient unit is divided into modules or districts and the same team of caregivers is assigned consistently to the same geographic location. Each module has a team leader and team members including professional and non professional members are accountable for patient care.

Advantages
- Continuity care is improved
- There is geographic closeness and efficient communication
- Opportunity to learn and teach
- Nurses are more involved in planning
- Every nurse has the opportunity to contribute to care plan.

Disadvantage
- Unstable staffing pattern makes team nursing more difficult
- Increased cost to stock each module
- All personnel must have complex skills and knowledge.

Primary Nursing

Primary nursing was developed in early 1970 and uses some concepts of total patient care. It involves total nursing care, directed by a nurse on 24 hour basis as long as patient is under the care. The nurse assesses, plans, implements, co-ordinates, monitors and evaluates patient care and services. The primary nurse assumes 24 hr responsibility for planning the care of one or more patients from the time of admission till the discharge. The associated nurses care for the patients by plans developed by the primary nurse. Research suggests that patients have fewer complications and shorter hospitalization when cared by a primary nurse.

An integral responsibility of the primary nurse is to establish clear communication among patients, the physicians, the associate nurses and other team members.

Advantages
- Job satisfaction is high
- Gives opportunity for nurses to see client and family as a system
- Accountability and responsibility for primary nurse is more
- High quality care to patients.

Disadvantages
- Difficult to implement as the degree of responsibility and autonomy required of the primary nurse
- Nurse may be isolated from other nurses
- Time consuming
- High cost.

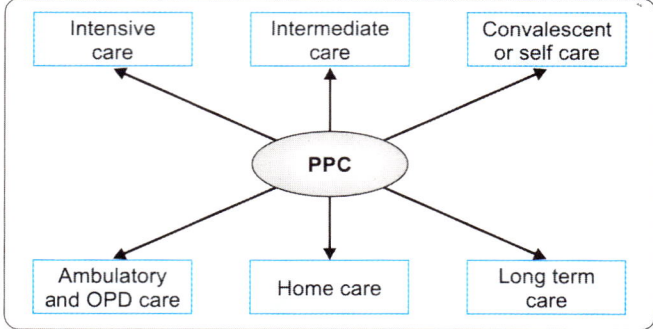

Figure 4: Elements of PPC

PROGRESSIVE PATIENT CARE

The progressive patient care (PPC) is a system of nursing care in which patients are placed in units on the basis of their needs for care as determined by the degree of illness rather than on the basis of a medical specialty.

Progressive patient care is the systematic grouping of patients according to their degree of illness and dependency on the nurse rather than by classification of disease and sex. It is a method of planning the hospital facilities, both staff and equipment, to meet the individual requirements of the patient.

—*Raven. RW, 1960*

PPC has been defined as "the right patient, in the right bed, with the right services, at the right time"

—*Haldeman JC, 1964*

The elements involved in progressive patient care are (Fig. 4):
- Intensive care units for critically ill patients
- Self-care units for convalescent patients or those requiring investigation.
- Intermediate care units for those patients who do not requir to be housed in either of the foregoing, and who would constitute approximately 60% of all patients in a hospital
- Beds attached to out-patient departments for "one day" patients.
- The elements can also be named as intensive care, intermediate care, self-care, long-term care and organized home care.

FACTORS INFLUENCING THE QUALITY PATIENT CARE

Many variable factors influence the number of nurses needed in a ward in order to render a high quality of patient care.
- The total number of patient to be nursed
- The degree of illness of patients (physical dependency)
- Type of service: medical, surgical, maternity, pediatrics and psychiatric
- The total needs of the patients
- Methods of nursing care
- Number of nursing aids and other non professional available, the amount and quality of supervision available

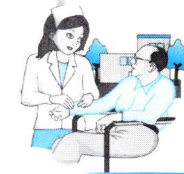

- The amount, type and location of equipment and supplies
- The acuteness of the service and the rate of turnover in patients according to the degree or period of illness.
- The experience of the nurses who are giving the patient care.
- The number of non-nurses who are involved in the patient care, the quality of their work, their stability in service.
- The physical facilities
- The number of hours in the working week of nurses and other ward personnel and the flexibility in hours
- Methods of performing nursing procedures
- Affiliation of the hospital with the medical school
- Methods of assignment-individual, team or functional method
- The standards of nursing care.

DUTY ROSTER

Duty roster is a plan of duty of nurses working in wards of a hospital. The main goal of duty roster is to ensure that the ward is adequately staffed with nurses of all categories during day and night.

Purpose

- To provide holistic patient care services over 24 hours per day
- Duty roster gives a detailed picture of staffing in the ward for a particular period of time
- To make nurses aware of their duty hours
- Help to achieve good ward management.

Principles in Planning Duty Roster

- Distribute adequate number of nurses of different category to provide quality patient care
- Ensure equal distribution of nursing hours to individual nurses
- Consider special days as admission day, inventory day etc
- Give special attention to request and needs of individual staff member
- During planning patients need to be given priority
- Use accepted symbols only while planning
- Duty roster should be approved by supervising staff
- Write full name and designation of each staff member.

Steps in Planning Duty Roster

- Prepare duty roster for one complete month
- Lists the names and designations of staff in the order of seniority
- Check the special request of staff for duty off, night duty, holiday off etc.
- Distribute nurses of different category and non professional workers equally considering special days
- Ensure that there is a senior nurse on duty to take charge during each shift
- Nurses should be encouraged to plan ahead their holidays
- Insert weekly off, holidays, permitted leave of staff clearly with consideration to their request
- The duty roster prepared should be circulated among staff
- Get approval from higher authority.

JOB ANALYSIS

Job analysis is a process to identify and determine in detail the particular job duties and requirements and the relative importance of these duties for a given job. The process results in collecting and recording two data sets including job description and job specification. Both job description and job specification are essential parts of job analysis information. Writing them clearly and accurately helps organization and workers cope with many challenges (Fig. 5).

Concept of job analysis is that the analysis is conducted of the job, not the person. While job analysis data may be collected from incumbents through interviews or questionnaires, the product of the analysis is a description or specifications of the job, not a description of the person.

Purpose of Job Analysis

- To establish and document the 'job relatedness' of employment procedures such as training, selection, compensation, and performance appraisal
- Determining training needs
- To identify or develop skill levels, compensable job factors, work environment (e.g., hazards, attention and physical effort) and responsibilities (e.g., fiscal or supervisory)
- To identify the required level of education (indirectly related to salary level)
- To identify duties that should be included in advertisements of vacant positions, appropriate salary level for the position to help determine what salary should be offered to a candidate.

Methods of Job Analysis

- Structured questionnaire/inventory
- Direct observation
- Logbooks/work diaries
- Interviews

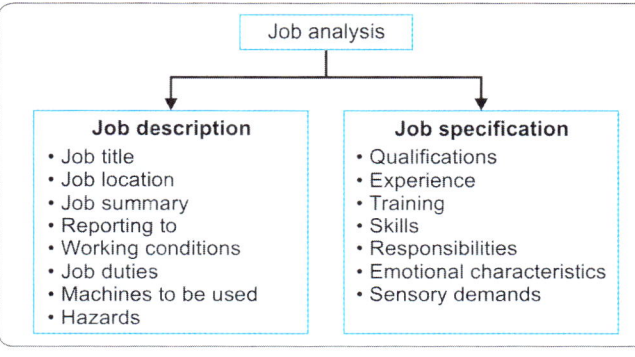

Figure 5: Job Analysis

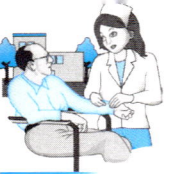

JOB RESPONSIBILITIES OF DIFFERENT CATEGORIES OF NURSING PERSONNEL

Staff Nurse

Staff nurse is a first level professional nurse who provides direct patient care, assist in ward management and supervision. The post of staff nurse is directly proportional to the Head Nurse or ward in charge nurse. All staff nurse should be in uniform at the time of marking their attendance, and should keep punctuality in duty and time.

Direct Patient Care

- Carry out the procedures of admission and discharge of the patients
- Maintain clean and safe environment for the patient
- Responsible for personal hygiene and comfort of the patient
- Attend the nutritional need of the patient and supervise dietary services
- Attend doctors rounds and carry out all the treatment and instructions
- Maintain safety of the ward equipments and supervise cleanliness of hospital utensil such as sputum cups, urinals, bedpan, kidney trays etc
- Perform various technical duties related to nursing care
  - Administration of medications
    Administer injections and intravenous infusions
    Administer intravenous blood transfusion under supervision of medical officer in emergencies
  - Assist doctors in various medical and surgical diagnostic procedures by preparing patients and getting ready with required things
  - Performing simple diagnostic procedures viz., urinalysis and estimation of hemoglobin percentage etc
  - Collecting and sending of specimens for diagnostic procedures
  - Recording of vital signs, i.e. temperature, pulse, respiration and blood pressure
  - Performing gastric lavage, giving enema etc.
  - Prepare patients for operation and see that he/she is sent to operation theater with all necessary documents and medications
  - Takes care of eyes, ears, back, bowel, bladder, perineum, etc when ever needed
  - Observes all patient conditions and take suitable actions accordingly and/or report changes to ward-in-charge/ or the doctor
  - Give expert bedside nursing to all patients
  - Dressing of surgical wounds according to the direction of medical officer
  - Accompany very ill patients sent to other departments
  - Impart health education and discharge advices to patient and his family members
  - Meeting emergency situation promptly. Keep every drug, maintain emergency tray and equipment in the ward
  - Administration of oxygen, Ryle's tube insertion for feeding and aspiration and other problem based care to patients
  - Filling and maintaining all records such as case sheets, temperature charts, intake output chart, diet sheet, doctors order sheet, nurses records
  - He/She gives the last care to patient after death, recording death in the register and arranges ambulance.

Operation Theater Management

- Maintain aseptic environment of the operation theater
- Ensure autoclaving of articles
- Prepare anesthetic trolley for surgery
- Assist the surgeon and anesthetist in every step skillfully while performing various types of surgery.

Labor Room Management

- Render comprehensive antenatal care
- Conduct normal delivery
- Attend and assists doctors in all obstetrical emergencies
- Take care of newborn and premature babies

Management of ICU's

- Intent *and* procure of all necessary equipment, drugs, oxygen cylinder which are required for the unit
- Operate ECG, cardiac resuscitation and other sophisticated high tech machines whenever needed or assist the doctor in operating such machines

Psychiatric Unit

- Assists the doctors in admission and discharge of patients
- Prepares patient for ECT and other procedures and therapies
- Assists in management of aggressive, suicidal and grief as other symptoms of patients

Ward Management

- Helps the ward in-charge to carry out the work during her absence
- Maintains general cleanliness of the ward
- Supervises the duties of subordinates
- Maintains the scheduled poisonous drug registers
- Supervises nursing care and other tasks carried out by the student

Educational Responsibilities

- Helps in orientation of new staff and students.
- Extends co-operation and participates in clinical teaching.
- Participate in in-service education program.
- Plans and implements formal and informal health education program.

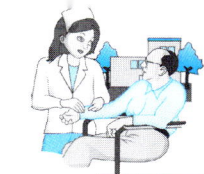

- Assists and extends co-operation in nursing research program
- Accomplishes other duty assigned by nursing superintendent.

Duties and responsibilities of a staff nurse gr. I remains same as above duties along with

- Duties of Head Nurse in the absence of Head Nurse
- Any other duties assigned by the Nursing Superintendent.

Head Nurse

Head Nurse is directly responsible to the Nursing Superintendent Gr. I. She/he is accountable for the nursing care management of a ward or a unit assigned to her/him. She/he is responsible for safety and comfort of the patients in the ward unit to provide high quality of nursing care both in terms of efficiency and effectiveness of service.

Duties and Responsibilities

Responsibilities of a Head Nurse will be broadly classified as follows:

- Supervising the performances of staff and managing the unit efficiently.
- Supervises/attends patient care
- Teaching of staff and students

Direct Patient Care

- Ensures proper admission and discharge of patients
- Assists/Attends direct care of patient as and when required
- Assigning duties to the staff
- Takes nursing round with staff and students
- Accompany the doctors rounds and ensures that doctors' instructions concerning patient treatment are carried out promptly
- Co-ordinates patient care with other departments
- Ensures that all nursing procedures are carried out promptly and see that total health needs of patient are met
- Ensure accurate recording of vital signs and observations
- Responsible to ensure therapeutic diet to patients as per doctor's order and supervise dietary services
- Ensures that emergency medicines/emergency trolley etc are. kept ready
- Ensures safety, comfort and good personal hygiene of patient
- Ensures smooth healthy communications between nurse-patient, nurse-doctor and other superior officers
- Ensures prompt recording of death and any unusual incidents
- Ensures timely filling of daily census records
- Ensures safe and clean environment for the ward and ascertain the quality of care rendered

Supervision and Ward Management

- Implements ward policy
- Makes the duty schedule and work assignment
- Indenting and procurements of ward supplies, medicines, equipments etc. and keep records
- Does regular inventory checking
- Prepares the list of articles for repair or for condemnation
- Acts as a liaison officer between ward staff and hospital administration.
- **Makes duty** arrangements and forward leave application of subordinate staff to the Nursing Superintendent with specific remarks
- Maintains all the records and registers promptly and correctly
- She/he will see that the unit ward is properly stocked with necessary equipment in good working condition and there is adequate supplies required in the ward
- Maintains good public relation in the ward
- She/he will go through the Nursing Superintendent's inspection notes maintained in the ward unit and see that the same are carried out promptly
- Maintains discipline among the staff working in the ward, supervise their work to see that all the staff are doing their work properly
- Ensures cleanliness of the ward and proper disposal of the waste after segregation
- Attends sanitary rounds
- Keeps the record of performance appraisal of nursing staff and submit their confidential report for considering meritorious awards/higher studies.

Educational Functions

- She/he will arrange health talk to patients
- Organizes formal and incidental ward teaching, bed side clinic, demonstration procedures etc. to the students and staff
- Conducts ward conferences and meetings
- Organizes orientation programs for new staff.
- Ensures that the students are getting desired learning experience in the ward
- Evaluates the performances of staff and students.
- Encourages staff developmental program.
- Gives incidental teaching to patients, relatives, staff nurses, students and auxiliary staff
- Helps in medical and nursing research.

As Night Supervisor

General Duties

- All the calls of medical officer should be routed through the night supervisor except in emergency
- Every death that occurs should be correctly entered in the death register in the order of occurrence and the death certificate entrusted to the relatives and their signature obtained on the copy available there
- He/she will see that enough IV fluids, emergency medicines and vene section trays etc. are readily available
- He/she will see that every ward has enough oxygen cylinders and suction apparatus which are in good working condition

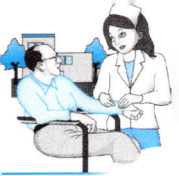

- He/she will give all assistance to the medical officer at night when required
- He/she should take appropriate action against the misbehavior and malpractices of the staff during night.

Responsibilities

- The night supervisor will be responsible for the efficient nursing care of patients at night
- He/she will see that all the night duty staff are present for duty in uniform, if any rearrangements of staff is required then the same may be done
- He/she will make planned and surprise inspection rounds in each section of the hospital during night in addition to attending the calls
- Any patient who needs special attention should be brought to the notice of the duty medical officer
- Ensures that all the night instructions given by the night duty doctor is carried out within that period
- Restricts the entry of strangers in to the ward with the assistance of night sergeant
- She/he will visit all dangerously ill list (post operative patient, accident cases, poisonous cases etc
- She/he will visit pay ward patients
- She/he should make supervision of work done in the casualty
- Ensures that the service of staff nurse and other staff in emergency situation in operation theater if it is required
- Receives all the reports from the wards/departments, compile and prepare a detailed night report of the whole hospital
- If any untoward incidents happened during night that should be reported to the Medical Superintendent in person.

Nursing Superintendent Gr. II

In hospitals where there is no post of Nursing Superintendent Gr.I, the Nursing Superintendent Gr. II will have to carry the duties and responsibilities connected with the nursing service. In hospitals where there are Nursing Officers, Nursing Superintendents Gr. II, the latter will be responsible for the nursing service administration section of the hospital if there are more than one post.

Duties and Responsibilities

- Taking attendance of the staff at the proper time and making daily duty posting as required
- She/he should see that all nursing staff, students, auxiliary staff are in specified uniform at the time of duty
- Maintenance of record of Nursing Service Section
- Making daily inspection rounds for giving guidance and directions to the staff in their work. Report of inspection will be recorded in the register kept for that purpose in each ward/section
- During ward round he/she will specially supervise the following:
  - Ensure the quality of nursing care received by the patients and doctors instructions are promptly carried out
  - Monitors/checks the quantity and quality of food served and keeps a check that there is no pilfer of dietary articles
  - Ensures that the staff and students are prompt in their duties and courteous to patients and their relatives
  - The ward and varandas are not crowded with bye-standers
  - Cleanliness of patient's unit, ward, varandas. side-rooms, stairways, bathrooms, lavatories and premises
  - Ensures that medicines are administered as per the instructions from medical officer
  - Ensures that patients records and ward reports are maintained properly
  - Ensures that the equipment is in good working conditions and sufficient supplies are available for emergency use
  - No unauthorized persons are engaged by the hospital staff to do their duties
- He/she acts as a liaison officer between Nursing Superintendent Gr. 1 and staff. In the absence of the Nursing Superintendent Gr. I he/she will be a liaison officer between the administration and nursing services staff
- Making arrangements for physical verification of stock of government articles supplied to various sections and wards twice in a year
- Making arrangements for condemnation of unserviceable articles
- Making arrangements for meetings of staff and students examination etc
- Preparing reports to be sent to the Superintendents
- Will be a member of the hospital development committee in the absence of Nursing Officer
- Ensures the welfare of the subordinate staff

In institutions where there are no Nursing Superintendent Gr. I, the Senior Nursing Superintendent Gr. II will have to look after all responsibility of the Nursing Superintendent Gr. I and the second Nursing Superintendent Gr. II will carry out the above responsibilities as guided by the former.

Nursing Superintendent Gr. I

Duty time: 8 a. m to 3 p. m.

Nursing Superintendent Gr. I will be directly responsible to the Nursing Officer or Medical Superintendent of the hospital and she/he is accountable for the safe and efficient running of the various nursing departments in the hospital. Nursing Superintendent Gr. I will be assisted in carrying out her/his duty by the Nursing Superintendent Grade II.

Duties and Responsibilities

Nursing Service

- Participates in the formulation of philosophy of the hospital in general and those specific to the nursing.
- Determines goals, aims, objectives and policies of nursing services in the hospital.

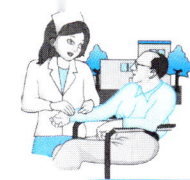

- Implements hospital policies and rules through various nursing units.
- She/he will be in-charge of all nursing and auxiliary staff and will guide and supervise their services.
- Decides and recommends personnel and material requirements for running various nursing service units of the hospital.
- Prepares duty roaster and duty arrangements according to the policies of the hospital or make rotation plan for nursing and auxiliary staff.
- She/he will see that the manpower is properly utilized and the staff has no room for complaint on the ground that they do get equal treatment from administrative side.
- She/he will grant casual leave, day off and holidays to the staff under her/his supervision without hindering the normal functioning of the hospital.
- She/he will forward daily reports to the Hospital Superintendent and discuss day-to-day activity, in the absence of Nursing Officer.
- Makes regular rounds in hospital wards and other specialty departments.
- Takes sanitary rounds with the Medical Superintendent, Nursing Officer and RMO.
- Maintains discipline among nurses and other auxiliary staff.
- Participate in hospital and inter hospital meetings/conferences.
- Investigates complaints against nursing and auxiliary staff and take necessary action/report to Medical Superintendent.
- She/he will write the confidential reports of the staff and recommends for promotion, higher studies or meritorious awards.
- She/he will submit indent in time for purchasing instruments, linen, equipment and other supplies required for running nursing service and see that they are obtained.
- She/he will prepare the list of articles for repair and replacement and give to the store section/Superintendent.
- She/he will be a member of the condemnation committee and will co-operate with the store section to arrange for regular condemnation.
- She/he will be a member of the hospital development committee in the absence of nursing officer.
- She/he will arrange for monthly/periodical meeting of staff and discuss about ways and means to improve the nursing service efficiently.
- She/he will bring to the notice of the Superintendent all problems relating to the staff equipment, hospital policies, standing orders, personal and inter-department relationship etc. which seems to effect adversely the standard of nursing care and will give suggestions for solving the same.
- She/he will maintain register for anecdotal reports/incidental reports.
- He/she will be the warden of the Nurse's hostel attached to the hospital and supervise the discipline in the hostel.
- Ensures the quality of nursing care rendered by the subordinate staff.
- Responsible for the welfare of the nursing and other auxiliary staff.
- Inspects the hospital kitchen and supervise the dietary services.
- She/he will be the custodian of the death register and keys of various departments.
- Assists Nursing Officer in her/his work and officiate in her/his absence.
- He/she will arrange for regular periodical orientation programs for the new comers.
- He/she will make arrangements for in service program whenever possible.

Nursing Officer (More than 500 Bedded Hospitals)

Duties and Responsibilities

- Nursing officer is directly responsible to the Medical Superintendents in the hospitals having 500 bedded and above.
- Participation in the formulation of the philosophy of the hospital in general and those specific to the nursing services.
- Determines goals, aims, objectives and policies of the nursing service.
- Implements hospital policies and rules through various nursing units.
- Nursing Officer will be responsible for planning, organizing and implementing the entire nursing service in the institution.
- Nursing Officer will be the reporting officer to the head of the institution on all matters of nursing service.
- He/she is in-charge of all nursing staff and will guide and supervise their services.
- **He/she is** assisted in earning out her duties, by the Nursing Superintendent Gr.I and Nursing Superintendent Gr II.
- All correspondence, leave application and transfer request from the subordinate staff will be routed through Nursing Officer.
- She/he decides and recommends personnel and material requirements for running various nursing service department of the hospital.
- Prepares budget for the nursing service department.
- Will be a member of the selection committee of students.
- Ensures the safe and efficient care rendered in the various nursing department of the hospital.
- Takes daily hospital round and weekly sanitary round with Medical/Nursing Superintendent, RMO and submit sanitary round report to the head of the institution for necessary action.

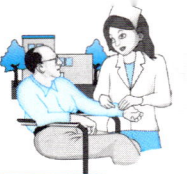

- Functions as member in the condemnation board for linen and other hospital equipment.
- Supervises/verifies the duty roster and sanction leave for Nursing Superintendent Gr. I and Nursing Superintendent Gr. II.
- Gives counselling and guidance to the subordinate staff and students whenever necessary.
- She/he will see and forward the daily report to the Medical Superintendent.
- She/he will maintains discipline among nurses and auxiliary staff, discuss nursing problems, initiate necessary action and submit report to the head of the department.
- Participates in hospital and inter hospital meeting/conferences.
- Investigates complaints of nursing and other auxiliary staff and recommend for necessary steps/action.
- Evaluates confidential report of staff and recommends for promotion higher studies and meritorious awards.
- Plan staff developmental programs and arrange for in-service education and orientation programs in consultation with District Nursing Officer and Principal, School of Nursing.
- Surprise inspection of nursing departments and kitchen.
- Arrange clinical experience for students and supervise them.
- Conducts monthly meeting with the nursing/auxiliary staff discuss problems, initiates necessary action and submit report to head of the institution and District Nursing Officer.
- Maintains necessary records concerning the nursing and auxiliary staff, confidential reports, health records and sanitary reports etc.
- Submits annual report of the nursing service department to the Medical Superintendent District Nursing Officer/concerned authority.
- Participates in professional and community activities.
- Will be a member of the hospital development committee.
- Will be a member of the nursing school management committee.
- Initiates participation in Nursing Research.

District Nursing Officer

Duties and Responsibilities

- District Nursing Officer will be directly responsible to the District Medical Officer of Health for providing efficient nursing service and entrusted to ensure efficient nursing service in the entire district.
- She/he will plan the nursing manpower requirement, ensure welfare measures and discipline of staff and organize induction/in-service education program in the District.
- She/he will be a touring officer and reporting officer to the District Medical Officer of Health in the matter of nursing administration in the district.
- She/he has to submit advance tour program to District Medical Officer for approval and submits tour diary report for necessary action.
- Orders/correspondence regarding the promotion, transfer and posting of nursing and auxiliary staff should be routed through District Nursing Officer.
- All correspondence/file related to nursing service will be routed through District Nursing Officer.
- She/he will be a member of the committee in the selection of nursing staff and students.
- She/he will inspect the dietary services in hospitals.
- She/he will ensure adequate supply of equipment and other supplies in all institutions, checks periodically that they are properly maintained.
- She/he will submit annual requirement budget proposal for the improvement of nursing service in the District.
- She/he will organize CME classes for nursing personnel in consultation with District Medical Officer, Nursing Officer, Principal School of Nursing and voluntary organization.
- She/he will conduct periodical/surprise visit in the institutions and inspect/assess the quality of Nursing Service.
- She/he will arrange monthly meeting with Nursing Superintendent/Nursing Officer of all the institutions to discuss problems related to nursing service and submit report to District Medical Officer and Assistant Director of Nursing Services.
- She/he will formulate proposals for the improvement of the nursing service in the district.
- She/he will take necessary steps to fill up the vacancies in time and monthly reports regarding the vacancy position of nursing staff which should be forwarded to Assistant Director of nursing services.
- She/he will participate in research activities.
- She/he will evaluate confidential report of the nursing staff and recommends for promotion, higher studies and awards for meritorious services.
- She/he will investigate complaints related to nursing service in the district subjected to the orders of DMOH and submit report to DMOH and copy to DHS for further action.
- She/he will be a member in the committee for Nurses' week/Nurses' day celebration.
- She/he should be included as member of the hospital development committee in major hospitals such as district hospital and general hospital etc.
- She/he is responsible for ensuring discipline among the nursing and auxiliary staff in the district.
- Any other duty entrusted by the District Medical Officer as and when required.

Assistant Director of Nursing Service

Duties and Responsibilities

- The Assistant Director of nursing service will assist in planning, supervising and coordinating the activities related to the nursing service and education in the State.

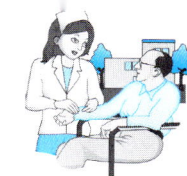

- She/he will be a reporting officer to the Additional Director of nursing services in the matter of nursing administration and education in the State.
- She/he will conduct periodical surprise inspection of institutions of the department and inspect situation, discuss with Nursing Superintendent/Nursing Officer and the Head of the institution on nursing problems and submit report to Director or Health Sciences through Additional Director of nursing services.
- She/he will formulate proposals for the improvement of the nursing and auxiliary services in the State.
- All the files related to Nursing Service and Nursing Education will be routed through Assistant Director of Nursing Services.
- Organize/assist in service education program/s for nursing staff.

Deputy Director of Nursing Services

- Deputy Director of Nursing Services will assist the Additional Director, Nursing Services in planning, supervision and co-ordination of the activities relating to the nursing administration in the state.
- She/he will conduct periodical inspection of the teaching institutions under the department and make proposal for improvement and submit report to the Director of Health Services through Additional Director of Nursing Services.
- Files related to Nursing Service and Education will be routed through Deputy Director of nursing Services.
- Organize in service training for nurses with the assistance of Assistant Director of Nursing services.

Additional Director of Nursing Services

- She/he guides, supervise and co-ordinates Nursing Service and Nursing Education in the State.
- Additional Director of Nursing Services will render necessary assistance to the Director of Health Services in the matter of Nursing Administration and Nursing Education.
- Additional Director of Nursing Services will conduct surprise inspection of the nursing institutions of the department, investigate complaints, problems of nursing service/education and submit report to the Director of Health Services.
- Formulate proposals for the development of Nursing Services in the state with assistance of Assistant Director and Deputy Director of Nursing Services.
- Files related to Nursing Service, Nursing Education transfer and posting Nursing Personnel shall be routed through Additional Director of Nursing Services.
- Additional Director of Nursing Services will be responsible for appointments, transfer and posting of non–gazette, nursing personnel.
- Conduct periodical meeting with the District Nursing Officers Principal School of Nursing.
- Attend Departmental conference/meeting in the state and outside the state.

Principal

Principal, the administrative head, of the nursing school will be responsible to the District Medical Officer. As the head of the institution she/he will be responsible for the smooth implementation of the Indian Nursing Council syllabus and school administration.

Administrative Responsibility

- Selection of students through the set up committee.
- General administration of school of nursing.
- Administration and overall supervision of teaching programs.
- Distributing teaching work load to each tutor along with teaching materials.
- Supervision and guidance of teaching staff including organization of in-service education of staff.
- Carrying out correspondence with other departments, agencies of individuals in connection with the program.
- Will be the drawing and disbursing officer
- Seeing to the supply of audiovisual aids, teaching materials as required.
- Supervision of students' welfare, health and security.

Extended and Expanded Role of Nurse

Nursing is the pivotal health care profession highly valued for its specialized knowledge and caring in improving the status of the public and ensuring, safe, effective quality care (ANA 2002)

Extended Roles of Nurses

The practice of nursing takes place in multiple settings and many nurses select their area of specialization based on interest and job satisfaction. Extended roles of nurses are:

- **Caregiver:** As a caregiver the nurse provide care to patients in various settings. Nurses work in a wide range of setting as hospitals, homes, schools and occupational health settings, etc. The various settings in which the provides caregiver.
- **Hospital/clinics:** As a nurse he/she provides comprehensive quality nursing care to patients in clinical settings that is giving direct care to patients attending hospitals or clinics. It includes preventive, promotive, curative and rehabilitative services to patients.
- **Home health care:** Nursing services provided to patients at their home. Home health care also give opportunity to provide patient care to patients during rehabilitative period of illness or to patients with disability. The nurse can teach and demonstrate caregivers and patients in meeting their needs and nursing services. She also assists patients for self–care that promotes physical, psychological and spiritual health.
- **Occupational health services:** Occupational health nurses provide emerging care, direct health/nursing care to injured or sick, preventive health care as assessment and screening of employees working in factories and industries and referral services to higher health care facilities, if

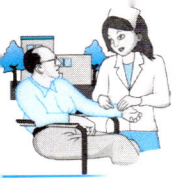

needed. They also provide health education mainly safety education and prevention of occupational hazards. Occupational Health Nurses also conduct inspection of occupational safety services in industries.

- **Hospice and palliative care nursing:** Hospice care can be associated with an agency that provides care to patients. In hospice care centers, nurses provide care to make the patient as comfortable as possible.
- **Ambulatory care:** There are many types of ambulatory care settings such as clinics, ambulatory diagnostic center etc. and this is a growing area for nursing service.
- **Communicator:** As a communicator the nurses are aware that effective communication techniques can help to improve the health care environment. The nurses has to communicate effectively with the patient and family members as well as other members of health team to provide holistic care to patients.

Expanded Role of Nurses

- **Advanced nurse practitioner:** Advance Nurse Practitioner is a registered nurse who has acquired expert knowledge base, complex decision making skill and clinical competencies for expanded practice, the characteristics of which are shaped by the context and/or country in which he/she is credentialed to practice (ICN).
    - Advanced Nurse Practitioner is a registered nurse with additional educational preparation and experience who possesses and demonstrates the competencies to autonomously diagnose, prescribe pharmaceuticals and perform specific procedures within the legislated scope of practice. (Canadian Nurses Association).

    They provide direct care focusing on health promotion, treatment and management of health conditions.
- **Clinical nurse specialist:** Clinical Nurse specialist is a registered nurse who holds a Masters Degree or Doctoral Degree in Nursing with expertise in a clinical specialty, uses in-depth knowledge and skills, advanced judgments and clinical experience in a specialty to assist in providing solution for complex health care issues. They are eligible to provide care in specialty areas as cardiac, pediatrics, obstetrics and gynecology practice.
- **Nurse midwife:** Nurse midwives are certified by council to provide independent care for women during pregnancy, labor, and delivery and postnatal care. The nurse midwives manage normal vaginal delivery independently. They also do antenatal and post natal management and referral services if needed.
- **Certified registered nurse anesthetist (CRNA):** Nurse Anesthetist is having advanced training in Anesthesiology. They are responsible for their patient through entire operative process in inducing sleep, monitoring vital signs, adjusting anesthesia levels and waking the patient after surgery. They can work in every situation in which anesthesia care is delivered.
- **Nurse researcher:** Nurse Researchers are registered nurses with Doctoral degree in nursing, investigate nursing problems to improve nursing care, develop new nursing models and theories and expand the scope of nursing practice. Nurse researchers can involve in nursing research and can guide nursing research conducted by other health care providers.
- **Nurse educators:** Nurse educators teaches and prepare registered nurses. They are responsible to teach and guide various nursing program as Diploma in nursing, Degree in nursing and Master's program, PhD program, Post Doctoral degree program, specialty nursing program etc.
- **Nurse managers:** Nurse Managers directs and co-ordinate nursing service department to provide quality nursing care to patients. They are also responsible to manage nursing service department by planning, organizing, budgeting, supervising and also ensure quality improvement, staff development.
- **Legal nurse consultants:** Legal Nurse Consultants are registered nurses who has had additional qualifications related to legal issues and health care. They also provide advice regarding health issues, reviews nursing records and also assists in planning response to legal issues and cases.
- **Nurse Entrepreneur:** Nurse entrepreneurs serve as consultants or own a health care related business.
- **Nurse advocate:** Nurse acts as an advocate for the patients' problems. The Nurse advocate give suggestions and alternative solutions to patient's problems and help them to manage health care related issues.

STEPS IN BUDGETARY PROCESS

Budget is a formal plan for managing financial resources and it is the document of expected income and expected expenses of an organization. Preparation of departmental budget is a major responsibility of a nurse manager. The steps of budgetary process include,

- **Assessment of needs:** For assessment of needs, the nurse manager must review and assess previous budgetary documents. The nurse manager has to plan the activities of nursing for the next financial year and also review organizations goals and new projects. Also invite participation of middle level and lower level nurse manager in the process development of nursing budget. While preparing budget include items as manpower expenses, expense for materials and equipment, operative expenses etc. Develop goals, objectives and budgetary estimates with support from collegue and subordinates and get approval and advice from top level management.
- **Develop a plan:** Prepare budget plan for the coming fiscal years (12 months). To deal with fluctuating patient census and needs the nurse manager need to develop a viable and comprehensive budget. In the Budget items that need to be included are salaries of staff, linen supplies and equipments,

office supplies, stationeries, maintenance and repair, conveyance etc. Prepare budget worksheet which include columns including columns for historic information with old budget actual numbers with comments explaining the variance, revenue and costs.
- **Implementation:** During implementation of budget ongoing monitoring and analysis's necessary to avoid inadequate or excess fund.
- **Evaluation:** Review budget periodically and modify budget plan if needed.

Critical pathway is one of the best method of planning, implementing and evaluating cost effectiveness of patient care.

Types of Budgetary Process

- **Capital budget:** Capital Budget is the plan for Purchase a major equipments, building etc. Capital budget composed of longterm planning and short-term planning methods. The long-term component include organizational expansion, future replacement etc which will exceed ne year. eg: renovation or construction of new block. The short-term component include purchase of equipment's within the annual budget cycle. eg: gurnitures, bed etc. for hospital
- **Operational budget:** It is a significant component of Budget. Operational budget shows expenses that change in response to quality of services. eg: electricity charges, expenses for maintenance, house keeping expenses, supplies and equipments etc.

MATERIAL MANAGEMENT

Introduction

The practice of managing materials was started by the armed forces who termed it as logistic management. At the time of war, lot of goods like guns, ammunition etc needed to be provided to the war front. There has to be efficient means of procuring the items, stocking the items, transportation of the items and using the items in the war front. It is important here that in order to support the forces fighting the war, the items should be made available in adequate quantities in the right time. Hence a scientific practice of managing the goods was evolved.

The types of activities in the hospitals are quite different from the activities in the war front. However the availabilies of the items in the hospitals in the right time is very important because hospital is a place managing the emergencies related to human lives. Therefore the hospital administrators have imbibed the spirit of logistic management for applications in hospitals.

- Material management is a scientific technique, concerned with planning, organizing and controlling the flow of materials from their initial purchase through internal operations to the service point through distribution.
- Material management is the integrated functioning of an organisation dealing with supply of materials and allied activities in order to achieve the maximum coordination and optimum expenditure on materials.

Aims of Material Management

- Ensuring adequate stock of items required to have a continuous supply.
- Proper storage and controlling of items.
- Items need to be stored in such a way that the items are easily retrievable.
- Mechanism should be available for distribution to the point of usage as per requirement.
- Ensuring efficient and effective utilization of available resources.
- Right quantity, Right quality, Right price, Right place, Right time

Objectives of Material Management

- *Primary objectives:* These objectives are connected directly with the purchasing department.
  - **Low purchase price:** This mechanism should ensure that the items are purchased at the lowest price.
  - **High inventory turn over:** The stocking of items should be restricted to minimum, so that the turn over of the items is more and there is minimum blockage of the capital.
  - **Low storage cost:** In order to stock the items, the hospital has to spend money for the storage space, air conditioning if required, security of the stores etc. Therefore it is important to minimize the stock of items and thereby minimizing the storage cost
  - **Maintenance of uninterrupted supply:** As already mentioned, it is important to have the availability of the items of the patient services at all times.
  - **Maintenance of quality of purchase:** At the time of purchasing the item it is important to have a standard specification for the items. The quality is to be maintained at the time of selection and also at the time of receipt and inspection.
  - **Cordial relation with suppliers**

  Suppliers of different items to the hospital are its external customers. Therefore maintaining a good relation with them will help in ensuring the availability of items and to orient the hospital staff with the newer introduction of hospital items in the market.
  - **Low pay roll cost:** The salaries and wages constitute the major expenses in any organization. Therefore it is important to minimize the manpower required for managing the materials.
  - **Development of vendors:** Depending on the cost of items, frequency of usage of items and various other factors, quotations are invited for purchasing the items. In order to have the quality in purchase, it is Important to have a panel of vendors for supplying the items to the hospital.

- **Good records:** Documentation about the procurement, receipt of items, stock of items, distribution, usage and disposal of items is important for calculation of budget, expenditure, annual consumption, ordering of the items, legal purposes, etc.
- *Secondary Objectives:* This deals with the contribution of the purchase department in achieving the primary objectives of some other departments.
  - **Favorable reciprocal relations:** Mutual interaction between the user department and purchasing department to exchange views about the stock of items, quality of items etc. will ensure efficiency in management of materials.
  - **New materials and products:** Whenever the purchasing department receives information about some newer products in market, the information can be passed on to the user department.
  - **Economic make or buy:** The purchasing department can advise the user departments in buying the products at cheaper price.
  - **Standardization:** It is a step towards ensuring the quality of items purchased.
  - **Product improvement:** There is a need to continuously improve the quality of the products for which the feedback of user department is important.
  - **Inter departmental harmony:** It is important to have a harmonious relationship between the user department and the purchase department and also between the user departments for the efficient management of materials.

Functions of Material Management

Keeping in view the objectives described the various functions of materials management can be listed as:
- Material planning and budgeting
- Purchasing
- Receiving and inspection
- Inventory control
- Stocking and distribution
- Cost reduction
- Disposal

Material Management System (Fig. 6)

- **Material planning (Demand Estimation) and budgeting:** Various factors need to be considered while estimation of demand of the items and other planning requirements. The required budget for purchase also needs to be ear marked. Factors for consideration are:
  - Previous year's consumption.
  - Changing pattern of usage of item.
  - Services newly started
  - Stock available in the store.
  - Lead time (Time required for purchasing the item) Considering the above factors, the quantity of the items to be purchased, specification etc. can be estimated and the budgetary provision can be arranged.

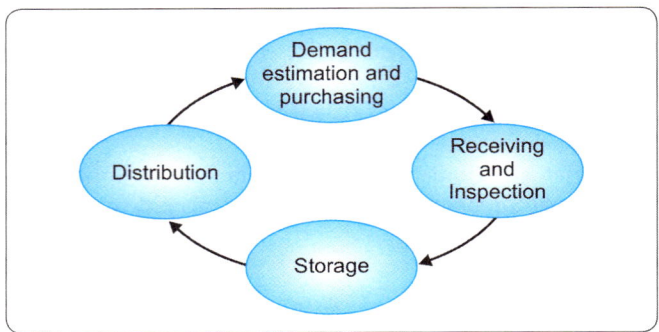

Figure 6: Hierarchy of material management

- **Purchasing:** Depending on the quantity of the items, frequency of usage, availability etc various methods of purchasing can be adopted, which can vary from centralized purchasing to decentralized purchasing or global tender to limited tender or local purchase. It includes sending enquiries, receiving quotations, tabulation of quotations selection, issuing purchase order and arranging payment to the firms.
- **Receiving and inspection:** This is another important function of material management. At the time of receipt of items, inspection of the items is to be arranged depending on the item. Inspection can be by an inspection committee also. Generally the quality and quantity of items supplied are compared with the terms of the purchase order in order to ensure compliance of the purchase conditions. With regard to medicines, shelf life of the drug and condition of the item supplied are also inspected at the time of receipt. The payment to the firms is arranged once the competent authority has duly certified the receipt of items as per the purchase conditions.
- **Inventory control:** Inventory is the quantity of goods or materials in hand. There are scientific methods of controlling the inventory to maintain an economic minimum investment.
- **Stocking and distribution:** The items are stocked in the hospital store. Special storage facilities like refrigeration, air conditioning etc. has to be arranged depending on the item.

  The items can be distributed to the various areas based on requirements. There are scientific methods for optimum storage and distribution of item.
- **Cost reduction:** Since the materials are consuming a good percentage of the hospital budget, measures for cost reduction should be instituted at various stages of managing materials like tendering, selection, storage, distribution usage etc. Measures for prevention of pilferage is also required for reducing the cost.
- **Disposal:** Most of the items are consumed for patient services. Some of the items like equipment, furniture which are obsolete and beyond economical repairs undergo the process of condemnation before disposal.

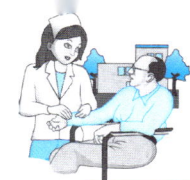

INVENTORY CONTROL

Introduction

Inventory means "the quantity of goods or materials in hand". Management of the inventory is one of the important functions of materials management. From the time of receipt of items in the store till its disposal, the items in the stock forms inventory. During this period, the items need to be stocked scientifically, distributed to various areas and feed back is given to the purchase division for replenishing the stock. Measures should also be in place for preventing decay or excess storage etc. When there is high inventory in hand, there is more capital blocked. When there is low inventory, less capital is blocked but it can result in stock out position. So there is a need to keep the optimum inventory for efficient patient care services.

Definition

Inventory control is the tool of management which is used to maintain an economic minimum investment in materials and products for the purpose of obtaining a maximum financial return.

Functions

- To provide optimum supply, consistent with maximum efficiency and optimum investment
- To provide cushion between the forecasted and actual demand for a material

Techniques of Inventory Control

- ABC analysis
- VED analysis
- SDE analysis
- FSN analysis
- HML analysis
- SOS (Seasonal and offseasonal)
- GOLF (Government, ordinary, local and foreigns)

ABC Analysis

This technique is based on the cost criteria where the following principle is applied. *When the inventory is analyzed based on the cost of the items:*

- Approximately 10% of the drugs or material value 70% of the total cost of items.
- Approximately 20% of the drugs or material value about 20% of the total cost of items.
- Approximately 70% of the drugs or material value about 10% of the total cost of the items.

It can be seen that the major chunk of resources is spent for purchasing a small percentage of the total items. Therefore strict control is exercised for the high value items and better financial control is possible.

Procedure of ABC Analysis

The list of all items stocked is obtained from the records. Unit cost of each item and annual consumption is also taken. From this data, total expenditure of each item for one year is calculated and represented in a tabular form. The items are arranged in descending order based on the total cost of items. Then the cumulative cost is calculated column wise. The items in the list at the level when the cumulative cost in the column falls at or above the 70% of the total cumulative cost constitute "A" category of items. The items falling between 70% and 90% of the cumulative cost can be categorized as "B" items and remaining items are "C" items.

Summary of ABC Analysis (Tables 3 and 4)

Table 3: ABC analysis helps in selective inventory control. The guidelines followed for it are– given in table

Policy guidelines for ABC Analysis

A items high consumption value	B items moderate value	C items less consumption value
Very strict control	Moderate control	Loose control
No safety stock (or very low)	Low safety stock	High safety stock
Frequent ordering or weekly deliveries	Once in 3 months	Bulk ordering, once in 6 months
Weekly control statement	Monthly control report	Quarterly control report
Maximum expediting and follow	Periodic follow up	Follow up and expediting in exceptional cases.
Rigorous value analysis	Moderate value analysis	Minimum value analysis
As many sources as possible	Two or more reliable resources	Two reliable resources for each item
Accurate forecasts in material management	Estimated based on past data on present planning.	Rough estimates for planning
Minimization of waste obsolete and surplus	Quarterly control over surplus and obsolete items.	Annual review over surplus and obsolete materials.
Individual posting	Small group posting	Group postings
Central purchasing and Storage	Combination purchasing.	Decentralized purchasing
Maximum efforts to reduce lead time	Moderate	Minimum clerical efforts
Must be handled by Senior Officer	Can be handled by middle management	Can be fully delegated.

Table 4: ABC classification

Classification	Percentage of items	Percentage of value	Controls
A	10	70	High level, low safety stocks, frequent physical verification, minimum EOQ orders, close schedule control and review
B	20	20	Controls not as tight as for "A" but more than for "C"
C	70	10	Expensive items, purchase in large quantities, at lesser intervals, minimize clerical effort to control large safety stock

(The ABC analysis helps in selective inventory control.)

VED Analysis

This analysis is based on the criticality of the items for use in the hospital. By using this analysis, the items can be classified as vital, essential and desirable.

Vital Items

These items should not have any stock outs and should be available for immediate use in the hospitals.

For example: injection adrenaline in a cardiac setup.

The top level management should ensure the availability of these items.

Essential Items

These are the items for which the shortage can be tolerated for a short period but has to be made available immediately.
For example: antibiotics.

Desirable Items

Desirable items those items where its shortage will not adversely affect the patient care services.

For example: enzymatic preparations.

The lower level of management can exercise the control of these items.

The ABC items and VED items can be combined to form a matrix as shown in Fig. 7.

The category 1 items combine the expensive and the vital items and the control of these items has to be exercised by the top level management so that there is strict financial control and availability of vital items are ensured.

The category 2 items are less expensive and less vital and can be controlled by the middle level management.

The category 3 items are unimportant items which are neither vital nor expensive and can be controlled by lower level management.

SDE Analysis

SDF analysis stands for scarce, difficult and easy to acquire items

This analysis is based on the difficulty in procurement of the item. i.e. scarce to procure, difficult to procure and easy to procure. This is useful for the lead time analysis and higher safety stock of "S" items can be kept.

FSN Analysis

FSN analysis stands for three groups of items based on rate of consumption:
- F– fast moving
- S– slow moving
- N– non–moving

This analysis is based on the speed of consumption of items i.e. fast moving, slow moving and non moving items. Special precaution should be ensured regarding "N" items.

HML Analysis

HML analysis categorizes the items as:
- H– high
- M– medium
- L–low

This analysis is based on the unit cost of the item i.e. high cost, medium cost and low cost. This helps in controlling the purchase of items.

- **Lead time:** This is the average duration of time required to make the items available in the hospital store. This can be classified into internal lead time and external lead time.
- **The internal lead time** is the administrative lead time from the time of requisition to placing the purchase order. This incorporates the time required for framing the specifications, intending, sending enquiries and obtaining quotations, comparative statement or tabulation, selection of the items, negotiation with the company and placing the purchase order.

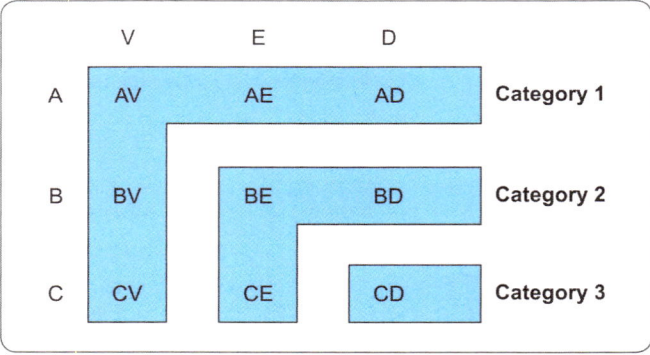

Figure 7: Matrix of ABC and VED items

- **The external lead time** is the time between placing the purchase order to the supplier and receipt of material in hospital store. Lead time is to be considered while framing the purchasing strategy. An average lead time of 2-6 weeks within the country is in the acceptable range.

Economic Order Quantity (EOQ)

EOQ is that quantity at which the cost of ordering the requirement of an item and the inventory carrying cost are nearly equal. This is useful in striking a balance between purchase cost and the cost of holding inventory. In order to arrive at the figure of EOQ, inventory carrying cost and the ordering cost need to be considered.

$EOQ = \sqrt{2AC/PI}$

A = Annual consumption of item in unit
C = Ordering cost
P = Purchase price per unit
I = Inventory carrying cost

This will help in maintaining optimum inventories and reduction in carrying cost.

- **Inventory carrying cost:** Whenever the items are stocked there are expenses for storage, maintaining temperature, avoiding pests and pilferage etc. The cost incurred for holding the inventory is termed as the inventory carrying cost. It includes:
  - Storage space
  - Stationary
  - Salaries and wages
  - Security
  - Pest control
  - Power/electricity
  - Air conditioning
  - Obsolescence
  - Pilferage etc

Approximately 1-5% of the total inventory cost will be required for maintaining the inventory. In order to minimize the inventory carrying cost, it is advisable to keep minimum inventory with higher turnover.

- **Procurement Cost/Ordering Cost:** This is the cost incurred to get the materials in to the inventory of the hospital. The cost is comprise of
  - Postal, telephone, fax, internet charges etc.
  - Advertisement
  - Stationery
  - Salaries and wages.
  - Travel
  - Incidental expenses

It is convenient to work out the ordering cost in common. Ordering cost will not be altered based on the value of the purchase order.

- **JIT (Just in time):** Now a days it is possible to order the item whenever required. Therefore, there is no cost involved in carrying the inventory. For example, whenever a particular specialized surgery is planned, the item can be ordered specifically meant for the surgery to be delivered few hours before scheduled time of surgery.

- **Buffer stock:** It is the quantity required for managing emergency/unexpected needs. It is calculated by multiplying the difference between maximum and average consumption rate per day/week/ month by the lead time for the item. It is at this level that the reordered quantity is meant to be received.

- **Re-order level:** It is the stock level at which a fresh order is to be placed. This reorder level can be calculated by multiplying the lead time with the average consumption per day and then adding the buffer stock.
  i.e. re-order level = (A x L) + BS
  A = Average consumption of the item per day
  L = Lead time
  BS= Buffer stock

At present through the hospital information system the re-order level can be displayed automatically and fresh orders can be placed based on that.

DELEGATION

Delegation is a major element of directing function of nursing management. It is an effective nurse management competency by which nurse managers get the work done through their employees. Delegation is part of management; it requires professional training and development to accept the hierarchical responsibilities of delegation.

Delegation of duties makes accomplishment possible through a division of labor. The head nurse, who delegates certain aspects of her administrative functions, frees herself for activities which she may be better prepared to perform than others. When duties are specifically delegated to certain individual's, opportunity is provided to place responsibility for getting the quality of results.

Delegation can be defined as getting work done through others, or as directing the performance of one or more people to accomplish organizational goals. The person who delegates is called superior and whom delegated is subordinate.

Delegation is the process of assigning responsibility and authority to co-worker and ensuring his accountability. It is giving the employee an appropriate authority to act alone and providing the necessary tools for achieving success. The manager should not dictate every detail about how the job should be done.

Authority-Responsibility-Accountability

Principles Underlying the Delegation of Responsibility

- **Principle in terms of results expected**: A clear cut outline of duties, responsibilities, relationships and assigning duties in terms of expected results.

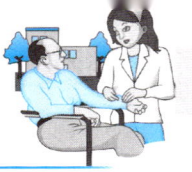

- Establishment of definite objectives and suitable measures for determination of satisfactory performance: By these means the nurse knows exactly what is expected of her. She has specific goals toward which to aim and is able to evaluate her own work. The head nurse has a basis for judgement and an opportunity to stimulate improvement.
- **Authority level principle:** Clarification of limits of authority
- **Principle of parity of authority and responsibility:** While assigning duties to subordinates, there should be equality of authority and responsibility.
- **Unity of command:** As employee should receive orders from one superior only. So subordinates should always be placed under the guidance, control and supervision of one supervisor who will set up work priorities and will arrange for co-operation.
- Once the limits of responsibility and authority have been designated, the head nurse should make no decisions in that area: She may give advice and counsel

Nature of Delegation

- Delegation implies transfer of certain specified functions by the superior to the subordinates. The subordinate acts as an agent of superior authority and the superior always retains the right to issue directions to revise decisions. Delegation of responsibility always lies with the superior.
- One person constitutes only one man power. Wherever a person's job grows beyond his capacity, his success lies in his ability to multiply himself through others. Here superior shares his duties with his immediate subordinates. Managerial work is by supervisors and operating work by operators.
- It is when an organization grows that the need for delegation arises, because one person or group of persons can no longer make all the decisions.
- Authority and responsibilities along with duties must therefore be divided. So in delegation authority is divided and distributed.
- The extent of delegation of authority is inversely related to the size and complexity of the organization.
- The degree of delegation depends on individual requirements of the situation, structure and judgement of the delegator.

Types of Delegation

- General or specific delegation
- Formal or informal delegation
- Written or oral delegation
- Downward and sideward delegation

General or Specific Delegation

In general delegation, the subordinate is granted authority to perform all the functions in his department or division. The subordinate exercise this authority under overall guidance and control of supervisor.

Formal or Informal Delegation

- When authority is delegated as per the organization structure, it is called formal delegation. Here subordinate has no option other than obeying the superior.
- Informal delegation takes place when an individual or a group agrees to work under the direction of an informal leader. This occurs when there are procedural delays so as to perform the task quickly.

Written or Oral Delegation

- Delegation made by written orders and instructions is known as written delegation.
- Unwritten or oral delegation is based on customs and conventions.

Downward and Sideward Delegation

- Downward delegation occurs when a superior assigns duties and grants authority to his immediate subordinate.
- Sideward delegation takes place when a subordinate assigns some of his duties and authority to another subordinate of the same.

Benefits of Delegation

Delegation offers many benefits to the organization and to the staff who work in the organization.

- **Cost effectiveness** is one of the benefits when resources, including staff are used appropriately. There is a potential cost savings.
- **Time saving** as activities are allocated among others, thereby multiplying the ability to get work done more efficiently.
- **Professional growth** can occur when staffs are challenged to develop new skills as they take on new opportunities. The delegator who might be a manager, team leader or staff nurse has an opportunity to grow, as new skills are learned more time is available to do other activities and so on. When delegation is done in a thoughtful manner the environment is typically one in which staff feel valued and trusted.

Five Rights of Delegation

National council of state board of nursing (NCSB 1995) recommended the five rights of delegation and these are written below:

1. **Right task:** One that is delegable for a specific patient or situation.
2. **Right circumstances:** Appropriate setting, available resources and other relevant factors considered.
3. **Right person:** Right person is delegating the right task to the right person to be performed by the right person.
4. **Right direction/communication:** Clear, concise description of the task, including its objective, limits and expectations.
5. **Right supervision:** Appropriate monitoring, evaluation, intervention (as needed) and feedback.

Steps in Delegation
- Selecting and assigning task
- Selecting the appropriate subordinate
- Instructing the subordinates
- Maintaining feedback and control

Reasons for Delegating
- Assigning routine tasks
- Assigning tasks for which the nurse manager does not have time
- Reduces the managers workload
- Renders continuity and permanency
- Problem solving
- Changes in the nurse manager's own job emphasis
- Capability building
- Motivates and develops subordinates
- Promotes expansion and development of organisation

Strategies for Effective Delegating

Although some managers balk at the idea of sharing enough information or authority for delegation to be effective, a variety of strategies can be implemented to ensure effective delegation. They are as follows:

- **Plan ahead:** Plan ahead when identifying tasks to be accomplished. Assess the situation and clearly delineate the desired outcomes.
- **Identify necessary skills and levels:** Identify the skill or educational level necessary to complete the job. Often legal and licensing statutes determine this. The manager should know the official job description, expectations from each worker and classification in the organization.
- **Select the most capable personnel:** Identify the qualified person who is proficient to complete the job in terms of capability and time to do so. Managers should ask the individuals to whom they are delegating if they are capable of completing the delegated task but should also validate this perception by direct observation. It is also important that the person to whom the task is being delegated considers the task to be important.
- **Communicate the goal clearly:** Managers should encourage employees to attempt to solve problems themselves; however employees often need to ask questions about the task or to clarify the desired outcome. When this happens, the manager should clearly communicate what is to be done, including the purpose for doing so and verify comprehension. The manager should also include any limitation or qualifications that have been imposed. Although the desired product should be specified, it is important to give the subordinate feedback and appropriate degree of autonomy in deciding exactly how the work can be accomplished.
- **Set deadlines and monitor progress:** Set time lines and monitor how the task is being accomplished through informal but regularly scheduled meetings. This shows an interest on the part of the manager, provides for a periodic review of progress and encourages ongoing communication to clarify any questions or misconceptions.
- **Model the role and provide guidance:** If the subordinate is having difficulty carrying out the delegated task, the manager should be available as a role model and resource in helping to identify alternative solutions. The manager should also convey a feeling of confidence and encouragement. Reassuming the delegated task should be a manager's last resort, because this action fosters a sense of failure in the employee and demotivates rather than motivates.
- **Evaluate performance:** Evaluate the subordinate's performance after the task has been completed. Include positive and negative aspects of how the person has completed the task. Specific feedback can provide a chance for personal and professional growth. Without this feedback, delegators and subordinates are unable to have a mutually trusting and productive relationship.
- **Reward accomplishment:** Be sure to appropriately reward a successfully completed task. The more recognition team members receive, the more recognition will be given to their leader.

Common Delegation Errors

Delegation is a critical leadership skill that must be learned. Frequent mistakes made by managers in delegating include underdelegating, overdelegating and improper delegating.

- **Underdelegating:** This usually stems from the manager's false assumption that delegation may be interpreted as a lack of ability on his or her part to do the job correctly or completely. Another important cause of underdelegating is the manager's desire to complete the whole job personally due to lack of trust in the subordinates; the manager believes that he or she needs the experience or that he or she can do it better and faster than anyone else. Manager feels that subordinates will resent having work delegated to them. The manager lacks experience in the job or in delegation itself or because he/she has excessive control on need to be perfect. Novice managers underdelegate because they find it difficult to assume the managerial role.
- **Overdelegating:** In contrast to underdelegating which overburdens the manager, some managers overdelegate, burdening their subordinates. Some managers overdelegate because they are poor managers of time, spending most of it just trying to get organized. Others overdelegate because they feel insecure in their ability to perform task. Employees may become overworked and tired, which can decrease their productivity.
- **Improper delegating:** Improper delegation includes such things as delegating at the wrong time, to wrong person or for the wrong reason. It may also include delegating tasks and responsibilities that are beyond the capability of the

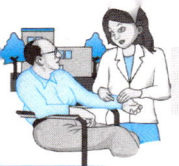

person to whom they are being delegated or that should be done by the manager. For example, delegating decision making without providing adequate information.

Barriers in Process of Delegating

Barriers in the Delegator

- Preference for operating by oneself
- Demand that everyone Knows all the details
- Super–nurse syndrome: Feeling that others cannot do what you can do so you try to do it all
- Feeling of overburdening the sub-ordinates
- Lack of experience in the job or in delegating.
- Lack of role models
- Lack of self confidence
- Insecurity: Manager thinks that they are incapable if they delegate to others and lack of trust in others to do the job right way
- Fear of being disliked
- Fear of criticism
- Refusal to allow mistakes
- Lack of confidence in subordinates
- Perfectionism, leading to excessive control
- Lack of organizational skill in balancing work loads
- Poor relationship with the staff will block effective delegation

Barriers in the Delegate

- Lack of experience
- Lack of competence
- Avoidance of responsibility
- Overdependence on the boss
- Disorganization
- Overload of work

Barriers in the Situation

- One-person show policy
- No toleration of mistakes
- Criticality of decisions
- Urgency, leaving no time to explain
- Confusion in responsibilities and authority, lack of position description
- Understaffing
- Poor communication

SUPERVISION

Supervision is one of the most important management functions in an organization. In every organization there is provision of supervision.

Supervision means overseeing the employee at work. It is a necessary concomitant of their hierarchical organization in which each level of subordinate to the one immediately above it are subjected to its orders. Workers at the intermediate level of the organization supervise as well as supervised.

Concept of Supervision

The term "supervision" has its origin in two Latin words: super meaning "above"; vision/video, meaning "seeing ". It is an act of a superior person to see the work of the personnel working under him/her.

Overseeing means:
- Directing
- Investigating
- Guiding
- Helping and
- Advising the subordinate in performance with the purpose of achieving the established objectives.

It is essential and important aspect of administration.

Therefore, supervision is a teaching learning process which provides:
- Constant observation
- Monitoring
- Evaluation
- Guidance
- Perform their activity effectively and efficiently maintaining the required standards.

Supervision is two fold process i.e., one fold guiding process and another fold superintending the work of subordinates.

Supervision is defined as the authoritative direction of the work of one's subordinates.

- Terry and Franklin meant supervision as "guiding and directing efforts, employees and other resources to accomplish stated work outputs."
- Williamson defined supervision "as a process by which workers are helped by designed staff members to learn according to their needs, to make the best use of their knowledge and skills to improve their abilities so that they could do their jobs more effectively and with increasing satisfaction to themselves and the agency.
- Supervision may be defined as:
- A two way dynamic and social process
- Undertaken for the specific purpose of fulfillment of organizational goals
- By striving to maintain the required quality of performance
- Through constantly supporting and assisting the workers to perform their best
- Supervision has been defined as the cooperative relationship between a leader and one or more persons to accomplish a particular purpose. Supervision is a kind of teaching which involves advising, helping inspiring leading and liberating. (Jean Barrett).

Basic Tenets of Supervision

- Supervision is an ongoing process invariably interwoven with motivation, performance appraisal, staff development and leadership.

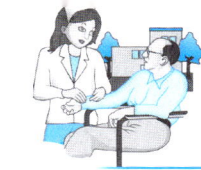

- Supervisors are always accountable for the performance of the subordinates under her/ his span of control.
- Supervisors are to help the workers improve, develop and reinforce knowledge and skills according to their individual learning needs.
- Supervisors are required to help the workers develop the right attitude.
- It includes assisting the workers to perform in the best possible way to yield the best results in terms of realization of the organizational goals.

Objectives of Supervision

- Help employees to develop their abilities and skill so that they can function effectively.
- Promote team spirit which create a positive work culture
- Help to increase employee morale
- Through supervision the supervisor can identify the factors or problems which disturb quality care.
- Supervision helps to appraise the performance of individual employees
- It helps to improve attitude of employees
- Guides or helps to achieve organizational goals or targets
- Enable employees to identify their own problems
- Motivation to subordinates
- Helps to improve performance of workers and development of employees

Principles of Supervision

- Good supervision generates and guaranties quality of services rendered.
- Good supervision coordinates and unifies efforts of the nursing staff.
- Supervision fosters the ability of each staff member to think and act for herself/himself, i.e it promotes effectiveness of individual staff member.
- It is based on the needs of the individual.
- It respects the individuality of the staff members.
- Supervision of graduate staff nurses differs from that of students.
- Supervision strives to make the ward a good learning situation.
- Supervision is well planned.
- Good supervision helps the individual nurse set up objectives which are for her dynamic, reasonable and worthwhile and helps her to attain her objectives.
- Supervision stimulates staff to continuous self-improvement. Stimulator results when the individual interests are aroused, so she responds with enthusiasm. Supervision creates in the staff member a desire for help in the attainment of her objectives.
- Good supervision helps the nurse to make a pattern for analysis and to analyze continuously her success in reaching her objectives.
- Supervision needs to be exercised without giving the subordinates a sense that they are being supervised.
- Supervision encourages a workers participation in decision–making.
- Supervision needs good communications.
- Supervision is a process of cooperation and coordination.
- Supervision should create suitable climate for productive work.
- Supervision should give an autonomy to workers depending on their personality, competence and characteristics.
- Supervision should respect the personality of the staff.
- Supervision should focus on continued staff growth and development.
- Supervision is responsible for checking and guidance.
- Good leadership is a part of good communication.

Principal Duties of a Supervisor

- To understand the duties and responsibilities of his own position
- To plan the execution of the work
- To divide the work among sub-ordinates and to direct and assist them in doing it
- To improve his own knowledge and technical expert and leader
- To improve his work methods and procedures
- To train the personnel
- To evaluate the performance of the employees
- To correct mistakes, solve employee's problems and develop discipline
- To keep subordinates informed about policies and procedures of the organization and above the changes to be made
- To co-operate with colleagues and seek advice and assistance when needed
- To deal with employee suggestions and complaints

Types of Supervision

Direct Supervision

This is done through face to face talk with the workers. This can be exercised at the ward/unit level in the hospital or PHC or sub center. These considerations are essential in direct supervision.

- Do not loose temper or abuse
- Use democratic approach and avoid autocratic methods
- Reprimand if necessary in private and do it promptly
- Give workers a chance to reply
- Do not talk too much and too fast
- Be human in behavior
- Do not take it granted that the worker has understood everything told to him
- Do not give instructions in a haphazard way

Indirect Supervision

It is done with the help of record and reports of the workers and through written instructions or through some agency between the supervisor and supervisee. This includes:

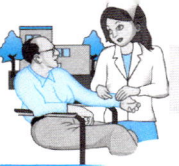

- Ensuring that every worker is carrying out allotted work in accordance with the plan of operation and with the prescribed methodology and in keeping pace with the time as far as possible.
- Analyzing the monthly progress reports to know the input of efforts and the achievement of the workers and their relation with each other.
- Analyzing what amount of work allotted for the month has been done with reasons for non-performance and providing suitable guidance for the same.
- Providing suitable guidance and support to all the workers in implementation of various activities.
- Analyzing the stage of program or job in each sector and to plan for future months on the above basis.
- Ensuring that the worker is utilizing his/her fullest capacity in the program.

Functions of Supervision

- **Administrative:** Assigning duties or preparing duty roster, providing materials and supplies to facilitate the staff's performance.
- **Educative:** By sharing knowledge, providing technical guidance, a supervisor plays the role of supervisor.
- **Helping:** The supervisor offers help by solving problems faced by the staff and to complete her work particularly in emergency.
- **Communicative:** The supervisor acts as a communication link between the staff and higher authorities and other members of the team.
- **Evaluative:** Each supervisor is supposed to carry out performance appraisal of all their staff working under her in unit and provide feedback for their efficiency.

Styles of Supervision

- **Task centered:** When the supervisor emphasizes the task more than the performer whom he supervise. This type of supervisor probably believe that 'ends' are important than the 'means'. Her concern for the task is high than the human aspect in dealing with the staff. The staff may view her as tough master.
- **Employee centered supervisor:** Such supervisors are people oriented. They believe that the concern for the staff, their needs and welfare is more important. Therefore if the staff is being cared well, work efficiency increases and staff will be able to take more responsibilities. However at times this style leads to inefficiency. And the Worker takes for granted as a lenient supervisor. The effectiveness of this style depends on various factors like nature of task, nature of employees and the situation.
- **An autocratic or critical supervisor:** It is one who cannot tolerate any deviation from the norms and/or lack of discipline. The decisions are always taken by her and such supervisor acts like Hitler who wanted all commands to be followed.
- **A benevolent supervisor:** They are very protective of her subordinates, keep guiding them what they should do and what they should not do, thus providing constant direction. Such supervisors are usually liked by their workers but are effective as long as they are physically present and they tend to develop the subordinates as dependent staff.
- **A democratic supervisor:** It is one who believes in style of "let's agree on what we are to do in dealing with the subordinate. Such supervisors provide guidance only when requested by subordinates. They are quite independent and cooperate with others and work together.

Thus, we can't say this style is best. In fact no style is best. Supervisor has to adapt a style depending upon the complexity of job and nature of job and its effect on the patient.

Qualities of a Good Supervisor

Some personal qualities are inherited e.g. attractive personality, good health, loyalty but in addition to these there are some qualities which have to be acquired. According to Halsey, a good supervisor must possess the following qualities:

- **Thoroughness:** A supervisor must have detailed knowledge of all the information relevant to the task and must care of every necessary detail.
- **Fairness:** A supervisor should exhibit a sense of justice, consideration and truthfulness towards subordinates.
- **Initiative:** Includes qualities of courage, self confidence and decisiveness.
- **Tact:** Saying and doing things in a way which gives subordinates a feeling of playing an important part in whatever is being done.
- **Enthusiasm:** It is an intense and eager interest in and devotion to the organizational goal.
- **Emotional control:** It means an emotional maturity which controls and channelize emotions in the right direction.
- **Personal qualifications:** Which include integrity, honesty, ability to cooperate, ability to attract, motivate and unite others to work.
- **Teaching ability:** Ability to communicate with the workers.
- **General outlook:** The supervisor should show liking of and be absorbed in it.

Over and above these qualities other qualities like leadership, approachable, stability of character, good communicator, problem solving or decision making ability and human aspect of supervision should also be there.

Techniques and Tools of Supervision

- **Observation**, for example, through field visit, spot checking.
- **Supervisory rounds:** Should be constructive in criticism and may be followed by group discussions or conference.
- **Individual and group conference** are valuable and effective method of supervision.
- **Check list**.
  - **Check-list:** It is one of the most important and common tool of supervision that can be used both in direct or indirect type of supervision.

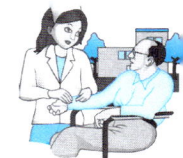

- **What is a check-list?** Check-list is an essential component of a task, skill or activity against which a performance as well as a performer is being supervised.
- **Why is it necessary**:
  o It helps in effective and systematic supervision.
- It avoids duplication.
  o It includes essential components of a task, skill or activity being supervised.
  o It ensures objectivity by providing factual data.
- **Rating scales:** It is a set of categories designed to elicit information about a quantitative or a qualitative attribute. It helps in assessing the performance of tasks, skill levels, procedures etc. These are judged at a defined level within a stated range. One prepares 3 point/ 5point/7 point rating scale. e.g., good (3), satisfactory (2), poor(1) etc. to judge a defined level
- Written policies, manual, bulletin boards etc.
- Report written/or verbal.
- Follow up visit and evaluation.
- Staff meeting: Monthly and periodic meeting are included in this method. These meeting are used by the supervisor to review their performance and jointly plan medical and nursing actions according to the need.
- Anecdotal records of employees kept by supervisor
- In service education.

Responsibilities of the Nursing Supervisor

Upward Responsibilities

- Identifies the activities of the hospital authorities
- Arrange to carry out these activities
- Keep your higher authorities informed about what is being done
- Suggest measures for improving efficiency of workers
- Act as liaison between higher authorities of the health management and the nursing personnel, interpreting the requirements of the district health authorities and the hospital authorities to workforce and vice versa
- Refers matters to supervisors for their timely and appropriate interventions without bothering them unnecessarily at the same time

Downward Responsibilities

- For selecting, orienting and training new staff nurses and new students
- To demonstrate them concerned decorum, manners, tact and courtesy in their working areas in day to day dealing
- Help them in effectively, humanely communicating with their client and all others concerned
- Build good interpersonal relationship among the workers
- Help nurse performers in performing different procedures effectively and in assessing the efficacy of their performance
- Assign duties and responsibilities to nurse performers
- Arrange for their day offs and plan for their rotation
- Making contingency plans for emergency in advance
- Appraise the nurses performance, give feedback guide and counsel them
- Help the workers make adjustments and guide them as necessary
- Assist the nurses to take pride in their work, urging them to do their best with dedication, human concern and sense of involvement.
- Help them to develop a value system that would be beneficial to the clientele, to the management and to concerned as well as themselves.
- Develop a spirit of dedication, teamwork, cooperation and harmony among the workers.

To be a good and effective supervisor he or she must have adequate knowledge and experience in the area in which supervisor is working.

STANDARDS IN NURSING

Standards of nursing are guidelines that help the nurses to practice the profession safely and provide quality care to patients. The objectives of nursing professionals are to provide safe, competent and ethical nursing care with compassion, comfort and collaboration with the patient, the families, the communities and the clinical care team. Standards are pre-requisite promotions of safe, effective, competent and ethical nursing care.

According to ANA, standard is described as a criterion used by general agreement as an acceptable level of practice for an established norms for the practice of nursing. Nursing standards provide a guide to the knowledge, skills, judgement and attitude that are needed to practice safety. They provide direction to nursing care and assess a foundation and baseline for nursing practice.

Standards are bench mark of achievement which is based on described level of excellence. In nursing practice standards are established criteria for practice of nursing.

Characteristics of Nursing Standards

- Standards outline what the profession expects from its members
- Standards must be realistic, acceptable and attainable
- Standards must be broad statements which can be applied to variety of settings and must be developed by experts from nursing profession itself
- Standards are dynamic and must be based on current knowledge and scientific practice and it should be reviewed periodically
- Standards must be revised periodically
- Standards must be understandable and unambiguous
- Standards create enhanced professional responsibility and accountability towards nursing care

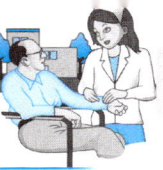

Purposes

- Standards promote, guide and direct professional nursing practice
- Standards help to improve quality of nursing service
- Standards provide a guideline for the nursing performance and activities
- Standards acts as a bench mark to evaluate quality of nursing practice in any setting
- Standards may help to determine the degree to which nursing care standards are maintained
- Standards can be used by supervisors to guide and evaluate staff nurses
- Standards help to determine nursing negligence and malpractice
- Standards help to provide legal protection for nurses

Standards are established by licensing bodies (for example, Indian Nursing Council) Professional associations (for example Trained Nurses Association of India), accrediting agencies (for example, NABH), Nursing Department of Hospitals, Govt. Institutions etc.

Types of Standards

There are different types of standards. They are:

- **Normative standards:** Normative standards describe nursing practices and are considered as good or ideal by authorities. Usually professional organizations as TNAI formulate normative standards.
- **Empirical standards:** Empirical standards are set and fixed based on empirical evidence. It describes practices actually observed in a large number of patient care settings. Regulatory bodies as INC usually prepare empirical standards.
- **End standards:** The ends standards are patient oriented standards which describe the changes as desired in a patients status/behavior. End standards require information about the patients.
- **Means standards:** These are standards framed to describe the nursing care activities specific for each patient procedure and is nursing care oriented. They describe the activities and behavior designed to achieve the end standards. Mean standards required information about the nurses performance.
- **Structure process and outcome standards:** These standards are formulated according to frame of reference related to the nursing structure process and outcome. Structure standards are related to framework i.e. care providing system, process standard describe the behavior of nurses at desired level of performance and outcome standards are descriptive statements of desired patient care results are the outcome standards. They reflect the effectiveness of care.

Frames of Reference for Standards/Elements of Standards

Frames of reference for standards are:
- Structure standards
- Process standards
- Outcome standards

Structure Standards

Focus on the settings of the organization such as facilities in hospital, nursing colleges etc. and environment in which nursing is practiced. These standards includes;

- Goals, philosophy and objectives of the organization
- Policies, rules and regulations and nursing standards
- Structure of institutions as building, infrastructure facilities, supplies and equipments
- Staffing in various departments, job descriptions, administrative setup and organization
- System of communication and interpersonal relations
- Documentation system etc.

Process Standards

These standards focus on the activities carried out in delivering care. It describes the behaviors of the nurses at the desired level of performance, the criteria that satisfy methods for specific nursing interventions and process standards activities concerned with delivery of patient care. These standards are measured or stated in action verbs as assessment of needs and problems of patient, plan nursing care according to priority, implementation of care etc. for example, nurse assess vital signs.

Outcome Standards

Outcome standards focus on the end results of nursing services and activities carried out and changes which occurred. They are related to both the quantity and quality of care given and are used to evaluate the outcome of patient. Descriptive statements of desired patient care results are termed as outcome standards because patients' results are outcomes of nursing interventions. Outcome standards reflect effectiveness of care or changes in health status of individuals. This change may be due to medical and nursing care offered to patients.

For example, ability of patient to do self care activities, morbidity and mortality rate, absence of complications etc.

Steps in Setting of Standards

- Identify an area of nursing practice in which there is need for setting standards
- Do a detailed review of literature, about the needed standards and the philosophy, objectives and goals
- The next step is writing the statements
- Discuss with experts in nursing profession about the framed standard of care and get approval of the standard
- Develop a protocol for each procedure
- Evaluate and check the validity of protocol
- Implement developed standards
- Update the standards periodically

Standards have a basis by which quality of service can be judged. It is necessary that nursing department has to develop

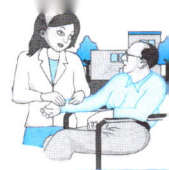

standards of patient care and appropriate evaluation tools so that professional aspects of nursing involves intellectual and interpersonal standards.

Sources of Nursing Standards

Some of the Indian Organizations that framed the standards of nursing care are:
- Joint Commission International (JCI)
- National Accreditation Board for Hospitals and Health Care Providers (NABH)
- National Accreditation Board for Testing and Calibration Laboratories (NABL)
- Professional Organizations as TNAI
- Universities and health care agencies

NURSING MANUALS

It is a good practice to compile all the rules/guidelines concerning the management and procedure in a manual that can be made available for reference. These directives generally fall under the following 3 headings:
- Procedure issued by the administrative office and referring mainly to regulations. This is essential for maintaining discipline.
- Procedure manuals, e.g., lab procedure manuals, nursing procedure manuals
- Unit procedure - Outline the procedure to be used in unit

The contents of the manual, particularly in relation to the specific procedure, will be more acceptable if compiled following a group discussion. It is important that manual should be kept up to date and old procedure should be removed when new material is issued.

Purpose of a Procedure Manual

- To serve as training material
- To ensure consistency
- To help reduce variation within a given process
- To gain employee cooperation, or compliance, and provide sense of direction and urgency

ROLE OF HEAD NURSE IN CLINICAL TEACHING

In nursing it is in the hospital clinics that the students get opportunities to apply theoretical knowledge in the real life situation. Clinical teaching helps to develop the clinical competencies, professional accountability and a good attitude to wards nursing profession.

Importance

Clinical teaching is important in nursing profession because of the following results/benefits:

- Developing clinical competencies as reasoning interpersonal communication skill
- It provides clinical experience to nursing students
- It helps students to attain skills in critical thinking and problem solving ability
- It helps to develop professional value system
- Clinical teaching provides real life experience
- It provides opportunity to students to practice nursing care procedures with confidence
- Develop ability for self evaluation with confidence and improve overall performance

Some of the clinical teaching methods are nursing care study, bedside clinic, nursing care conference, nursing rounds, patient assignments etc. The head nurse can utilize different methods to improve clinical skills.

It is in the ward, the students learn relationship between symptoms and treatment, cause and effect of illness, and prevention and cure of disease. Ward teaching is the teaching program conducted in the ward by head nurses or clinical instructors. It is in the ward that student nurse best learns attitude and management skills, skills in caring, sick and worried. The clinical area provides a rich field of learning opportunities. The students experience stress and anxiety in clinical situation. The head nurse who is in-charge of the ward should recognize this fact and be patient and flexible when working with students in clinical setting. She/he should also create a safe learning environment in the clinical area for students to learn and demonstrate. The ward in-charge can organize ward teaching program by observing the following steps.

- **Planned teaching program:** Ward teaching should be planned in advance to avoid time lags and prepare sessions in advance so that it can be conducted without disturbing functions of the ward.

  Formulate goals and objective for clinical education. The head nurse with the help of clinical instructor and senior nurses formulate definite goals and objectives for clinical teaching. The content of teaching and method of teaching depends upon the student's knowledge.

  Knowledge of basic science and nursing arts is important to understand the clinical condition and nursing care of patients. So before organizing clinical teaching, the head nurse has to assess the level of knowledge and skills of students and recognize the individual differences, so that she can concentrate more to those are which are needed by students. After preparing content, she has to organize ward teaching program.

- **Organizing clinical teaching:** The head nurse is responsible to develop teaching strategies according to the level of students that encourage students to think critically in clinical situations. During the session communicate the objectives clearly to the students and create interest among them. Allow time for discussion and demonstration of clinical skills. The class room teaching should be parallel

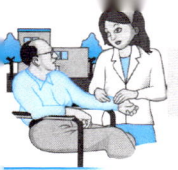

with the ward experience. The ward sister should be flexible and provide support, encouragement and direction to students to achieve goals.

The conclusion of clinical teaching is as important as introduction and provides opportunity for students to clarify their doubts and ask questions. After 'ward teaching' provide timely useful feedback to students. Encourage them to evaluate the session and keep a record of the program.

As a clinical teacher, the head nurse should be an expert in the care of patients' families and communities. She needs to keep herself updated in concepts and theories about new technologies and their use in nursing. Clinical knowledge derived from other fields of research are also applicable to the practice of nursing. She should demonstrate clinical teaching and judgement. So while planning clinical teaching the head nurse should:

- Assess the learning needs of students, recognizing and accepting individual differences
- Communicate objectives to students
- Plan and organize content of teaching by considering students objectives
- Explain and demonstrate theories, concepts and clinical skills effectively
- Provide opportunities to practice the same to get adequate clinical experience for the students
- Provide specific timely feedback and evaluation and encourage the students to evaluate their performance
- Acts as a role model to students

For effective organization of the program cooperation between head nurse and clinical instructor/nursing teacher is important. The head nurse should be knowledgeable and be able to share her knowledge to subordinates and students. She should be an effective teacher and should serve as a role model for the students.

NURSING ROUNDS

Nursing rounds are conducted by the nurse manager or the head nurse with active participation of staff nurses and nursing students in the ward. In nursing rounds, the adequacy of treatment and nursing care or services provided to a group of the patients are discussed and verified. The head nurse, staff nurses and student nurses as a team go to the bed side of each patient and discuss the patient's condition, medical care and nursing management. Through these discussions the administrator can make a judgment of the treatment received by patients and caregivers. It is good, if it is conducted at the beginning of the day. Nursing rounds are intended to teach and discuss briefly about nursing management of patients in the ward.

Before starting the nursing rounds, the head nurse has to explain the purpose of nursing rounds to the patient and make the patient feel comfortable. She introduces each patient to the group, explain patient's condition and related nursing care.

For each patient 2-3 minutes can be spent with a maximum of 30–45 minutes. The charge nurse explains briefly about patient's condition. The students or staff who are assigned to these patients can also contribute to the discussion. Patient's treatment record can also be verified. The group then discusses the nursing care aspects in brief and the head nurse concludes the discussion with necessary guidance and discussions. After discussion the nurse head concludes the discussion by giving necessary suggestions. Record all the suggestions.

During nursing rounds if situation arise the head nurse can demonstrate the procedure. Nursing rounds provides opportunity to monitor quality of nursing care service rendered by nurses. It also provides patient an opportunity to discuss their problems. Through nursing rounds, the students develop an ability to provide comprehensive nursing services to patients.

Advantages

- Nursing rounds provide opportunity to discuss nursing care in real situation.
- There is facility to learn problem based care under the guidance of experienced nurses.
- It helps to develop a positive attitude towards nursing service.
- It helps to promote team spirit.

Disadvantages

- Conducting of nursing rounds is time consuming
- When there is unexpected emergency or busy schedule, it is difficult to conduct nursing rounds

BEDSIDE CLINIC

It is an organized clinical instruction or discussion of nursing problems of patient. This is a teacher centered method for a small group of students. The usual duration is 30 minutes. Bedside clinic is a planned clinical teaching that can be conducted by ward incharge or clinical instructor. The conduct of bedside clinic should be informed to students prior enough so that they can also get prepared. Bedside clinic improves the nurse's ability to collect the information about patient, assessment of needs and problems of patients and implement nursing care appropriately. It is preferable to conduct bedside clinic at the bed side of patient or when patient is brought to clinical examination room attached with the ward itself. Head nurse or charge nurse usually co-ordinate the clinic.

Bedside clinic is an informal/formal discussion regarding patient's problems and sharing of knowledge and experience about the same or, identifying management strategies using problem solving techniques.

Purposes

- Bedside clinic provides an opportunity for understanding the condition of each patients in real life situation.

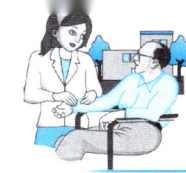

- Improve the ability of health care workers to solve patient care problems in an organized way.

The major steps in conducting bedside clinic are:

- **Preparation phase:** During this phase, the head nurse has to explain the purpose of clinic to the group. Select the patient and get consent from patient or relatives. Before patient is brought to the examination room or the group goes to the bedside, the nurse who is assigned to the patient collects the details of personal characteristics of patient's, family history, socio-economic background and past and present medical history. The students who are assigned to that patient can also contribute their observations.
- **Conduction phase:** This phase can be conducted at the bedside of the patient. During this phase, the charge nurse describes the details of the patients. The number of students can be limited to 10–15. Allow the patient verbalize his needs or problems. It is a discussion method which focuses on total care of patient, specific nursing care, observations and recorded data and their implications. During this phase explain patient's condition, signs and symptoms, past and present medical history, treatment and nursing management. Students clarify their doubts and they are allowed to interact with patients to clarify their doubts. The group can interact with the patient for further clarification about the disease aspects, needs and problems. The clinic may lasts about 20–30 minutes.
- **Conclusion phase:** After discussion the group comes to a conclusion about the management of patients and prepare the summary of the clinic.

Advantages

- Provides learning in situations where patients with different disease conditions are there.
- Enhances critical thinking and problem solving skills of staff and students
- Develops skill and confidence in providing need based nursing service. Bed side clinic provides opportunity for critical thinking and problems solving skill
- All members in group can actively participate in discussion
- It provide learning in real practical environment
- Helps to develop skill in providing care
- Enhances confidence of student nurses in giving nursing care.
- Enables to recognize practical aspects of care and the students become aware of new technologies
- Provides opportunity for students to evaluate patients

Disadvantages

- Time consuming and high personal cost
- The number of participants are limited to 10–15
- All communications should be made consciously
- It is difficult if number of students exceeds more than 20

NURSING CARE CONFERENCE

A nursing care conference is a method of clinical teaching that provide opportunity for informal discussion of problems and free exchange of ideas and experiences about the problem. It consists of a group discussion with problem solving technique. It is a meeting of a group of people to discuss a particular topic. Conference is a two way process where teaching and learning occurs simultaneously. The nursing care conference is a meeting of a group of nurses where innovative ideas are discussed and a new information is exchanged among the experts or it is a discussion of nursing care problems by a group of expert nurses and arriving at possible solutions. Conference contributes to the development of creative potential and problem solving skill. A nurse administrator or the nurse in-charge usually coordinates nursing care conference.

The main purpose of nursing care conference is to identify the common nursing care problems, to discuss problems and issues and suggest approaches or measures to solve the problems. Experts from related specialty as dietitian, occupational therapists etc can also participate in nursing care conference.

The nurse administrator in consultation with the hospital authority can plan to conduct the clinic. The venue and time should be informed to the participants. The nurse in charge with the help of subordinates collects information regarding the issue or the problem from the concerned.

The steps in conducting nursing care conference are:

- **Introduction phase:** The nurse-in-charge of the conference introduces the theme or problem of conference to the group for discussion. The task here is to make a commitment to work on a problem relating to a particular area. All members who are participating in nursing care conference should be actively involved in the discussion.
- **Working phase:** During working phase the members discuss issues, identify problems and arise suggestions, identify the solution and discuss. The members can clarify their different opinion and the possible solutions are listed down by the charge of the conference. She co-ordinates and directs discussion and record all the solutions.
- **Closing phase:** Once the members of the group decide the solution the next phase is closing phase.

Advantages

- It provides opportunity to formulate possible solutions of problems in a creative way.
- It fortifies critical thinking of staff in the conference thereby the skill of creativity and judgment can be enhanced.
- There is an opportunity for active participation of all members.
- Provide opportunity to find out solutions to the particular problems
- It provides opportunity to think.

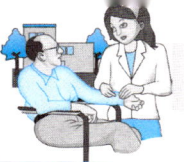

Disadvantages

- Nursing care conference is time consuming
- Arranging group participants and experts are difficult due to busy schedule of the hospital.

Nursing care conference is a formal meeting of a group of nurses to discuss the problems and issues related to nursing care and services. In nursing care conference experts from other specialty areas of care as doctors, occupational therapists etc can also be involved. Nursing care conference provide good learning experience to nurses. Student nurses can also be involved in conference which will also provide opportunity for learning.

Nursing care conference can also be organized to discuss nursing problems associated with disease conditions, identify needs and problems and nursing interventions to solve the problems. The charge nurse directs and controls the discussions and registers all suggestions or remedies. After discussions, possible solutions can be formulated and the issues/problems can be identified.

WARD MANAGEMENT ROLE OF HEAD NURSE

The head nurse or ward in-charge is responsible for management of ward and has 24 hours accountability. The head nurse should set nursing care standards etc. In accordance with organizational policies, organize resources, plan educational programs, supervise and evaluate policies of nursing care. Ward is that area of hospital or a block where patients experiencing similar conditions or receiving similar treatments are admitted, for example, medical ward, surgical ward etc. A nursing unit/ward is an area where patients with similar needs are grouped to facilitate the delivery of care by health care professionals trained in that specialty.

Objectives of Ward Management

- To provide comprehensive quality service to patients admitted in the ward
- To create a therapeutic environment for comfort of patient and staff
- To ensure optimum use of resources to provide quality patient care
- To make available adequate material resources at all time
- To protect patients from infection, accidents and occupational hazards
- Develop and implement good communication system and human relations
- To encourage utilization of ward resources to provide maximum patient care services
- To help nursing staff in achieving high degree of job satisfaction
- Develop and initiate proper evaluation and periodic monitoring system
- Encourage nurses to participate in research activities

Components of Ward Management

- **Patient care:** Patient care services include admission and orientation of patient to ward routines, assessment of needs or problems of patient, planning patient assignment, management of emergency, ward teaching, appraisal of nursing service, supervision and evaluation of nursing care services etc. She is accountable for excellence in clinical practice and delivery of patient care. She has to plan and implement strategies and programs consistent with organizational policies, goals, objectives.
- **Admission and orientation:** Formulate ward policies and ward routine for admission of patient, introduce rules and regulations, and see whether they are provided with comfortable patient care area.
- **Assessment of needs and problems:** Ensure that need based/priority based nursing services are provided to each and every patient after assessment and planning. Ensure quality nursing care to patients with proper documentation.
- **Patient assignment:** According to area of service and hospital policy different methods of patient assignment can be ensured. For that she should provide orientation to new staff, Orientation of job description, their duties and responsibilities etc.
- **Planning time:** In order to provide 24 hour patient care services, time schedules and ward routines are to be prepared. Ensure good working relationship between professionals and non professionals working in the ward, ward round and clinical teaching. Regularly conduct ward rounds and bedside clinics to equip nurses with updated knowledge about assigned patients for providing better nursing services.
- **Maintenance of records and registers:** As records are important legal documents, ensure that all records and registers are properly maintained.
- **Supervision and appraisal of nursing service:** Being supervisor or manager of ward, the head nurse should conduct regular evaluation or appraisal of nursing care services rendered by staff.

Personal Management

For proper management of human resources, the head has to observe the following:

- Orientation to newly appointed staff
- Establishment of good interpersonal relations
- Supervision and evaluation of staff working in ward
- Conduct regular staff development program and nursing care conferences
- Implement hospital policies and ensure safety and welfare of nursing staff
- Conduct staff meeting regularly
- Do performance appraisal of staff working in the unit and provide necessary guidance

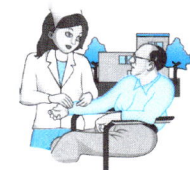

Management of Unit Environment or Maintenance of a Therapeutic Environment

The head nurse is responsible for maintaining a safe and caring environment that promotes effective care to patients and provide comfortable area for staffs to function effectively in order to maintain optimum environment for patients and family members. The head nurse has to observe the following points:

- Provisions of adequate lighting—natural or artificial.
- Maintaining adequate temperature and humidity (40-60) that promotes normal body function.
- Prevent unnecessary noise to prevent irritability and fatigue.
- Provision of safe water supply and adequate facilities for biomedical waste management etc.

The ward in charge should consider factors to prevent hazards and injury. The head nurse should make sure that safety precautions are there to prevent patient's injury from fall. Keep furniture and equipment in good working conditions, prevent injury from chemicals and keep environment free from chemicals dust and insects etc.

Management of Equipment and Supplies

Material management is one of the important responsibilities of ward in charge to provide adequate supply in right quality and quantity for patient care. There should be provision for proper supplies and equipment for effective functioning of ward. All equipment and materials should be conveniently arranged with good inventory control. There should be adequate facilities for storage of articles. The registers and records should be maintained properly.

ACCOUNTABILITY

Accountability is a legal obligation and in health care it is also an ethical and moral responsibility.

Accountability and responsibility are two important parts of delegation. Nursing is a strong and respected professional group which has significant influence in health care. Nurses are not only caring, compassionate, competent practitioners, they have concern for their profession, patients and the health care system head.

Accountability is defined as, "being responsible and answerable for actions or inactions of self or others in the context of delegation" (**National Council of State Boards of Nursing, Resources section**). This refers to the nurse's legal liability for her actions and patient outcomes

Accountability refers to (individual) answerability for ones own actions. Accountability refers to individual being
A nurse is answerable to:

- Herself/himself
- The client
- The profession
- The employing institution such as a hospital and society for the effectiveness of nursing and care performed.

Professional accountability means that the nurses are directly responsible to their patients for the quality of care they provide. It involves follow up and a reflective analysis of ones decision to evaluate their effectiveness.

Purpose of Professional Accountability

Accountability calls for an evaluation of nurse's effectiveness in practice
It serves the following purposes

- To evaluate
- Non professional practices and reassess existing ones
- To maintain standards of health care
- To facilitate personal reflection, ethical thought and personal growth on the part of the health care professional
- To provide a basis for ethical decision making.

The nurse balances accountability towards the client, the profession, the employer and the society. To remain accountable to society, nursing professionals agree to evaluate practices and to take action to preserve nursing excellence. The joint commission on accreditation of healthcare organization (JACHO), A national accreditation association, recommends standards for the delivery of the nursing care. The following activities serve to support standards of the JACHO, 2002 and ANA in the nursing profession as follows.

- Evaluation of new professional practices and reassessment of existing ones
- Maintaining of standards of health care
- Facilitation of personal reflection, ethical thoughts and personal growth
- Provision of a basis for ethical decision making

QUALITY ASSURANCE

Quality assurance refers to a program for the systematic monitoring and evaluation of the various aspects of a project, service, or facility to ensure that standards of quality are being met.
Quality refers to all those features of a product (service) that are required by the customer —*ISO*

In health scenario, quality is **proper performance** of interventions that are safe, affordable to the society, and have an ability to produce an impact on morbidity, mortality and disability.

"Refers to a system for monitoring outcomes of professional interventions and departmental activities which are compared with established standards to evaluate and document appropriateness and effectiveness of practices"

WHO defined QA, as making sure that the services provided by the hospital are the best possible in given existing resources and current medical knowledge.

The Institute of Medicine (IOM) defines quality as the degree to which health services for individuals and populations increase the likelihood of desired health outcomes and are consistent with current professional knowledge and the three elements of quality assurance are structure, process and outcome.

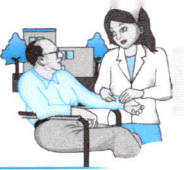

Quality defined as the degree to which the patient care services increases the probability of defined outcomes and reduce the probability of undesired outcome given in the current state of knowledge.

—*Joint Commission for Accreditation of Health care organization*

Quality Assurance in Health Care

Quality assurance is the monitoring of the activities of client care to determine the degree of excellence attained to the implementation of the activities. (**Bull, 1985**)

In essence, quality assurance is which set of activities that are carried out to set standards and to monitor and improve performance so that the care provided is as effective and as safe as possible.

Contributors in the Field of Quality

Dr. W A Shewhart: American physicist, engineer and statistician, emphasized the Statistical Process Control (SPC).

Shewhart Cycle _ PDSA Cycle showed a new approach to Quality Management.

Juran's Trilogy defines three management principles for improvement of quality – quality control, quality improvement, quality planning. He was an American engineer, known as "Quality Guru" He was one of the 'Big Four' (Deming/Juran/Crosby/Ishikawa) contributed to the body of knowledge
—*TQM*

Dr. Avedis Donebedian introduced the three measures - structure, process and outcome and emphasized the importance of considering these measures when monitoring and assessing the quality of care.

Bill Smith introduced Six Sigma methodology in quality management. six sigma aimed at reduction of variation to the level Six SD.

Edward Deming introduced the concept of Total Quality Management(TQM). He is known as Father of TQM. He proposed 14 quality principles. It is also know as

Deming 's Wheel – PDSA Cycle or plan –do– study –act.

Florence Nightingale introduced the concept of quality in nursing care in 1855 while attending the soldiers in the hospital during the Crimean war. Nightingale wrote notes on Nursing, which was published in 1860 that served as the cornerstone of the curriculum at the Nightingale School and was established in other nursing schools established.

> In 1947, **ISO** (International Organization for Standardization) came into existence
> ISO 9001: 2008
> ISO 9001:2015
> In 1952, joint commission on Accreditation of Hospitals (JCAH) was formed, which published the first accreditation/standards for hospitals.
> In 2006 NABH was established.
> In 2013, Govt. of India introduced National Quality Assurance Standards for Public Health Institutions

Objectives of Quality Assurance

- To maintain an ongoing process of quality nursing care
- To integrate reviews and evaluations of patient care
- To establish priorities to solve problems
- To improve cost-effectiveness by using resources more effectively
- To provide technical assistance in designing and implementing effective strategies for monitoring quality and correcting systemic deficiencies.
- To refine existing methods for ensuring optimal quality health care through an applied research program (**Decker, 1985 and Schroeder, 1984**).

Objectives of quality assurance according to Jonas (2000) are:
- To ensure delivery of quality client care
- To demonstrate the efforts of health care providers
- To provide the best possible care
- Evaluate achievements of nursing care.

Key questions for QA in a health care setting
- How many patients do providers expect to see per hour?
- What laboratory services are available to patients, and how accurate, efficient, and reliable are they?
- What referral systems are in place when specialty services or higher technologies are needed?
- Do patients receive care as per the standards of medical/nursing profession?
- Are the physical working conditions adequate and sanitary, ensuring the privacy of patients and professional environment?
- Does the pharmacy has a reliable supply of all the needed medicines?
- Are there opportunities for continuing medical/nursing education?

Quality Assurance Vs Quality Control

Quality control (QC) emphasizes testing of products to uncover defects, and reporting to management who make the decision to allow or deny the release whereas **quality assurance (QA)** attempts to improve and stabilize production, and associated processes, to avoid, or at least minimize issues that led to the defects in the first place.

Quality assurance in nursing

Quality assurance is a dynamic process through which nurses in both academic and clinical practice assume accountability for quality of care they provide

George, Veigas and Isaac, 1984.

Quality assurance is the defining of nursing practice through well written nursing standards and the use of those standards as a basis for evaluation on improvement of client care **Maker 1998.**

Why is quality assurance in nursing education a necessity?

QA has been reported to assist nurse educators to define educational and clinical guidelines and standards, operating procedures as well as take tangible steps towards improving

program. QA promotes confidence, improves communication and fosters a clearer understanding of educational and practice needs and expectations (cost effective).
(Peterson, Kovel- Jarboe and Schwartz, 1997).
- QA provides the tools to the nurse educational institutes
- QA is found to assist the nurses' satisfaction and motivation (Quinn, 2001).
- QA can also be seen as a logical approach for conveying the importance of excellence to individuals who are nursing care recipients.

Quality Assurance Cycle

In practice, QA is a cyclic process that must be applied flexibly to meet the needs of a specific program (Fig. 8).

1. **Planning for quality assurance:** This phase prepares an organization to carry out QA activities. Planning begins with a review of the organization's scope of care to determine which services should be addressed. For most organizations, it is impossible to improve the quality in all areas at once. Instead, QA activities are initiated in a few critical areas. Once the organizational leaders have decided where the QA effort will begin, they must select a quality improvement approach. The organization can then determine QA priorities based on the program mission and vision.

2. **Setting standards and specifications:** To provide consistency, high quality services, an organization must translate its programmatic goals and objectives into operational procedures. In its widest sense, a standard is a statement of the quality that is expected. Performance standards are specific deliveries and the activities that support it.

Guidelines, standard operating procedures, and performance standards should be developed for both clinical and management areas. Program staff should periodically review guidelines and standard procedures. Health workers at all the levels should participate in developing guidelines and setting standards because health workers often understand local conditions better than high level managers, the resulting guidelines are more likely to be appropriate and effective. Also staff participation will generate commitment to quality because health workers are more likely to implement and support an effort that they has helped to develop. Finally, staff members are more likely to accept QA activities if they have been involved in defining quality. Their standards will become the measures for judging the quality of their services.

3. **Communicating guidelines and standards:** Once practice guidelines, standard operating procedures, and performance standards have been defined, it is essential that staff members communicate and promote their use. This will ensure that each health worker, supervisor, manager and support person understands what is expected of him or her. Managers and the health center team share a mutual responsibility for quality. The notion of this partnership should be communicated along with the guidelines and standards.

4. **Monitoring quality:** Monitoring is a routine collection and review of data that helps to assess whether program norms are being followed or whether outcomes are improved. By monitoring the key indicators, managers and supervisors can determine whether the services delivered follow the prescribed practices to achieve desired results. The monitoring system is central to QA program. It is necessary to choose an indicator for every standard or specification.

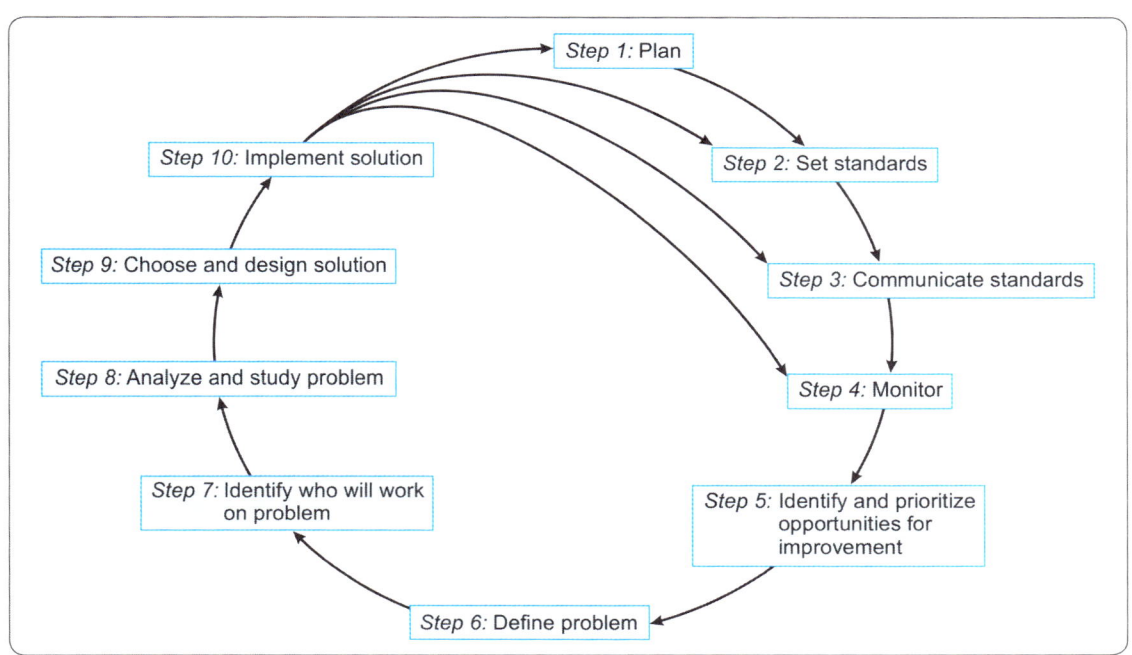

Figure 8: Quality assurance cycle

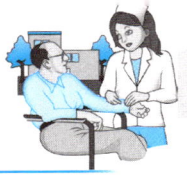

5. **Identifying problem and selecting opportunities for improvement:** Program managers can identify quality improvement opportunities by monitoring and evaluating the activities. Once a health facility team has identified several problems, it should set quality improvement priorities by choosing one or two problem area on which to focus. Selection criteria will vary from program to program.
6. **Defining the problem:** Having selected a problem, the team must define it operationally as there may be a gap between the actual performance and the performance prescribed by guidelines and standard. The problem statement should identify the problem and how it manifests itself. It should clearly state where the problems begins and ends, and how to recognize when the problem is solved.
7. **Choosing a team:** Once the health facility staff has employed a participatory approach to selecting and defining a problem, it should assign a small team to address the specific problem. The team will analyze the problem, develop a quality improvement plan, implement and evaluate the quality improvement effort.
8. **Analyzing and studying the problem to identify the root cause:** Achieving a meaningful and sustainable quality improvement efforts depends upon understanding the problem and its root cause. Given the complexity of health services delivery, clearly identifying root cause requires systematic in depth analysis. Analysis tool such as system modeling, flow charting, and cause-and-effect diagrams can be used to analyze a process or problem.
9. **Developing solutions and actions for quality improvement:** The problem solving team should now be ready to develop and evaluate the potential solutions. Unless the procedure in questions is the sole responsibility of an individual, developing solutions should be a team effort. It may be necessary to involve personnel responsible for processes related to root cause.
10. **Implementing and evaluating quality improvement efforts:** Implementing quality improvement requires careful planning. The team must determine the necessary resources and time frame and decide who will be responsible for implementation. In-depth monitoring should begin when the quality improvement plan is implemented.

Team should modify the solutions as needed and should fully document results and lesson learned. Once the solution has proved to be effective, program managers should codify and disseminate the new process so that others can learn from the experience. The QA team should also make plans to identify a new problem, either through data generated by an existing monitoring system or the team may repeat the quality improvement cycle.

Approaches for a Quality Assurance Program

General Approach

It involves large governing of official body's evaluation of a person's or agency's ability to meet established criteria or standards at a given time.

- Credentialing
- Licensure
- Accreditation
- Certification

Credentialing

It is generally defined as the formal recognition of professional or technical competence and attainment of minimum standards by a person or agency. According to Hinsvark (1981) credentialing process has four functional components
- To produce a quality product
- To confer a unique identity
- To protect provider and public
- To control the profession.

Licensure

Individual licensure is a contract between the profession and the state, in which the profession is granted control over entry into and exists from the profession and over quality of professional practice.

The licensing process requires that regulations be written to define the scopes and limits of the professional's practice.

Licensure of nurses has been mandated by law since 1903.

Accreditation

Accreditation and/or Certification is the process of requesting an independent review of an organization's performance against national quality and safety requirements.

In the part the accreditation process primarily evaluated on agency's physical structure, organizational structure and personal qualification.

Certification

Certification is usually a voluntary process with in the profession. A person's educational achievements, experience and performance on examination are used to determine the person's qualifications for functioning in an identified specialty area.

Specific Approaches

Quality assurances are methods used to evaluate identified instances of providers and client interaction.
- *Peer review*
- *Audit*
- *Utilization review*
- *Evaluation studies*
- *Client's satisfaction*
- *Incident review*
- *Standard as a device for quality assurance*
- *Audit as a tool for quality assurance*

Peer Review

To maintain high standards, peer review has been initiated to carefully review the quality of practice demonstrated by members of a professional group.

- One centers on the recipients of health services by means of auditing the quality of services rendered.
- The other centers on the health professional by evaluating the quality of individual performance.

Standard as a device for quality assurance

Standard is a pre-determined baseline condition or level of excellence that comprises a model to be followed and practiced. The ANA standard for practice include

Standard 1: The collection of data about health status of the patient is systematic and continuous. The data are accessible, communicative, and recorded.
Standard 2: Nursing diagnosis are derived from health status data.
Standard 3: The plan of nursing care includes goals derived from the nursing diagnoses.
Standard 4: The plan of nursing care includes priorities and the prescribed nursing approaches or measures to achieve the goals derived from the nursing diagnoses.
Standard 5: Nursing actions provide for patient participation in health promotion, maintenance, and restoration.
Standard 6: Nursing actions assist the patient to maximize his health capabilities.
Standard 7: The patient's progress or lack of progress towards goal achievement is determined by the patient and the nurse.
Standard 8: The patient's progress or lack of progress towards goal achievement directs re-assessment, re-ordering of priorities, new goal setting, and a revision of the plan of nursing care.

Audit as a tool for quality assurance

A good QMS will not function or improve without adequate audits and reviews.

Audits are carried out to insure that actual methods are adhering to the documented procedures, whilst system reviews should be carried out periodically and systematically.

An audit is a systemic and official examination of a record, process or account to evaluate performance

Auditing in health care organization provide managers with a means of applying control process to determine the quality of service rendered

Clinical audit is a process that has been defined as "a quality improvement process that seeks to improve patient care and outcomes through systematic review of care against explicit criteria and the implementation of change.

Types of clinical audit

Retrospective audit

Conducted after patient discharge or deaths. Post care questionnaire and patient interviews, patient charts and care plans can be used.

Concurrent/ Prospective audit

Evaluates as the care is being administered and includes:
- Observation of staff
- Inspection of patients
- Open chart auditing
- Staff and patient interviews
- Group conferences (patients, families, staff)

Method to develop criteria of audit tool

- Define patient population and the problem to be audited.
- Identify a time framework for measuring outcomes of care.
- Identify commonly recurring nursing problems presented by the defined patient population.
- State patient outcome criteria.
- State acceptable degree of goal achievement,
- Specify the source of information.
- Design and type of tool

Nursing Audit Vs Performance Appraisal

Nursing audit

- Effects of care on patient.
- Purpose is to maintain and promote quality care (Administrative job)
- Evaluated through Research methodology.

Performance appraisal

- Focus on performance of the nurses
- Purpose is educational, growth and development of staff (managerial job)
- Evaluated based on job description or set performances.

Quality Assurance Model

Purpose of Quality Assurance Model in Nursing

To ensure quality nursing care provided by nurses in order to meet the expectations of receiver, management and Regulatory Body. It also intends to increase the commitment of provider and the management.

- It lays the standards for quality in nursing education and nursing care.
- INC believes that nurse will
- Do good for person/ receiver of care, do no harm, maintain respect for life and human dignity, believe in justice and fairness to individuals in terms of access to resources and case, and protect the vulnerable
- Have moral obligation to provide services as per the prescribed norms of the regulatory body/organization/ institution
- Be responsible and accountable for providing quality care in line with set standards
- Be committed to understand of the dynamic nature of her/ his role in interdisciplinary health team
- Be obliged to create public awareness and consider social expectation before making decisions for providing nursing care
- Be obliged to include receiver in making choices in planning and implementation of care

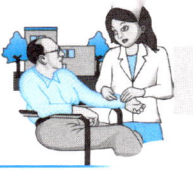

- Work in conjunction with legislation, accreditation and political system
- Have obligation to promote education of self and others
- Be committed to advancement of the profession

Goals of Quality Assurance Model

- Develop confidence of the receiver(s) that quality care is being rendered as per assurance
- Develop commitment of the management towards quality care
- Increase commitment of providers to adhere to set standards for nursing practice and strive for excellence
- Strengthen documentation of nursing care
- Promote optimum utilization of resources in providing cost-effective nursing care

Deming Model (PDCA)

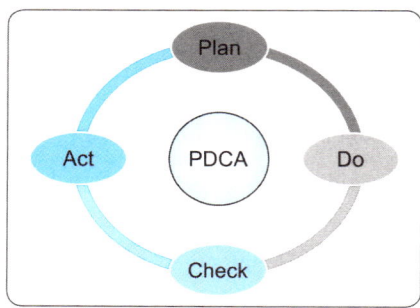

Plan – establish objectives and process need to deliver desired results.

Do – implement the process developed.

Check - monitor and evaluate the implemented process by testing the results.

Act – apply action necessary for improvement.

PDCA analyze the existing conditions and methods for improvement.

PDCA is repeated through out the life time of the product or the service

Donabedian Model (Dr. Donabedian)

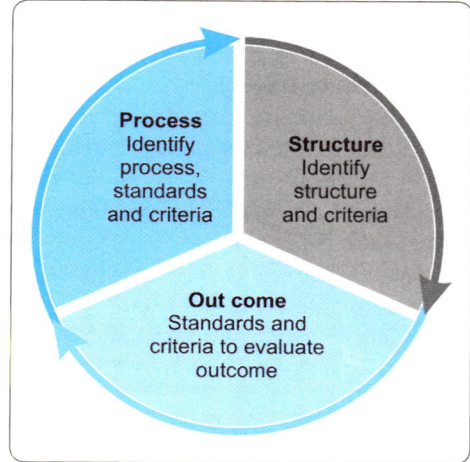

Structure–physical, organizational and other characteristics of system.

Process–Action and behaviors required in nursing care and interaction between nurse and patient. This include assessment, care plans, technical performance, documentation.

Out come–Relate to the recipients of nursing care.

ANA Quality Assurance Model (Dr. Norma Lang)

- identify values.
- identify standard and criteria.
  Evaluation and .8 documentation
- secure measurement.
  Implementation .7
- make interpretation.
  Select appropriate action.6
- identify possible actions

Six Sigma

It refers to six standard deviations from the mean and is generally used in quality improvement to define the number of acceptable defects or errors produced by a process. By achieving six sigma, failure rate is minimized to 3.4 defects per million opportunities (99.9996% success rate). Motorola company adopted Six sigma model.

5 steps (DMAIC)

Define, Measure, Analyze, Improve, Control

In health care six sigma is used to develop a system of care that provide quality care to all clients to all times. This technique was first used by Motorola Company to improve quality of their products.

Six sigma refers to six standard deviation from the mean and is generally used in quality improvement to define the member of acceptable defects or errors produced by a process. In Six sigma curve, there is a mean in the center of the highest point of the curve. From the mean the curve slops down on both sides and is divided in to standard deviations and is designated by σ(sigma) and is given a number, that is plus one σ, minus one σ. Six σ deviation from the mean is considered a total lack of error, statistically 3.4 defects per million opportunities (99.9996% success rate). To Implement six sigma, the staff/employee need to be given special training. Trained staff are designated as Black belts, who serve as consultants for hospitals.

Principles of six sigma

- Training is needed from top to the bottom to improve efforts
- Include the preference and needs of customers
- Create an infrastructure that integrate six sigma method
- Formulate short-term projects with specific goals
- Process improvement should be maintained by ongoing six sigma quality control
- Six sigma needs a clean and consistent methodology
- Focus on people and process.

Six Sigma uses a process similar to the PDCA cycle and the process include plan, measure, analyse, improve and control

Lean Methodology

Lean methodology is used to accelerate the velocity and reduce cost of any process by removing any type of activity that absorbs resources and yet creates no value. Toyota Production systems adopted Lean methodology.

Quality defined as the degree to which the patient care services increases the probability of defined out comes and reduce the probability of undesired outcome given in the current state of knowledge.

—*Joint Commission for Accreditation of Health care organization*

10 step Quality assurance process of Joint commission

- Assign responsibilities
- Delineate scope of care/ Service
- Prioritize aspects of care or service as high volume, high risk, problem solving.
- Establish indicators for identified project
- Establish threshold for evaluation based on customer expectations.
- Collect and analyse data
- Evaluate effectiveness of action and document level of improvement.
- Determine and implement appropriate actions
- Communicate result
- Continues monitoring/Improving on the process.

Basic Quality Tools for QA/TQM

- Flow chart
- Fish bone diagram
- Pareto chart
- Bar chart
- Control chart
- Histogram
- Scatter diagram

Basic Quality tools for Quality Improvement / Total Quality Management

In quality management we can use different tools to analyze problems during implementation and to improve performance

- Flow chart – Flow chart is a graphic representation of sequence or events. It gives a visual view of all steps in the process of CQI and how each step is related to the other. It shows the way to complete a process or attain objectives and also help to identity where errors are likely to be found in the process.

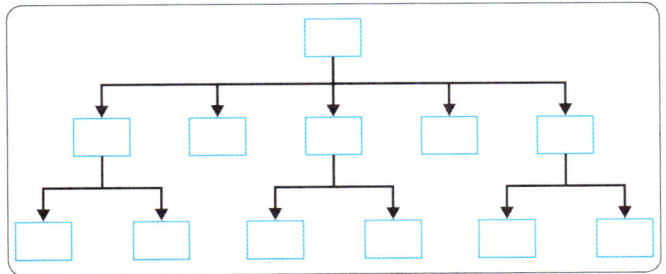

- **Pareto charts:** Pareto chart can be used to identify the factors that have more cumulative effect on the system and so we can screen out less significant factors on analysis. Pareto chart can be formulated by plotting the cumulative frequencies or relative frequency data in descending order. It also help QA team to identify quality problems based on degree of importance and to decide where improvement may be started.

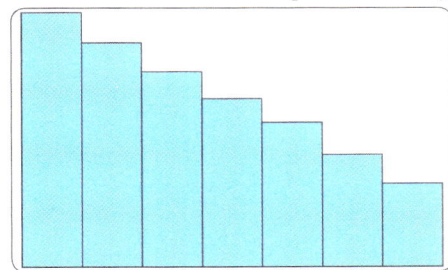

Pareto chart

- **Scatter diagram:** Scatter diagram help to show the relationship between occurance, situations or actions, to find out variables and how they affect out comes.

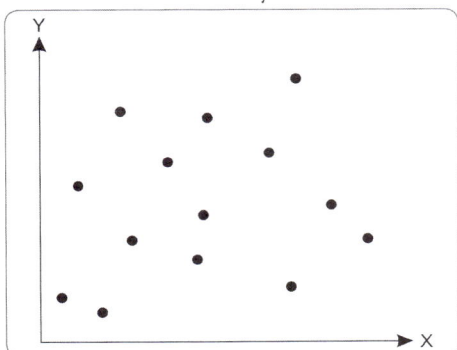

Scatter diagram

- **Control chart:** Control chart give an idea of expected range of variation from selected task. The control chart is marked by upper and lower control limits, which are calculated by statistical formulas to data from the process. Pints which fall outside shows variation due to some causes and that can be eliminated. It helps to identify the causes that change the process.

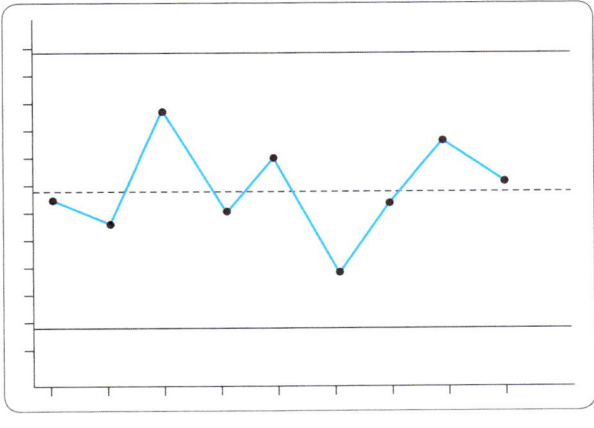

Control Chart

- **Histogram:** Histogram is simple graphical representation of accumulated data with its dispersion and central tendency. Histogram helps to evaluate distribution of events.

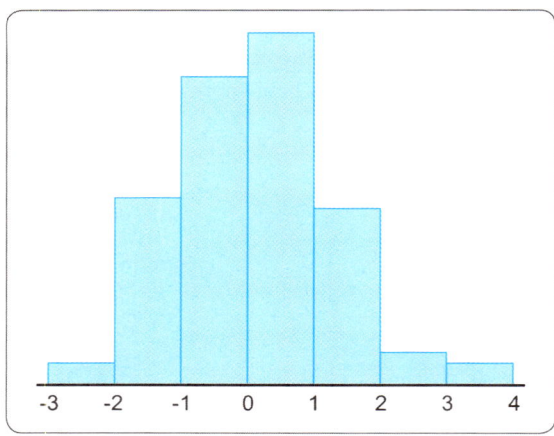

Histogram

- **Ishikawa/ fish bone diagram:** Fishbone diagram is also termed as cause effect diagram. It is used to associate multiple possible causes with a single effect. The primary branch represent effect and the branches represents the causes that directly relates to the effects.

CONTINUOUS QUALITY IMPROVEMENT

Continuous quality improvement (CQI) is an integral part of quality healthcare. Quality is the result of high intention, intelligent direction and sincere execution of services.

CQI referred to as total quality and its based on the philosophy that encourages all members of the facility to identify better ways to do their work. CQI requires the co-operation of all staff in different Departments. The ongoing QI activities saves time. CQI process include identifying goals, formulation of objectives to establish policies, procedures and protocols and proper execution of activities. For effective CQI, support, commitment and involvement of staff and management are required.

CQI Process – Focus – PDCA model

F – Find out or identify process to be improved

O – Organize CQI team, that knows the process at hand and for that select staff members

C – The team members meet and assess the process and clarification of knowledge

u – Understand sources of variation

S – Select the improvement

P – Plan the improvement

C – Check and study result

A – Take steps to sustain any gain from improvement and continue improvement

TOTAL QUALITY MANAGEMENT

The concept of total quality management (TQM) was first introduced by Deming defined quality as a predictable degree of uniformity and dependability at low cost and suited to the market.　　　　　　　　　　　　　—*W. Edward Deming.*

TQM is a management approach in an organization, centered on quality based participation of all its members and aiming at long-term success through customers satisfaction. Total Quality Management is a management approach of an organization which is centered on quality based participation of all members of an organization and society.　—*ISO*

TQM is a systematic approach to the practice of management requiring changes in an organizational process, strategic priorities, individual beliefs, individual attitude and individual behavior.　　—*Oakland 1990*

TQM is the application of a number of activities and the important elements of TQM are:

- Customer driven quality
- Top management leadership
- Commitment
- Continuous improvement
- Fast response
- Action based on facts
- Employee participation
- TQM culture　　　　　—*Moghaddan and Moballeghi (2007)*

TQM is a management approach in an organization centered on quality based participation of all workers.

Elements of TQM

- TQM is customer focused which will bring satisfaction to clients
- TQM adopts the philosophy of continuous improvement which is an important element and it should start from top management. For that set realistic goals, provide resources, offer employee tool, opportunities and encouragement to employees.
- In quality process commitment and attitude of work force is an important element
- Encourage active participation of employees
- Develop leadership at top level management
- Education and training as the real work force
- Good communication networking
- Mutual respect and team work

TQM promotes innovation in an organization and it also motivates workers for better quality. It is a management approach in an organization centered on quality, based on participation of all workers.

Principles of TQM by Deming

- Create a constancy of purpose for improvement of service
- Adopt a philosophy of continual improvement

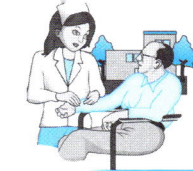

- Focus in improving process
- End the practice of awarding service on price alone
- Constantly improve every process of quality management
- Institute job training and retraining
- Develop leadership in the organization
- Encourage employees to participate actively in the process
- Foster inter departmental cooperation
- Eliminate target for the work force
- Focus on quality and not quantity
- Promote team work
- Educate and train employees to maximise personal development
- Charge all employees for carrying out the TQM package

Benefits of TQM

- Satisfaction for patients and relatives
- Improved job
- Less staff conflicts
- Continuous improvement of organization
- Increased organizational outcome and image
- Improvement in employee morale
- Good team work and work culture
- Motivated employees
- Good communication among employees and good relationship with patients and relatives

Barriers to TQM

- Lack of policy and administrative manuals
- Lack of motivation among employees
- Lack of proper leadership
- Deficient work culture dynamism
- Lack of adequate resources
- Poor evaluation system
- Lack of good hospital management system
- Lack of incident review procedures

Nurse Manager in Implementation of Quality Improvement in Health Care

The nurse managers have a unique role in implementation of TQM process. Implementation of quality management program is a commitment of top management. The responsibilities of nurse manager include formulation of quality management team and the team is further responsible for coordinating, facilitating and implementing all the activities.

Quality policy and manual is important document of quality management system which provides an overview of implementation. It includes general information about organization's top level management, departments and also patients' rights and infection control practices etc. The role of a nurse manager are as follows:

- Encourage all staff to involve actively in quality control process.
- Communicate goals and outcome to all staff
- Act as a role model for subordinates
- Actively involves in research activities related to quality assurance
- Organize continuing education programs
- Create a work culture. Support and actively participate in activities of QA process
- Develops a system for continuous monitoring of nursing service
- Develops QA tool and criteria for evaluation, teaching and training the nurses to use tool.
- Observe nursing care services and review nurses documentation.
- Participate in team activities
- Continuous evaluation of program is essential, for periodic and continuous appraisal of nursing care. Use findings to determine area for staff education
- Actively participate in implementation of program
- Regularly evaluate quality management system being implemented. Identify defects and its causes.

PATIENT RECORD SYSTEM/ DOCUMENTATION

Records and reports are effective sources of communication. Effective communication among health professional is vital to the quality of patient care.

A record is a valuable source of data that is used by all members of health care team. Patient record or chart are confidential, and these are permanent legal documentation of information relevant to the client health care. Clinical record is a formal legal document that provides evidence of patient care. Although health care organization uses different systems and forms for documentation, where all records have similar information.

Reports are oral, written or audio typed exchange of information between caregivers. All records basically contain the following informations.

DOCUMENTATION

Documentation is one of the important responsibilities of nurses which aim at facilitating communication and decision making. The different documentation system available are:

- Source oriented records
- Problem oriented medical records (POMR)
- Problem implementation evaluation
- Computerized documentation

Source-Oriented Records

Source oriented records are traditional patient records. In this type of recording each member in the health team who provides care to patients make recordings in each sections

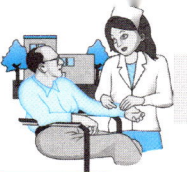

of patient record. For example, nurses write nursing care in nurse's records, doctors enter physician order in doctors order sheet.

Problem Oriented Medical Records

In POMR, the data are documented according to the problems of the patient. Each member of the health team who carries the patient as nurses, doctors etc,, contribute to the problems list and plan of care.

POMR has four basic components, they are:
- Database
- Complete problem list
- Plans of care
- Daily progress note and discharge summary

1. **Database:** Database consist of all the information about patients at the time of admission as findings of physical assessment, past medical history, socio–economic status, basic laboratory data etc. The data are updated constantly as and when these are important in patient's status.

2. **Problem list:** In problem list problems of patients are listed according to priority. All members who cares the patient as nurses, physician, nursing assistance etc must contribute the problem list. As far as nurses are concerned they must lists down problems of patients and related nursing diagnosis. For example, incontinence – urinary urgency related to immobility.

3. **Plan of care:** Most commonly health care professionals use the format SOAP for preparing the progress notes. SOAP – stand for subjective data, objective data, Assess and planning

   S– In subjective data, information obtained from patient's are written as what he says. Nurses can use patients words as such or they can be summarized later.

   O– Objective data: In objective data nurses may use informations that is measured or observed by the use of senses. For example, respiratory rate

   A– Assessment: Assessment is interpretation drawn from subjective and objective data. It is a brief paragraph describing what nurses think about the particular problem. It is a statement that describes severity of problem that has worsened condition which leads to admission of patients in a hospital.

   P– Plan: Plan is the plan of action that are going to be implemented to reduce the stated problems.

   Nowadays, SOAP format is modified to another format SOAPIER – by including I – Interventions, E – Evaluation and R – Revision or modification suggested by evaluation.

4. **Daily progress note and discharge summary:** In daily progress note the health care professionals who are involved in providing care, update the condition and progress of patient care and making summary of discharge.

Advantages of POMR
- POMR helps to organize information regarding patient care.
- It is found to be effective in providing nursing care
- There is consistency in documentation i.e. concise, complete and accurate record keeping.

Disadvantages
- Time consuming
- Training for health professionals are necessary for proper implementation
- It is found to be difficult to implement it in rapid turnover areas
- It results in lengthy progress notes.

Problems, Intervention, Evaluation (PIE)

PIE system was originally used in Crave Country Hospital in North Carolina in 1985. PIE stands for problems, intervention, evaluation. PIE is organized based on patient's problems and his informations. PIE is composed of 3 stages. In the first stage, problems of the patients are written in the nursing diagnosis form. In the second stage, nursing diagnosis is written. Finally patient's reaction to treatment is documented.

In PIE system a complete assessment and documentation is done at the beginning of each shift and is documented. Resolved problem are removed from daily documentation and continuing problems are documented and numbered each day.

Advantages
- PIE system ensure that record contains nursing diagnosis, intervention and evaluation i.e. there is proper application of nursing process.
- Saves times as there is no separate plan of ease.
- It promotes continuity of care
- Academic and practical dynamism for nursing students.

Computerized Documentation Electronic Medical Records

Charting by Exception (CBE)
CBE uses,
- Flow sheets – Flow sheets include graphic records of vital signs, fluid balance record etc.
- Standards of nursing care – CBE must develop its own standard of nursing practice, which identify the criteria for patient care. Recording as per standards of care involves check mark in the standard care format .

Computerized clinical record systems are being developed as a way to manage the huge volume of information required in contemporary health care. Nurses use computers to store the client's data base, add new data, create and revise care plan and document client progress.

Multiple flow sheets are not needed in computerized record system because information can be easily retrieved

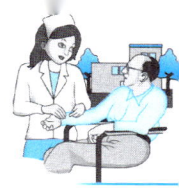

in a variety of formats. For example the nurse can obtain the results of a client's blood test, a suggested list of interventions for a nursing diagnosis, a graphic chart of client's vital signs. Many systems can generate a work list for the shift with a list of all treatments, procedures, and medications needed by the client.

Computers make care planning and documentation relatively easy. To record nurses action and client's response, the nurses either chose from a standardized list of terms or types narrative information into the computer. Automated speech recognition technology now allows nurses to enter data by voice for conversion to written document.

Pros and cons of Computer Documentation

Pros

- Computer records can facilitate a focus on client outcomes.
- Bedside terminals can synthesize information from monitoring equipment.
- Allows nurses to use their time efficiently.
- The system links various sources of client information.
- Client information, requests and results are sent and received quickly.
- Links to monitors improves accuracy of documentation.
- Information is legible
- The system incorporates and reinforces standards of care
- Standard terminology improves communication

Cons

- Client's privacy may be infringed on if security measures are not used.
- Breakdowns make information temporarily unavailable
- System is expensive.
- Extended training periods may be required when a new or updated system is installed.

Case Management

The case management model can incorporates a multidisciplinary approach to documenting client care. In many organizations the standardized plan of care is summarized into critical pathways for a specific disease or condition. The critical pathways are multidisciplinary care plans that include client problems, key interventions, and expected outcomes within an established time frame. The use of computerized charting system allows for the integration of chart by many disciplines. The nurse and other team members such as physicians, dieticians, social workers, physical therapist, and respiratory therapists use the same critical pathways to monitor the client progress during each shift or in the case of home care, every visit.

Along with critical pathways the case management model incorporates the graphic and flow sheets. Progress notes typically use some type of charting by exception. For example if goals are not met, no further charting is required. A goal that is not met is called a variance. Variations are deviations to what is planned on the critical pathway - unexpected occurrences that affect the planned care or the client's response to care. When a variance occurs, the nurse writes a note documenting the unexpected event, the cause, and actions taken.

Documenting Nursing Activities

Admission Nursing Assessment

A comprehensive admission assessment, also referred to as an initial data base, nursing history, or nursing assessment, is completed when the client is admitted to the nursing unit. The nurse generally records ongoing assessments or reassessments on flow sheets or nursing progress sheets.

Nursing Care Plans

Joint Commission on Accreditation of Healthcare Organizations (JCAHO) requires that the clinical record include evidence of client assessments, nursing diagnosis and/or client needs, nursing interventions, client outcomes and evidence of a current nursing care plan. Depending on the record system being used, the nursing care plan may be separate from the client's chart, recorded in progress notes and other forms in the client record or incorporated into multidisciplinary plan of care.

Kardexes

The kardex is a widely used, concise method of organizing and recording data about a client, making information quickly accessible to all health professionals. The system consists of a series of cards kept in a portable index file or on a computer generated forms. The information on kardexes may be organized into sections. e.g.

- Pertinent information about the client, such as name, room, age, religion, marital status, admission date, diagnosis, etc
- List of medications with the date of order and time of administration of each.
- List of IV fluids with the date of infusion
- List of daily treatment and procedures ordered such as X-ray or lab results
- Problem list, goals, and list of approaches to meet the goal and relieve the problems.
- Whether kardex is a written paper or computerized, it is important to have a place on it to record date and initials of the person reviewing or revising it. It is a quick visual guide to ensure that the information is current and updated on a regular basis.

Flow Sheets

A flow sheet enables nurses to record nursing data quickly and concisely and provides an easy to read record of the client's condition over time. Flow sheet includes graphic records of vital signs, fluid balance records etc

- **Graphic record:** This record typically indicates body temperature, pulse, respiration rate, blood pressure, etc.

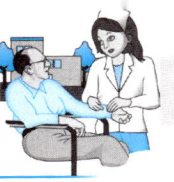

- **Fluid balance record:** All routes of fluid intake, and all routes of fluid loss or output are measured and recorded on this form.
- **Medication administration form:** Medication flow sheet usually include designated areas for the date of medication order, the expiration date, name and dose, frequency of administration and route, and the nurses signature.
- **Skin assessment record:** A skin or wound assessment is often recorded on a flow sheet. It may include categories related to stage of skin injury, drainage, odor, culture information and treatment.

Progress Notes

Progress notes made by nurses provide information about the progress, a client is making towards achieving desired outcomes. The format used depends upon documentation system used such as narrative notes, SOAP, PIE notes, charting by exception, and focus charting.

General Guidelines for Recording

- **Date and time:** Document the date and time of each recording. This is essential not only for legal reasons but also for client safety.
- **Timing:** Follows the agency's policy about the frequency of documenting, and adjusts the frequency as a client's condition indicates. No recording should be done **before** providing nursing care.
- **Legibility:** All entries must be legible and easy to read to prevent interpretation of errors.
- **Permanence:** All entries made in dark ink so that the record is permanent and changes can be identified.
- **Correct spelling:** It is essential for accuracy in recording. Incorrect spelling gives a negative impression to the reader and, thereby, decreases the nurse's credibility.
- **Signature:** Each recording on the nursing notes is signed by the nurse making it. The signature includes the name and title.
- **Accuracy:** The client's name and identifying information should be stamped or written on each page of the clinical records. Before making any entry, check that it is the correct chart.
- Do not identify charts by room number only, check the client's name. Notations on records must be accurate and correct.
- Accurate notations consist of facts or observations rather than opinions or interpretation. It is more accurate, for example, to write that the client "refused medication" (fact) than to write that the client "was uncooperative" (opinion).
- When describing something, avoid general words, such as large, good, or normal, for example, chart specific data such as "2 cm × 3 cm bruise" rather than "large bruise". When a recording mistake is made, draw a line through it and write the words <u>mistaken entry</u> above or next to the original entry, with your initials or name. Do not erase, or use correction fluid. Write on every line but never between lines.
- **Sequence:** Document events in the order in which they occur, such as record assessments, then the nursing interventions, and then the client's responses. Update or delete problems as needed.
- **Appropriateness:** Record only information that pertains as the client's health problems and care. Recording irrelevant information may be considered an invasion of the client's privacy.
- **Completeness:** Not all data that a nurse obtains about a client can be recorded. however, the information that is recorded needs to be complete and helpful to the client and health care professionals. Nurse's record need to reflect the nursing process, record assessment, dependent and independent nursing interventions, client problems, client comments and responses to interventions and tests, progress toward goals.
- **Conciseness:** Recording need to be brief as well as complete to save time in communication.
- **Accepted Terminology:** Use only commonly accepted abbreviations, symbols and terms as specified by the agency. Many abbreviations are standard and used universally.
- **Legal Prudence:** Accurate, complete documentation should give legal protection to the nurse, the client's other caregivers, the health care facility and the client. "*Complete charting for example by using the steps of the nursing process as a framework, is the best defense against malpractice.*"

RECORDS AND REPORTS OF THE CNO OFFICE

- Allocation register includes the name, and addresses of all the nursing staff
- Leave account register
- Deployment register
- Cumulative record
- Chief nursing office communication book
- Roll call book evening/ night
- Daily report of the hospital which includes:
  - Statistics register
  - EOPD Statistics
  - Emergency Ward Statistics
  - Labor room
  - Critical /private ward
  - VIP patient report

Standards for Nurses Note (Sample Recording)

- Monitor and record patients hemodynamic findings – febrile/afebrile

  (Temperature, PR, RR, BP) in case of patients with fever, post–operative cases, infectious disease and immunocompromised patients (Fig. 9).

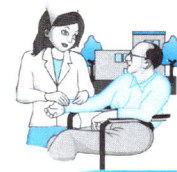

> Hemodynamic status
> Treatment prescribed
> Observation of patient's condition
> Intervention performed by the nurse
> Dietary pattern, sleep pattern, urinary output, bowel pattern etc.

Figure 9: Sample of recording

- Consciousness and orientation status in case of neurological deficit, psychiatric and cognitive deficit patients.
- Record the observations on the day of admission and changes occurred during the following days of admission.
- Record the major findings according to the condition.
- In case of neurological deficit patients, GCS and pupillary reaction to be noted. Note range of motion (ROM), sensory and motor deficits, stiffness or flaccidity of muscles.
- In case of cardiac and respiratory condition, monitor and record pulse rate, rhythm, volume, respiration rate, depth, lung sounds, presence of dyspnea, use of accessory muscles for respiration, distended neck veins.
- For any patients with renal problems, I/V fluids, urinary catheter or drains, nurse should maintain intake output chart.
- In case of bed ridden patients, ROM exercise is given/skin status at pressure point, position change every 2 hourly, chest physiotherapy.
- For gastrointestinal conditions, record for presence of nausea, vomiting, abdominal pain, distension, loose stools, constipation.
- Record nutritional/elimination/sleep status.
- Record the interventions performed by the nurse

TELEMEDICINE/TELE HEALTH

Information and communication technologies have great potential to address the challenges faced by different countries. Telemedicine is a rapidly developing field in health service arising out of effective fusion of information and communication technologies with medical science. It is a potentially miraculous method that promises improvement of health care delivery system and the practice of telemedicine is getting popular all over the world. Telemedicine literally means 'distance healing', 'tele' means 'distance' and 'mederi' means to heal. It is emerging as a viable and acceptable way to provide health care. Telemedicine was started with NASA's (National Aeronautics and space Administration) efforts in 1960.

Telehealth refers to remote non-clinical services as providing training, conducting administrative meetings, continuous medical service etc. According to WHO, telehealth includes surveillance, health promotion and public health functions. Telehealth uses electronic information and tele communication technologies to support long distance clinical health care patients and professional health related education and training, public health and health administration. It employs information technology through the use of computers, related software, telecommunication system comprising of compatible telephone lines and telephone lines, satellite linkups etc. to provide quality health care.

Telemedicine is the use of medical information exchanged from one site to another via communications to improve patient's health status   — *American Telemedicine Association*
Telehealth is defined as health information sent from one site to another by electronic communication.   —*Thobaben, 1998*
Telemedicine is the delivery of health care services, where distance is a critical factor by all health care professionals using information and communication technologies for the exchange of valid information for diagnosis, treatment, and prevention of disease and injuries, research and evaluation and for continuing education of health care providers, all in the interests of advancing the health of individuals and their communities.   —*World Health Organization.*

Telemedicine allows health care professionals to evaluate diagnosis and treat patients at distance using telecommunication facility. Health professionals providing telehealth service shall be fully licensed and registered with their respective regulatory or licensing bodies and with respect to the site where patient is located. They should be aware of credentialing requirements at the site where the consultant is located and the site where patient is located. They also should have necessary orientation.

Telemedicine software can help keep patients in touch with the health care provider and through telemonitoring medical specialists can suggest treatment measures. Telemonitoring software helps the medical specialists to monitor patient's blood pressure, heart rate, weight, haemoglobin, blood sugar level etc. and suggest treatment options. Through telehealth we can deliver patient care services as emergency medical assistance, long distance consultation, delivering patient education, transmission of medication remainders, diet planning for diabetes and other chronic diseases, etc.

Uses of Telemedicine

- Telemedicine helps to transmit images for assessment and diagnosis.
- It has easy access to remote areas.
- Transmit clinical data for assessment, diagnosis and management of disease
- Telemedicine helps to provide data for disease prevention and promotion of good health to school children, adolescent groups etc.
- It enhances health service or education via video conference.
- Telemedicine helps to conduct meetings among telehealth networks and health presentations including research activities.
- It is beneficial to people living in isolated areas.
- It helps to monitor patients with chronic disease at home.
- It is a tool of disease surveillance and program teaching.

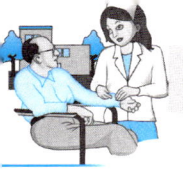

- It Facilitates continuous medical education and research activities.
- It is a tool for disaster management.

The three main categories of telemedicine transmission formats include

1. **Store - and - forward** health transmission (asynchronous)
   In store–and–forward transmission, the medical data is captured and stored in the device and at a convenient time the data are transmitted securely to the doctor or medical specialist. It does not require both the parties at the same time. It is more beneficial to patients living in remote areas. Dermatology, radiology and pathology are the common specialties for which this type of transmission is conducive.
2. **Real time or interactive telehealth** (synchronous). In real time telehealth there is live interaction between patients and providers of care through online communication and telephone conversation etc. Video conferencing equipment is one of the most common form of technology used in synchronous telehealth. Activities as history collection, physical examination, ophthalmology consultation etc. can be done through real time telehealth.
3. **Remote monitoring:** Through remote monitoring a medical specialist can monitor a patient remotely using technical devices. Usually this method is used for treatment of patient with chronic diseases as diabetes mellitus, cerebro vascular accident etc.

Advantages

- Telemedicine is accessible to people residing in rural areas and in isolated communities
- Telemedicine can be used as a tool so that expert medical specialists can give advice to those in another locations.
- Enhances quality of medical care by guidance from specialist medical practitioners.
- It facilitates access to patients and rural practitioners to specialist services and supports.
- Helps to reduce isolation of rural practice by upgrading their knowledge through telemedicine
- Continuing medical education and research.
- Telemedicine facilitates faster diagnosis and treatment and shorter hospital stay
- It is cost effective to patient and cost beneficial to society i.e. saves travel, time and money
- Telemedicine extends access to consultation from specialists
- Facilitates more informed decision making

Disadvantages

- As telemedicine is an emerging field there may be lack of trained manpower. Health care profession is not fully familiar with e- Medicine.
- Technical problems as failure of function of system due to interruption of power supply may occur
- Issues related to security, privacy and confidentiality of patient data
- Initial investment is costly
- Poor data communication infrastructure may interface functioning
- Possibility for malpractice and it involves medico legal concerns
- There is need to develop software solutions in health care

Application of Telemedicine

- **Telehealth care:** Tele health care is the use of information and communication technology for prevention and promotion of health and provide home health care to people through tele-consultation and tele follow up.
- **Tele education:** Education regarding health prevention, health promotion etc at different organizations, For example school, college etc.
- **Disaster management:** Telemedicine can play an important role to provide health care facilities to victims of disasters. Portable telemedicine system with satellite connectivity and customized telemedicine software is ideal for disaster relief.
- **Continuing medical education and public awareness**: Tele conferencing is the discussion and interaction between doctors during workshop, conferences, seminars, continuing education programs in a visual room environment, for example.

Eg: demonstration of live surgery or presentations.

Worldwide people living in remote areas struggle to access timely quality specialty medical care due to unequal distribution of health facilities. Tele medicine activities started in India from 1919 itself. The Indian space Research Organization has been deploying a SATCOM – based tele medicine network across the country with the support of various Govt. agencies. Also our country has taken initiative with the aim to provide quality health care facilities to rural and remote areas of the country. The government has planned and implemented various National Level Projects. Activities are organized in the field of medical e-learning by establishing digital medical libraries.

In India, TM programs are supported by Department of Information Technology, ISRO, NEC Telemedine program for north–eastern states, corporate hospitals like Apollo Hospital, Asian Heart Foundation and State Govt. Hospitals in the past 3 years, ISRO, TM network has expanded to connect 45 remote rural hospitals and 15 superspecialty hospitals.

TELENURSING

Telenursing is a branch of telehealth which uses telecommunication and information technology for providing nursing services in health care.

Telenursing is the use of telemedicine technology to deliver nursing care and conduct nursing practice —*ICN 2007*

The principal goals of International Council of Nurses–Telenursing networks are:

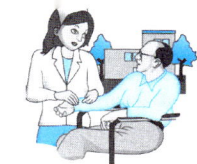

- To serve as a global resources for nurses working or interested in telenursing practice, technology development, policy, standards, education and research.
- To promote effective networking and linkages
- To enable the sharing of telenursing knowledge and expertise and stimulate reflection on the changing nature of nursing care delivery systems across the globe.

Telenursing is a component of telehealth which is a rapidly developing mode of health service delivery. Telenursing refers to the use of telecommunication and information technology for providing nursing service in health care. Through telenursing we can meet health needs of patients using information, communication and web based systems.

The most developing field of telenursing today is home health care. Telenursing can be used in giving home care to patients who are immobilized or living in remote places, patients with chronic disease like chronic obstructive pulmonary disease, diabetes, Alzheimer's disease etc. The practice of telenursing will provide opportunities to telenurses to become key players in care management across the health care continuum.

Purpose

- Telenursing is a e–health application in the field of nursing practice which is found to be used in Hospital based care, home care, hospices, rehabilitation centers etc
- Telenursing helps to improve access to health care to people living in remote places.
- Telenursing promotes health care consultation by medical specialists or experts.
- Facilitates video conferencing among professionals.
- Patients can contact nurses or medical specialists at any time.
- Continuity of care can be enhanced.
- Telenursing provides opportunity for continuing education for nurses.
- Through telenursing we can impart patient education and professional consultations.

Advantages

- Limited resources can benefit a large population
- Telenursing helps to solve increasing shortage of nurses
- Saves time and reduce distance to travel
- Telenursing helps to reduce length of hospital stay of home care patients.
- Enable nurses to share clinical information with professionals and colleagues.
- Telenursing provides facilities for teaching patients and relatives to control disease

Disadvantages

- There is possibility of technical failures
- Chances of misinterpretation of data and images being transmitted
- Inability to use electronic equipment
- Lack of confidentiality and security of electronic information.

There are possibilities of legal ethical and regulatory issues related to use of Tele nursing, as accountability and malpractice. Moreover staff nurses need training on proper use of the system. Also there are issues related to confidentiality and malpractice.

ELECTRONIC MEDICAL RECORDS

Definition

An electronic medical record is a medical record in digital format created in hospitals. This facilitates access to patient's data by nurses at any given location, making automated check for drug and allergy interactions, clinical notes and laboratory reports. The term electronic medical record can be expanded to include systems which keep track of other relevant medical information. Although an EMR system has the potential for invasion to patients' medical privacy.

Electronic patient records is a measure to put all patients records online so that any hospital have access to that. This would allow sharing of information between hospitals and health authority.

Types of EMRs

Following are different types of EMR:

- **Departmental EMRs:** It contains information entered by a single hospital department.
- **Inter-departmental EMR:** This type of record contains information from two or more hospital departments, e.g. records from department of cardiology, pharmacy etc.
- **Hospital EMRs:** It contains all or most of patient's information from a particular hospital.
- **Inter-hospital EMRs:** It contains patient's medical information from two or more hospitals.
- **Electronic patients record:** Contains all or most of patient's clinical information from a particular hospital.
- **Computerized patients record:** This record contains patient's clinical information from a particular hospital.
- **Electronic health care record:** Contains all patients' health information.
- **Personal health record:** These records are controlled by the patient and contains information at least partly entered by the patient.
- **Computerized medical records:** These types of records are created by image scanning of a paper based health record.
- **Digital medical record:** A web based record maintained by a health care provider.
- **Clinical data repository**

    An operational data store that holds and manages clinical data collected from health service providers.

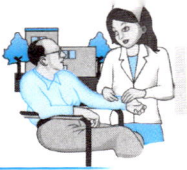

- **Electronic client records:** Scope is defined by health care professionals, For example by physiotherapist or social worker.
- **Population health record:** These records contains aggregated data.

Benefits of EMR

- It ensures speed and saves time. More time is available for patient care
- EMR is capable of carrying more information than traditional system
- EMR stores medical transcription subjective, objective, assessment and plan notes and medical codes
- Improved quality of care

Disadvantages

- High cost
- Legal issues
- Technical problems
- Security of information is a problem

PERFORMANCE APPRAISAL

Performance appraisal is a criteria for measuring performance of employee or group of employees and it includes behavior competencies, demonstration of skill and knowledge and achievements of objectives.

Performance appraisal is the process of obtaining, analyzing and recording information about the relative worth of an employee.

Performance appraisal is a systematic, periodic and so far as possible, an impartial rating of an employees excellence in matters pertaining to his present job and to his potentialities for a better job —*Flippo*

According to HEYEL, performance appraisal is the process of evaluating the performance and qualifications of employees in terms of other requirements for purposes of administration including placement, selection for promotion, providing financial reward and other actions, which require differential treatment among the members of a group as distinguished from actions affecting all members equally.

Performance appraisal is a control measure that the nurse manager uses to achieve organizational goals. Through regular evaluation of each employee's job performance the manager can achieve several purposes. She can help efficient workers to improve their performance, informs inefficient workers that their performance is inadequate and recommends methods for improvement, identifies employees who deserve salary promotion or salary increase, recognize employees who qualify for special assignments, improve communication between herself and subordinates, and establish a basis for coaching of employees who need special assistance.

BF. Skinner's experiments with classic conditioning revealed that person learn best (learning results in behavior change) when they receive immediate feedback concerning the adequacy of their performance. The information that is given to an employee during performance appraisal constitutes feedbacks that will guide the employee in improvement efforts.

Performance appraisals are necessary in an organization to understand each employee's abilities, competencies and relative merit and worth for the organization. Performance appraisal provides opportunity for the manager to observe the performance of employees. It should be carried out regularly in an institution and the evaluation of information should be shared with employees periodically.

Objectives

For Employees

- To evaluate the performance of employees in an organization
- To review the past performance of employees
- To improve communication between supervisors and subordinates
- To improve the quality of job performance of employees
- To assess training and developmental needs of employees
- To help managers to decide promotion, increment and other advancements
- To motivate employees and to give recognition for their accomplishment
- To provide an opportunity to the employees for self evaluation
- To improve organizational development

For Organization

- Assess or evaluate the achievement of goals of the organization
- Act as a tool for measurement of work standards
- Assess aspirations and talents of staff and efficiency of staff development program
- Performance appraisal serves as a tool for salary and other benefits
- Help to plan promotion, transfer and job rotation of employees
- Improve interpersonal relation and communication between management and employees

Principles of Performance Appraisal

- It must be based on objectives of organization
- There should be well defined criteria for evaluation and should be known to employees
- The method used for appraisal should be based on objectives and criteria
- The evaluations should be documented and discussed with employees

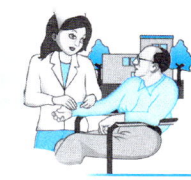

- Self-evaluation in performance appraisal promote development of employees which contribute to quality of care.

Performance Appraisal Process

Performance appraisal is a method of assessing the performance of workers by an experienced superior officer. The process of performance appraisal involves the following steps,

- **Establish criteria for performance standards:** The performance appraisal process begins with establishment of criteria and standards which should be based on goals and objectives. The standard should include the work performance of particular job, knowledge, skill, attitude, initiative and leadership, activities to improve scientific development of worker, ability to communicate, etc. The subordinates should also be included in the planning process.
- **The standard formulated should be communicated to workers:** The performance appraisal criteria established should be communicated to the employees and evaluators and it should be explained in detail.
- **Measure the performance using selected methods based on criteria:** In this stage select the appropriate technique or method of appraisal. Evaluation can be done annually or biannually. The evaluator should observe the basic principles of appraisal during evaluation.
- **Compare the actual performance against standards:** The findings of evaluation is compared with the pre determined standards and criteria.
- **Discus the evaluation:** The result of appraisal are communicated with the concerned employees. Discuss the strengths and weaknesses so as to assess training needs and provide necessary corrections.
- **Arrange follow up meeting and take corrective actions:** The management can arrange training, staff development programs, counseling services or corrective actions as and when necessary to improve performance.

Evaluation Principles

- The worker's evaluation should be based on **behaviorally oriented performance standards** for the position that she occupies. Since the job description and associated performance standards are presented to the employee during orientation as objectives towards which she should strive. Her performance should be evaluated with reference to those same objectives.
- An **adequate and representative sample of the nurse's behavior** should be observed in evaluating her performance. Care must be taken to evaluate her usual or consistent behavior and to avoid magnifying the importance of an isolated, atypical instance of superior behavior. Since exceptional behavior by a worker, whether good or bad, is more apt to attract a supervisor's attention than a more typical behavior, each supervisor should determine in advance the occasions on which she intends to observe each nurse in performance of specific job activities.
- The nurse should be given **a copy of her job description, performance standards, and evaluation** form to review before the scheduled evaluation conference so that the nurse and the supervisor can discuss the evaluation from the same frame of reference. Both the nurse and the supervisor should complete the evaluation form.
- In documenting an employee's performance appraisal, the manager should **indicate those areas in which performance is satisfactory and those in which improvements are needed.** The supervisor should refer to the specific instances of satisfactory and unsatisfactory behavior in order to clarify the base for evaluation comments.
- If there is **need for improvement** in several area of nurse's performance, the manager should **specify** which are to be given priority as the nurse attempts to upgrade job performance.
- The **evaluation discussion should be scheduled at a time that is convenient** for both nurse and manager, should be held in pleasant surroundings, and should also allow time for both to discuss the evaluation at length.
- The **evaluation should be structured** so that it is perceived as helpful by the nurse whose performance is being analyzed. An employee can withstand even strong criticism from a manager who shows consideration for her feeling and offers to assist her in improving job performance.

Methods/Tools of Evaluation

There are different kinds of performance appraisal methods. Performance appraisal system is effective only if tools developed are appropriate. Some of the important methods are:

Performance Appraisal Methods (Fig. 10)

- **Individual evaluation methods**
  - Confidential reports are mostly used in Govt. sector. It is a report prepared by the administrator about the employee at the end of every year which contains information about employee's work performances, strengths, weaknesses, achievements etc based on prepared criteria

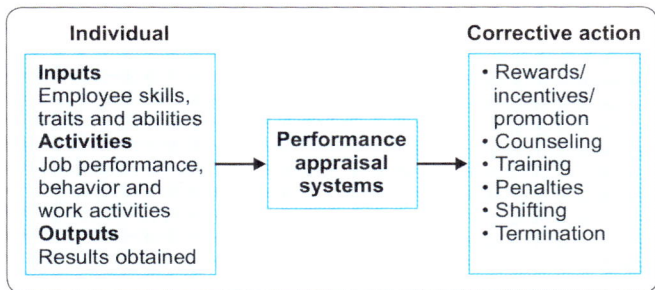

Figure 10: Performance appraisal system

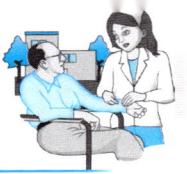

- Essay appraisal
- Critical incidence
- Checklists or rating scales
- Forced choice methods
- Management by objectives
- **Multiple person evaluation method**
  - Ranking method
  - Paired comparison method
  - Forced distribution method
- **Other methods**
  - Group appraisal method
  - Field review method
  - 360 degree appraisal

Some of the methods are described in detail below. They are:

Free Response Report

In the free response report the evaluator is asked to comment in writing on the quality of the nurse's performance in a particular position over a given period. Because the evaluator is given no direction concerning which aspects of performance are to be evaluated, the assessment is apt to be valid. The free response report may also lack objectivity if it concentrates only on those areas of the nurse's performance about which the supervisor entertains strong feelings.

Essay

Essay is a performance appraisal method in which the manager is required to describe in narrative forms the employees performance, strength and weakness and the area they need to improve. Quality of essay may be more reflective of the writing skill of appraiser than the performance. In this method there is possibility of personnel bias. This method is considered to be complex and time consuming

Ranking Method

- **Simple ranking method:** Some evaluation tools call for the evaluator to rank the employee in relation to his coworkers with respect to various aspects of performance. A particular staff nurse might be ranked by her superior as having demonstrated the highest performance among seven staff nurses in her unit with regard to patient care, as third highest in the same group with regard to the quality of her patient teaching, and lowest in the group with regard to the amount of her research productivity.
- **Paired comparison:** This method is suitable for large organizations. In this method each employee is compared with other employees taking only one at a time. The evaluator compares two employees and select an employee whom the evaluator considers as better employee. In the same way an employee is compared with all other employees who scored maximum. for being a better employee and is considered to be the best employees. Paired comparison is a simple and easier method. For example if there are three employees in an organization A, B and C, the employee A is compared with B and C, the employee Bis compared with A and C and C is compared with A and B. The results of comparison are tabulated and a rank is given to each employee.

Critical Incidents Method

In this method of Performance appraisal, the evaluator rates the employee on the basis of the performance of employee when a critical events occurred and how the employee behaved at that time. It includes both negative and positive reactions as unwilling to attend the same or handled the situation scientifically etc. The drawback of this method is that the supervisor has to note down the critical incidents and the employee behavior as and when they occur.

Field Review Method

In this method, manager assess the performance of employees through interviewing the immediate supervisor of a concerned employee. The evaluator asks questions to superiors about the performance of employees. A major drawback of this method is that it is time consuming. But this method helps to reduce the superiors' personal bias.

Performance Checklist

A performance checklist might consist of a number of questions related to his job performance and for which the answer may be yes or no.The evaluator indicate whether the answer to a question is positive or negative about a worker.. The evaluator indicates the answer against each questions..

Eg; Is the employee punctual ? Yes / No

The different types of check list are:
- Weighted check list; in which weights are assigned to different statements to indicate their relative importance. It is composed of many behavior statements which represent desirable job behavior,
- Forced choice check list; In forced choice checklist four or five statements are given for each trait.which the manager select an undesirable and desirable behaviors of worker.
- Simple check list: In simple checklist equal importance is given to each statement.

Forced Choice Comparison

In this method the evaluator prepare a group of statements both favorable and unfavorable items which describes the characteristics of employees. The evaluator is forced to rate any one of the statements either positive or negative.. The final ranking is done on the basis of all the statements.

Self Appraisal

In this method the employees are asked to submit their work related accomplishment. These self appraisal process gives details of their certificate, in service education, and continuing education details, awards etc.

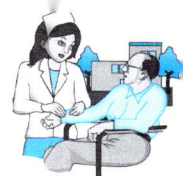

Rating Scale

Using rating scale workers quality and quantity of efforts can be evaluated. This method is more reliable.
- Forced choice rating: In forced choice rating, raters are asked to choose from groups of statements that according to their evaluation and then statements are scored.
- Critical incident review: The manager record the actual incidence in the personal records and use of actual of positive or negative behaviors.

Trait Rating Scale

It is one of the most widely used method of rating an employee against the set standards which may be the job description, desired behavior or personality trait.
Example of trait rating scale;

Knowledge			
Adequate	Satisfactory	Good	Excellent
1	2	3	4
Judgement			
Not adequate	Satisfactory	Good decisions	Excellent decisions
1	2	3	4
Attitude			
Not adequate	Satisfactory	Good	Excellent
1	2	3	4

Behaviorally Anchored Rating Scale

BARS is relatively a recent technique in which the rating scale method and critical incident approach are integrated. In this method the requirements for effective performance are identified and these requirements are anchored at each end of a vertical bar. The bar consists of a series of vertical scales - each scale identifying each important dimension of job performance. The bars are scaled from 1 to 9 where 1 is the lowest rating performance and 9 is the highest rating performance. The evaluator records the performance of each behavior of an employee on the appraisal form and score the performance. This method helps to reduce errors of performance appraisal as personal bias and prejudice.

Management by Objectives

MBO is an excellent method of performance appraisal which promotes individual growth and excellence because subordinates are involving in the process. In MBO the superiors and subordinates jointly discuss the goals and objectives to be accomplished during the appraisal period. The employees are also involved in setting goals and criteria used for evaluating performance. During the evaluation period both of them discuss together the problems and progress and finally the actual performance are compared with predetermined objectives. Modifications are made periodically by inviting suggestions of employees. Superiors assists the employees by giving corrections and if necessary training and counseling. There is good team spirit in this method as employees are involved in setting goals.

Peer Review Method

In peer review, the peers or co-workers do performance appraisal by monitoring the wok assessment or work performance. Peer review when reviewed properly, provide employee with valuable feedback. The disadvantages of this method is that sometimes peers feel uncomfortable to evaluate their coworkers with whom they work closely. There may be possibility of interpersonal conflicts due to unfair appraisal. Some workers have less idea regarding peer review Moreover this method is time consuming.

360 Degree Evaluation (Multi Rator Feedback)

360 degree appraisal is the most comprehensive method of performance appraisal where the employees are assessed by his or her peer workers, subordinates, superiors, patients, care givers etc. and also there is self evaluation of employees themselves. The evaluator gets feed back from multiple individuals which provide a broader and more accurate perspective of work performance of employees.

eg: 360° evaluation of a staff nurse include feedback from those who interact with the staff nurse as other staff nurse or peers, from doctors, staff from other department where the staff nurse interacts during her duty, from patients, their relatives etc

Advantages of 360 degree evaluation
- Evaluation is more accurate as it include self assessment, peer review, management review etc.
- Help to improve credibility of performance appraisal
- Employees get more accurate feedback regarding his strength and weakness
- Improve professional growth of employees

Advantages of Performance Appraisal

- To provide back-up data for management decisions concerning transfer, promotions, salary benefits.
- To serve as a check on hiring and recruiting practices.
- To motivate employees by providing feedback about their work.
- To improve communication between supervisor and employee, and to reach an understanding on the objectives of the job.
- To help the supervisors observe their subordinates more closely.
- To establish standards of job performance.
- To help the organization determine if it is meeting organizational goal.

Disadvantages

- This process is costly in terms of resources
- The evaluators must be trained
- This method is time consuming

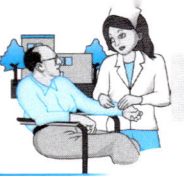

Problems in Performance Appraisal

- **Halo effect:** Tendency to overrate a subordinate's performance for the following reasons.
- An employee with the pleasing personality or high level of social skills is apt to receive a higher performance rating than her work quality would warrant.
- A subordinate who has performed well in the past but whose current work the manager has not closely observed may be assumed to be performing at the same high level, so may be given an unduly high rating by the manager.
- A subordinate who shares the manager's area of clinical expertise, research interests, or personality quirks is likely to receive higher than deserved ratings
- **Horn effect:** Tendency to rate an employee lower than her performance would warrant for one of the following reasons.
- An employee whose work is consistently above average but is inclined to disagree openly with her manager is apt to receive a lower rating than deserved
- An employee whose work is of high quality but fails to conform to the manager's ideal of proper behavior for an employee of the hospital is likely to receive a lower rating than deserved
- An employee whose performance is above average but associates with poor-performing employees is likely to receive lower than deserved ratings
- **Pitchfork effect:** Common tendency to rate the people on the basis of their most recent behavior and forgetting the events and their performance in the starting of the period.
- An employee who didn't performed well throughout the year but has delivered a spectacular performance or received an impressive award within a few days of her annual performance evaluation is often given a higher rating than overall annual performance deserves because the manager's attention is focused on the worker's recent success.
- An employee who has performed at above average level throughout the year but within a few days of her annual performance evaluation has committed an error in patient care or employee supervision is apt to receive a lower that deserved rating because her recent blunder remains fixed in the manager's memory.

Some of the other problems of performance appraisal are,

- Central tendency is the most commonly found error. It is the tendency of the rater to give average ratings to all employee without actually appraising or condemning them. This type of errors may due to the fact that a very high rating or low rating may lead to criticisms or further questions. So the evaluators may think that giving an average rating is safer.
- Stereotyping an employee on the basis of the performance of his/her team is another common error.
- Personal bias Personal bias or prejudices may affect performance evaluation.
- Stereotyping. Stereotyping means forming a mental picture of a person on thebasis of age, sex, religion, culture etc. may affect evaluation.

Qualities to be Evaluated

- Qualities of performance
  Quality of work, knowledge and skill, implementation of duties as orderliness, appropriateness of work and accuracy
- Quantity of work and promptness
- Mental abilities
  Abilities as adaptability, judgement, reasoning power etc.
- Supervisory and leadership abilities as organizational capacity, communication and interpersonal relations, co ordination and team spirit
- Personal qualities
  Appearance, attitude, initiative, self confidence, self control etc.
- Capacity for future development

Sample Performance Appraisal for Ward Incharges

Name: Review Period: Ward: Date:

Sl. No	Appraisal parameters	1	2	3	4	5	Rates	Score
I	**PATIENT CARE**							
1.1	Ensures proper delivery of patient care							
1.2	Monitor patient condition and makes plan of care							
1.3	Gives orientation to new admission cases							
1.4	Carry out the orders/sending investigations without delay or mistake							
II	**PROFESSIONAL BEHAVIOR**							
1.1	Shows interest in attending in-service education							
1.2	Maintains good interpersonal relationship							
1.3	Follows professional dress code							
1.4	Demonstrate good conduct							

Contd...

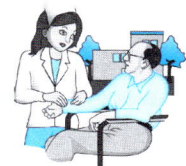

Sl. No	Appraisal parameters	1	2	3	4	5	Rates	Score
III	**RECORDS AND REPORTS**							
1.1	Maintains nurses record properly							
1.2	Maintenance of reports (IP register, Stock register, night reports etc) appropriately							
1.3	Documents and reports significant events to the higher authority							
IV	**COMMUNICATION**							
1.1	Communicates effectively with patients							
1.2	Communicates effectively with patients and their bystanders							
1.3	Communicates effectively with junior and senior staffs							
V	**EQUIPMENT AND SUPPLIES**							
1.1	Takes responsibility for the equipments and supplies in the ward							
1.2	Maintains inventory appropriately							
1.3	Ensures adequate supply and judicious use of materials							
VI	**MANAGERIAL SKILLS**							
1.1	Organizes and supervises patient care by ensuring adequate number of staff in each shift							
1.2	Ensures proper ward cleanliness and proper waste management							
1.3	Shows leadership /assertiveness skills							

Remarks:

Signature of the floor supervisor with Date

Remarks (Complementary/ Adverse):
Remarks by CNO
Key: 1. Unacceptable, 2. Marginal, 3. Satisfactory, 4. Commendable, 5. Superior

NURSING AUDIT

The word "audit" comes from the Latin word"auditus" a hearing. It originally meant the hearing of the facts and arguments about a situation to determine the truth.

- Nursing audit is a review of the patient record designed to identify, examine, or verify the performance of certain specified aspects of nursing care by using established criteria.
- Nursing audit is the process of collecting information from nursing reports and other documented evidence about patient care and assessing the quality of care by the use of quality assurance programs.
- Nursing audit is a detailed review and evaluation of selected clinical records by qualified professional personnel for evaluating quality of nursing care.
- A concurrent nursing audit is performed during ongoing nursing care.
- A retrospective nursing audit is performed after discharge from the care facility, using the patient's record.

Meaning

- Quality - a judgement of what constitutes good or bad.
- Audit - a systematic and critical examination to examine or verify.
- Nursing audit -
  - It is the assessment of the quality of nursing care.
  - Uses a record as an aid in evaluating the quality of patient care.
- Medical audit - the systematic, critical analysis of the quality of medical care, including the procedures for diagnosis and treatment, the use of resources, and the resulting outcome and quality of life for the patient.

Definition

"Nursing audit refers to assessment of the quality of clinical nursing" —*Elison*

Nursing Audit is an exercise to find out whether good nursing practices are followed.

The audit is a means by which nurses themselves can define standards from their point of view and describe the actual practice of nursing.- Goster Walfer

Purposes of Nursing Audit

- Evaluating Nursing care given,

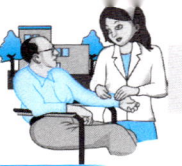

- Achieves deserved and feasible quality of nursing care,
- Stimulant to better records,
- Focuses on care provided and not on care provider
- Contributes to research.

Essential Characteristics of Nursing Audit

- Written standards of care against which to evaluate nursing care
- Evidence that actual practice was measured against such standards
- Examination and analysis of findings
- Evidence of corrective action being taken
- Evidence of effectiveness of corrective action
- Appropriate recording of the audit program

Methods of Nursing Audit

There are two methods:

- **Retrospective view:** This refers to an in-depth assessment of the quality after the patient has been discharged, have the patients chart to the source of data.

    Retrospective audit is a method for evaluating the quality of nursing care by examining the nursing care as it is reflected in the patient care records for discharged patients. In this type of audit specific behaviors are described then they are converted into questions and the examiner looks for answers in the record. For example the examiner looks through the patient's records and asks:
    - Was the problem solving process used in planning nursing care?
    - Whether patient data collected in a systematic manner?
    - Was a description of patient's pre-hospital routines included?
    - Laboratory test results used in planning care?
    - Did the nurse perform physical assessment? How was information used?
    - Were nursing diagnosis stated?
    - Did nurse write nursing orders? And so on.
- **The concurrent review:** This refers to the evaluations conducted on behalf of patients who are still undergoing care. It includes assessing the patient at the bedside in relation to pre-determined criteria, interviewing the staff responsible for this care and reviewing the patient's record and care plan.

Points to be Remembered

- Quality assurance must be a priority.
- Those responsible must implement a program not only a tool.
- A coordinator should develop and evaluate quality assurance activities.
- Roles and responsibilities must be delivered.
- Nurses must be informed about the process and the results of the program.
- Data must be reliable.
- Adequate orientation of data collection is essential.
- Quality data should be annualized and used by nursing personnel at all levels.

Audit Committee

Before carrying out an audit, an audit committee should be formed, comprising of a minimum of five members who are interested in quality assurance, are clinically competent and able to work together in a group. It is recommended that each member should review not more than 10 patients each month and that the auditor should have the ability to carry out an audit in about 15 minutes. If there are less than 50 discharges per month, then all the records may be audited, if there are large number of records to be audited, then an auditor may select 10 per cent of discharges.

Training for auditors should include the following:
- A detailed discussion of the seven components.
- A group discussion to see how the group rates the care received using the notes of a patient who has been discharged, these should be anonymous and should reflect a total period of care not exceeding two weeks in length.
- Each individual auditor should then undertake the same exercise as above. This is followed by a meeting of the whole committee who compare and discuss its findings, and finally reach a consensus of opinion on each of the components.

Audit Reports

- The audit objective
- The name of auditors
- Date of the audit
- The audit methods used, sample size and time frame
- The findings in relation to criterion
- Selected comments from questionnaires and suggestions for improvement

Audit Cycle

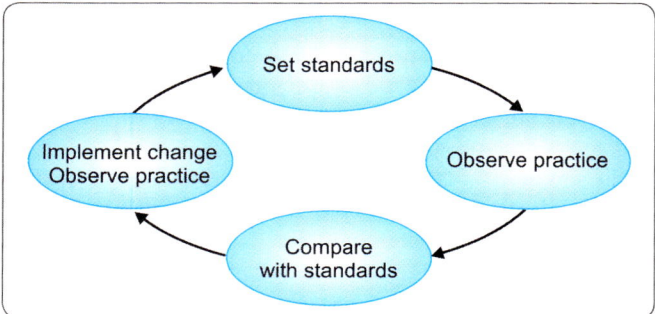

Audit as a Tool for Quality Control

An audit is a systematic and official examination of a record, process or account to evaluate performance. Auditing in health care organization provide managers with a means of applying control process to determine the quality of service rendered. Nursing audit is the process of analyzing data about the nursing process of patient outcomes to evaluate the effectiveness of nursing interventions. The audits most frequently used in quality control include outcome, process and structure audits.

- **Outcome audit:** Outcomes are the end results of care; the changes in the patients health status and can be attributed to delivery of health care services. These audits assume the outcome accurately and demonstrate the quality of care that was provided. Example of outcomes traditionally used to measure quality of hospital care include mortality, its morbidity, and length of hospital stay.
- **Process audit:** Process audits are used to measure the process of care or how the care was carried out. Process audit is task oriented and focus on whether or not practice standards are being fulfilled. These audits assumed that a relationship exists between the quality of the nurse and quality of care provided.
- **Structure audit:** Structure audit monitors the structure or setting in which patient care occurs, such as the finances, nursing service, medical records and environment. This audit assumes that a relationship exists between quality care and appropriate structure. These above audits can occur retrospectively, concurrently and prospectively.

For the effective quality control, the nurse manager has to play following roles and functions.

Advantages of Nursing Audit

- Can be used as a method of measurement in all areas of nursing.
- Scoring system is fairly simple.
- Results easily understood.
- Assesses the work of all those involved in recording care.
- May be a useful tool as a part of a quality assurance Program in areas where accurate records of care are kept.
- It gives a biographical index of quality of nursing each patient has achieved.
- Patient is assured of good services.
- It will give valuable and pertinent information for the staff, improvement in quality of nursing as well as strengths and weaknesses in nursing service are revealed.
- It will lead to better cooperation and communication among the nurses and health team members as a result of improved quality of nursing notes.
- It will help each professional nurse for her self evaluation.
- It helps the administration-better planning can be done through nursing audit. It enables the nurse administrator to uncover the inefficient service and point the ways to elevation of standards.
- It will reduce the incidence of medico-legal complications arising out of incomplete or inaccurate records maintained by nurses.
- It will broaden and strengthen nursing service in the hospital.

Disadvantages of the Nursing Audit

- Appraises the outcomes of the nursing process, so it is not so useful in areas where the nursing process has not been implemented.
- Many of the components overlap making analysis difficult.
- Is time consuming.
- Requires a team of trained auditors.
- Deals with a large amount of information.
- Only evaluates record keeping.
- It is considered as a source of punishment by the professional group.
- It is only served to improve the documentation not the nursing care.

Utilization of Results of Nursing Audit

For Nursing Care Services

- Modifying nursing care plans and the nursing care process, including discharge planning, for selected patient population.
- Implementing a program for improving documentation of nursing care through improved charting policies, methodologies and forms.
- Focusing supervisory attention upon areas of weakness identified, such as one particular nursing unit or specific employee.
- Focusing of nursing rounds and team conferences.
- Designing responsible orientation and in-service education programs.
- Gaining administrative support for making changes in resources including personnel.
- Using the evaluation based on nursing audit criteria to focus staff attention on individual patient outcome.

For Nursing Administrators

- Provide evaluations of particular program such as orientation of personnel or establishment of patient teaching program.
- Support requests for accreditation or for financing of a particular program.
- Serve as a basis for planning new programs or program changes.
- Serve to identify areas of strength and weakness in the total nursing programs, in specific areas of the program, and in various settings in which a program exists.
- Determine the influence of varied staffing patterns.
- It may be used as data in cost-effectiveness status. For example, studies comparing the quality of care received by patients in varied situations in which costs of staffing vary.

For Supervisor and Head Nurse

- Identify the areas of needed patient care improvement.
- Provide basis for planning in-service education program
- Identify teaching/supervision needs of staff members who give direct care to patients.

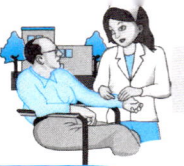

For Staff Nurse
- Provide self-examination of care in their specific nursing unit or settings.
- Identify particular types of care in which practice may be improved merely by increased attention and consciousness.
- Identify types of care in which improvement will depend on the staff's acquiring additional knowledge and skill.

CONCLUSION

Of all the technologies affecting the health care system in the future, the greatest impact will come from telemedicine. The field of telemedicine includes diagnostic software, record keeping and the communication of knowledge about health care observations to almost anywhere in the world. It has the capability of developing a client profile that includes biochemical definitions of Illness, health and wellness-for that person. Medical record keeping will continue to become more sophisticated, and systems will be able to monitor the outcomes of different modalities of care. Telemedicine will allow the consumers to be involved both in their own health care and in monitoring the outcomes produced by various health care providers.

DISASTER MANAGEMENT

Disaster is defined as any occurrence that causes damage, ecologic disruption, loss of human life or deterioration of health and health services on a scale sufficient to warrant an extra ordinary response from outside the affected community or area (WHO).

Every year millions of people all over the world are affected by disasters and result in damages to human lives and property

A disaster is sudden unexpected event that disrupts a community, causes premature death or alter health status of people.

A disaster is any occurrences that cause damage ecological disruption which leads to human material and economic or environmental loses.

Classification of Disasters

There are different classifications of disaster
- **Types of disasters according to cause**
  - Natural disasters—Natural disaster are caused by nature or emerging diseases
    E.g. Flood, storm, hurricane, tornado, earth quake, volcanic eruption, landslides, avalanche, epidemics etc.
  - Man made disasters—are emergencies, technological disasters and other disasters not caused by natural hazards. E.g. War, riots, chemical, biological, radiological and nuclear terrorism, accidents etc.
- **According to speed of onset**
  - Rapid onset Disaster—Disasters occurs suddenly with little warning. E.g.: Earthquakes, flood, storm, wind etc.
  - Slow onset Disaster—They occurs overtime or slowly. E.g. Droughts, famine, deforestation etc.

PHASES OF DISASTER

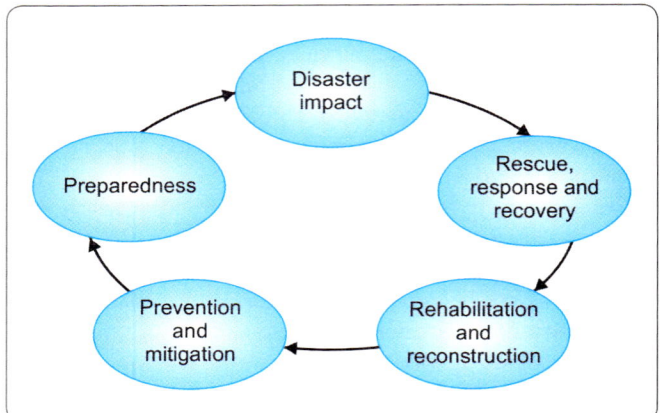

- **Disaster impact and response:** Disaster response are the activities of local people, health care institutions, public or voluntary agencies immediately during or after a disaster. In this phase the actions taken include search and rescue, first aid, triage and field care, tagging and hospitalization of victims. In the relief phase the major activities include vaccination, control and prevention of communicable diseases.
- **Search, rescue and first aid:** Field triage is important to manage mass causalities to save as many lives as possible.

  Triage must be initiated immediately after or along with Disaster. It is the process of rapidly classifying the victims on the basis of severity of their injuries. Triage is the sorting and allocation of treatment to patients and disaster victims according to a system of priorities designed to maximize the number of survivors.

  The main aims of triaging are to sort patients requiring emergency treatment during a disaster and to provide proper care according to degree of urgency to get maximum number of survivors and to utilize resources effectively.

  Triage may be of different types. They are:
  - Simple triage : It is done at the scene of a disaster to sort maximum number of patients who need immediate attention at the field itself. Followed by tagging by coloured tapes or triage tags to identify priority of patients need.
  - Continuous integrated Triage: This type of triage are applied in tertiary care centres where adequate resources are available.
  - Reverse triage: While discharge of victims /patients, triage can be applied,.

    Triage tag: is a label placed on each patients which help to identify victim who need prime attention or treatment or transportation to higher level centres. The following is an example of triage

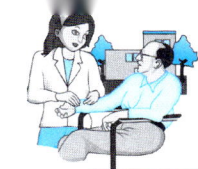

Type	Colour	Type of injury
Priority/emergent	Red	Critical – may survive if simple life saving measures are applied
Priority 2/urgent	Yellow	Likely to survive if care is given within hours
Priority 3/Non urgent	Green	Minor injuries care may be delayed while other patients are attended that is ambulatory patients
Priority 2/Priority 3	Blue	Catastrophic patients or those who need extensive care within minutes.
None	Black	Dead or severely injured and not expected to survive.

Different countries have different triage system. Some of the examples are

Australia and NewZeland – Australia Triage Scale (ATS)

Canada – Canada Triage and Acuity Scale (CTAS)

America – Emergency Severity index etc.

- **Relief phase:** The recovery phase is a prolonged period sometimes extend to months or years, so during this phase individuals and community attempts to bring their lives and activities to normal level. Relief phase starts when assistance from outside agencies starts to reach the disaster site. Following initial emergency phase, supplies are needed to treat causalities and to prevent further damage and rehabilitation of the victims. The needed supplies include food, clothing, shelter homes, sanitary measures, facilities for disposal of waste materials etc.
- **Rehabilitation and reconstruction:** Immediately after disaster start rehabilitative activities along with relief phase. In this phase attention to be given to the physical and mental health of survivors and material and logistic helps to sufferings of victims. The family must also be addressed. During this phase give special attention to the following activities:
- **Epidemiological surveillance and disease control:** Population displacement, overcrowding, poor sanitation, disruption and contamination of water supply, poor sanitation, ecological changes and disruption of control of programs may favour breeding of vectors, displacement of domestic and wild animals etc. These activities may disrupt normal healthful environment and lead to various health problems and communicable diseases. As soon as possible start rehabilitative measures to reduce risk of health issues and problems. Epidemiological surveillance and emergency reconstruction, acquisition, storage and proper distribution of supplies and equipment as food and clothing are utmost important. Nutritional status of affected population must be monitored with special attention to infants, children, pregnant women, lactating mothers, elderly and sick person. Ensure provision of safe water supply and adequate facilities for disposal of excreta and waste by temporary engineering measures. Personal hygiene and food hygiene must be given special consideration. Management of safety and hygiene of temporary shelters must be addressed properly. The survivors of the disaster which may be distressed due to the shock of disaster, loss of lives of relatives, loss of personal property etc, may lead to stress and sometimes post trauma stress disorders. Along with physical health, mental health should also be addressed and they should be given counseling to bring them back to normal life.

Disaster Preparedness

Disaster preparedness is a continuous and integrated process and is a key to effective disaster management. Prepardness refers to measures taken to reduce the impact of disasters. Disaster preparedness are development of activities to strengthen capacity of country to manage disasters. That is to predict disaster or whenever possible and where possible to prevent disasters, mitigate their impact on vulnerable population and respond to and effectively cope with their consequences.

Formulate effective disaster emergency response mechanisms through,

- Development of action plan
- Development of disaster warning systems and plan for evacuation,
- Education and training to officials and people at risk
- Establishment of emergency response policies and standards.
- Education and training to local population in the community.

Disaster preparedness strategies: Disaster preparedness include measures that we can taken to reduce the effect of disasters that is to predict disasters, mitigate the impact, respond and to cope with consequences.

Disaster preparedness measures include,

- **Hazard, risk and vulnerability assessment:** Hazard refers to the potential occurrence in a specified time period and geographic area of a natural phenomenon that may adversely affect human life, property or activity to the extent of causing a disaster. Eg. Flood, cyclone.

Risk – Risk is a measure of expected loss due to a hazard. So risk assessment is important to identify potential hazard and consequences.

Vulnerability: The extent to which a community or geographic area is damaged or disrupted due to a hazard. For disaster preparedness it is important to know the vulnerabilities of the particular area and try to understand the type of disaster most likely to affect in an area.

For Disaster preparedness:

- Assess the potential severity of hazards of a community and identify the areas that are susceptible to hazards and the population and the infrastructure that might be affected.

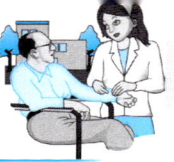

- Assess the disaster risk of the area
- Assess the status of health care facilities and potential areas for public shelters.
- Find out the available resources and assistance as personal, supplies, equipments and information system

- **Response mechanisms and strategies:** Response mechanisms and strategies include development and strengthening the emergency response mechanisms as evacuation procedures. Emergency management teams, emergency management systems in hospitals, preparation for emergency shelter centers, making arrangements for rapid acquisition of emergency relief supplies and equipment.
- **Preparedness planning:** Disaster preparedness planning involves identifying organizational resources and, planning preparedness activities for effective emergency response. The plan include Disaster preparedness plan, policy, co-ordination and communications with local organizations and NGOs. The type of response activities, include recruiting and training of volunteers in triaging and rescue, education and rehearsals for rescue and relief.
- **Coordination:** Disaster management requires coordinated efforts of people in the affected area and community based organizations, rapid response teams, civil, defense and Govt. agencies, various departments as revenue, health etc. and Non Governmental organizations. Proper coordination of all those teams are essential during disasters.
- **Information management:** Timely information before, during and after disaster are important for proper management of disaster. For that develop procedures and mechanisms for obtaining analyzing and responding to early warning system.
- **Early warning systems:** Early warning systems are necessary to detect, forecast and issue alert related to impending hazards. Early warning information usually comes from materiological departments, Ministry of Information and Technology, Disaster management authority etc. Early warning to public may help to reduce effect of hazards and impact.
- **Resource mobilization:** Disasterpreparedness measures include policies for acquisition and disbursement of funds and emergency funding strategies.
- **Public education and training:** The aim of education and training to public is to develop an alert and self-reliant community to support disaster management activities. It is important for each member in the family to get informed and increase awareness regarding disaster preparedness. So organize public education, training and reherssals of emergency rescue activities and mock drills to empower professionals, the public and NGO's.
- **Community based disaster management:** Local population, volunteers and organizations in the disaster prone and stricken areas should be empowered through education and training.

So the components of Disasterpreparedness include communitydisaster preparedness, field triage, preparedness in emergency department of hospitals.

Impacts of Disaster

The impacts of disaster can be classified as:
- **Physical and biological impact:** The physical hazards of the affected people may be different depending upon type of disaster. Some of the physical and biological hazards include disabilities, trauma and injury, fractures, deterioration of health, weakness, fatigue, burns and even death.
- **Social impacts:** Social impacts of disaster include loss of livelihood, loss of house andshelter, family disorganization, isolation, changes in lifestyle and cultural practices migration, risk for vulnerable population, interpretation in communication system etc.
- **Psychological impacts:** Psychological impact of victims may vary enormously in the ways they respond to disaster and the reactions include sadness, irritability, fear, anxiety, insecurity, stress, difficulty in sleeping, loss of trust, hopelessness, depression, feeling of withdrawn, insecurity feeling, sexual abuse and violence, lack of interest to live, stress and sometimes there are occurrence of post-traumatic stress disorders.
- **Environmental problems:** Poor environmental hygiene as lack of facilities for disposal of waste and excreta especially in shelter homes. Lack of adequate drinking water, presence of flies and vectors, inadequate hygiene, Interruptions of communication system are of the other impacts.
- **Community impacts:** The impact of disaster in the community include displacement of population, loss of loved ones and property, altered community structure, unemployment and all these disrupt community living.

Disaster Mitigation

Disaster mitigation activities are undertaken to lessen the severity of disaster or minimize the effect of disaster on human lives and property. Disaster mitigation refers to actions or measures that can either prevent the occurrence of a disaster or reduce the severity of its effects. Mitigation activities focus on measures for eliminating risks. (American Red cross).

Mitigation can be organized by making an investment of time, money and planning prior to occurrence of natural disaster.

According to United Nations International Strategy for Disaster Reduction (UNISDR,) Mitigation consists of a framework of activities that will help to minimize vulner abilities and disaster risks to avoid or to limit the adverse impacts of hazard.

Some of the mitigation measures include
- Hazard mapping
- Adoption and enforcement of land use
- Enforcement of building codes
- Public awareness
- Flood plain mapping etc.

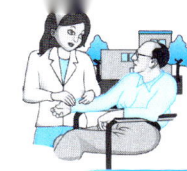

Mitigation activities include
- Non-structural mitigation and
- Structural Mitigation.

Structural Mitigation

Structured Mitigation. Structural mitigation is the act of protection from disaster or hazards by modifying physical construction of building to avoid possible impact of hazard. It includes construction of projects which reduce economic and social impact of activities as physical construction of building to reduce or avoid hazard, construction of disaster resistant infra-structure or construction of projects which reduce economic and social impacts of hazards. Common structural measures for risk reduction include dam flood levies, ocean wave barriers, earthquake resistant construction of building and evacuation shelters.

Non–structured disaster management activity include formulation of policies and practices, land use planning laws and their enforcement, having insurance schemes, planning education ,creating awareness and health education regarding local hazard and protection plan among public people, etc.

For Mitigation of disasters Government of India has initiated some preventive and mitigation activities. They are,
- National earth quake risk management project which aimed at strengthening structured and non structured management efforts and educing vulnerability in high risk areas by capacity building and public awareness.
- National building code which provide guidelines for regulating the building construction activities across the country.
- National cyclone risk management project. The aim of National Cyclone risk management to upgrade cyclone forecasting and warning system.
- National flood risk management project for reduction in diversity or consequences of flood, improve capability for relief and rehabilitation.
- Flood management scheme to provide financial assistance to state government for undertaking flood management activity.

Some of the other activities include measures to prevent road traffic accidents as design of road to enhance safety, public education, enforcement of rules and regulation, directions and training.

Disaster Management

India's geo-climatic conditions make it one of the disaster prone countries in the world and are facing many disasters which cause loss of life, damages and destruction of property. Disaster is an unpredictable event affecting a large number of population and cause disruption of normal life.

Disaster is defined as a catastrophe arising from natural or manmade causes results in substantial loss of life or human sufferings or damage to and disruption of property or degradation of environment.

India is prone to disaster due to many factors as geo – climatic conditions, population growth, socioeconomic conditions, deforestation, unplanned urbanization and so on.

Disaster management is the organization, planning and application of measures preparing for, responding to and initial recovery from disaster. Disaster management focuses or creating and implementing preparedness to reduce the impact of Disaster. (UNISDR – 2015)

Disaster management is a process of planning organizing measures focuses on to prevent hazards and consequences due to disaster, capacity building, proper formulation and coordination of activities of disaster preparedness, disaster mitigation, emergency rescue and relief, rehabilitation and reconstruction.

Objectives of Disaster Management

Identify individuals and department to act during disaster and specify their roles and responsibilities.

Plan and organize standard operating procedures for emergency response and relief during disaster.

Organize activities to reduce impact of disaster.

Principles of Disaster Management

- Well-developed disaster plan and trained disaster management team are essential for disaster management.
- Effective field triage is vital in reducing the impact of disaster.
- Establish command control centers and communication systems for proper management.
- Co-ordinated team work and emergency care of victim at the site of disaster are important for successful disaster management
- Maintenance of accurate communication of activities at disaster site are essential for disaster management.
- Health care facilities must be equipped with resources for emergency management of victims.

DISASTER NURSING: ROLE OF NURSE ADMINISTRATOR

The goal of disaster nursing is to provide best possible nursing service to promote the physical and emotional wellbeing of victims and community affected by disasters.

Nurses being member of disaster management team must have the qualities as confidence, good communication skill, co-ordination, leadership skill, responsibility and readiness to work in multi-disciplinary team, accountability and be able to do emergency first aid and resuscitation. They should be trained to manage emergency disasters. As members of disaster management team.

The nurse administrator are responsible to have emergency and disaster plan in the area in which she is working and knowledge regarding disaster prone areas and potential impact.

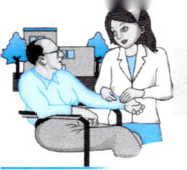

Awareness regarding disaster management policies, protocols and resources as disaster management agencies both (Govt. and NGO's) hospitals, ambulance services are essential.

The disaster management team must be adequately trained and know how to work together.

Plan to prepare individuals, family and community. Organize disaster drills with the help of Government and voluntary agencies to disaster management team members and also local volunteers.

Establish well-functioning communication system with modern technology to give early warning alerts to people prior to disaster.

Enhance public awareness through mass media communications.

During disaster initiate life saving measures, first aid, triaging and tagging the victim, care of injured and transportation of victims to higher level health care facilities.

In the hospital set emergency triage to provide emergency management to victims. In the emergency department it is the responsibility of nurses to receive the patent and according to risks or severity provide care.

Initiate immediate post disaster interventions as evacuation of victims and shelter. Areas for affected people management of shelter areas are important responsibility of nurses. Ensure adequate supply of safe drinking water, food, medicine, clothing etc. Population at riskbas mentally challenged, adolescents, elderly, under five children needs special care and attention.

Address physical needs of survivors . Approach survivors in a calm and quite manner .Provide food, shelter, water, clothing and immediate care of physical needs and problems.

In the rehabilitative phase the important activities that should be given considerations are epidemiologic surveillance and prevention and control of communicable diseases, environmental hygiene, proper disposal of waste and excreta.

Control of vector are important to provide a safe environment to prevent diseases. Be vigilant to avoid epidemic outbreaks by effective public education regarding healthy life style and hygiene. Nurses should encourage victims to overcome crisis. List in carefully to the victims and counsel them to return to normal life. Encourage them to share their feelings to prevent post traumatic distress syndrome. If necessary refer them to a psychologists or social worker.

In the rehabilitation phase a coordinated use of medical, social economic and vocational measures should be used. Training, counselling and education to each and every individual in the affected area is necessary to bring them to the highest possible level of functional ability.

Involve all government and non government agencies and resources to restore economic and civil life of the community.

Encourage people and family to resume normal activities and life. The interventions that nurses can do include acknowledgement of their perceptions and reality of the experiences, way to increase self carevand communication skill and referral of them to experts if necessary Establish trust and facilitate ventilation of feelings and refer those who need counseling and support.

Disaster survivors may display a wide range of anxiety and stress. Use therapeutic approach to address the needs of individual or family.

Development of community groups are necessary to facilitate support. Infection control team also have vital role in prevention of post disaster epidemics of communicable diseases, health of survivors who are in shelter homes etc.

At the end keep proper documentation regarding the situation, disaster management activities, issues and challenges faced and the lessons learned. Plan for disaster preparedness and mitigation.

Suggested Reading

- Billing MD, Halstead JA. Teaching in Nursing a guide for faculty. 3rd ed. Philadelphia: Saunders Elsevier Publishers; 2009.
- Heidger Ken LE. Teaching and learning in school of nursing. 4th ed. New Delhi: Konark Publishers; 2007.
- http://www.ncbi.nih.gov/pubmed/2601676.
- Kozier B, Erb G, Berman A, Burke K. Fundamentals of Nursing - Concepts, process and practice. 7th ed. Philadelphia: Pearson education; 2007. p. 201 - 03
- Stanhope M, Lancaster J. Foundations of nursing in the community. 2nd ed. Philadelphia: Mosby; 2006. P. 606
- Kishore J. Health programs in India. 7th ed.New Delhi: Century publications; 2007. P. 486 -87
- Lindeman CA, Mc Cathie M. Fundamentals of contemporary nursing practice. Philadelphia: Saunders; 1999. P.465
- Rosdahl CB, Kowalski MT. Textbook of basic nursing. 9th ed.Philadelphia: Lippincott W and W; 2008. P. 1597
- Nettina SM,. Manual of nursing practice. Philadelphia: Lippincott W and W; 2006. P. 20 -21
- Stone SC, Mcguire SL, Eigsti DG. Comprehensive community health nursing. 5th ed. USA: Mosby; 1998. p.724-25
- Hood LJ, Leddy SK. Conceptual basis of professional nursing. 6th ed. Philadelphia: Lippincott W and W; p.415
- http://www.cdacmohali.in S_Telenursing.aspx

Contd...

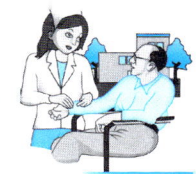

- http://wwww.crnns.ca/documents/telenursingpractice2008.pdf
- Katherine W.Vestal, Nursing management concepts and issues. J. B. Lippincott company 2nd Edn.
- Potter PA, Perry AG, Fundamentals of nursing, 6th ed:2006;Mosby an imprint of Elsevier; 477-87
- Roberta Straessle Abruzzesse. Nursing staff development: Strategies for success. Mosby year book.
- Nixon VY. Information technology in medical profession. Nightingale nursing times. 2007; 3 (6): 21-23
- www.americatelemed.org
- Health Employees Association of British Columbia. (1997). What an employer should know about performance evaluations. Revised November, 2002.
- Ashraf A. Constructing a nurse appraisal form: A Delphi technique study. Journal of Multidisciplinary Healthcare 2008: 1-14
- Introduction to management, Icfai center for management research: Hyderabad 2007: 285-298.
- Colmer Malcom R.Moroney's surgery for nurses.16th edn. Churchill Livingstone: Pearson professional limited; 1995. pp.110-12
- IGNOU.Nursing Audit.Nursing Foundation.New Delhi; 2004. 59-62
- Dhaulta P.Jaiwanti. Nursing Administration And Management; New Delhi: The
- Trained Nurses' Association Of India, 2007, Page 61-62.
- Basavanthappa B T. Nursing Adninistration.2nd edition. New Delhi; Jaypee brothers
- Marquis B L, Huston C J. Leadership roles and management functions in nursing- theory and application. 6th edition. Philadelphia: Lippincott William and Wilkins publications; 1996.
- Barett J. Ward management and teaching. 2nd edition. New Delhi: BS publications; 1967
- Finkelman W A. Leadership and management in nursing. 1st edition. Dorling Kindersley publications; 2009.
- Bessie L.Marquis, Carol J. Huston, Leadership roles and functions in nursing,theory and application, 2nd edition, Lippincott. p. 54-57
- Introduction to Management- Study Guide. The ICFAI Center for Management Research. Pno.21-27
- http://www.internationalbudget.org/resources/library/essentials.pdf
- http://www.entrepreneur.com/encyclopedia/term/82266.html
- http://www.economywatch.com/budget/budget-planning-planner.html
- http://www. Nursingdivision budgetinf pdf.
- BT Basavanthappa. Nursing Administration. New Delhi; Jaypee Brothers:152-159
- Evans, James R. (1994) Introduction to Statistical Process Control Archived October 29, 2013, at the Wayback Machine., *Fundamentals of Statistical Process Control*, pp 1–13
- The World Health Organization, Public Health Laboratory Quality Assurance: tools and training. http://www.euro.who.int/en/health-topics/Health-systems/laboratory-services/quality-tools-and-training
- "Managing Quality Across the Enterprise: Enterprise Quality Management Solution for Medical Device Companies". Sparta Systems. 2015-02-02
- *The Quality Assurance Journal*, ISSN 1087-8378, John Wiley and Sons
- *Quality Progress*, ISSN 0033-524X American Society for Quality
- *Quality Assurance in Education*, ISSN 0968-4883, Emerald Publishing Group
- *Accreditation and Quality Assurance*, ISSN 0949-1775

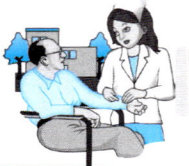

Assess Yourself

LONG ANSWER

1. Discuss in detail factors influencing ward management? Explain method of patient assignment with suitable examples.

SHORT NOTES

1. Job description
2. Methods of patient assignment
3. Duties and responsibilities of a head nurse
4. Four ethical concepts relating to nursing
5. Four factors affecting ward management
6. Role of head nurse in material management
7. Material management
8. Quality assurance
9. Nursing audit
10. Performance appraisal
11. Inventory control

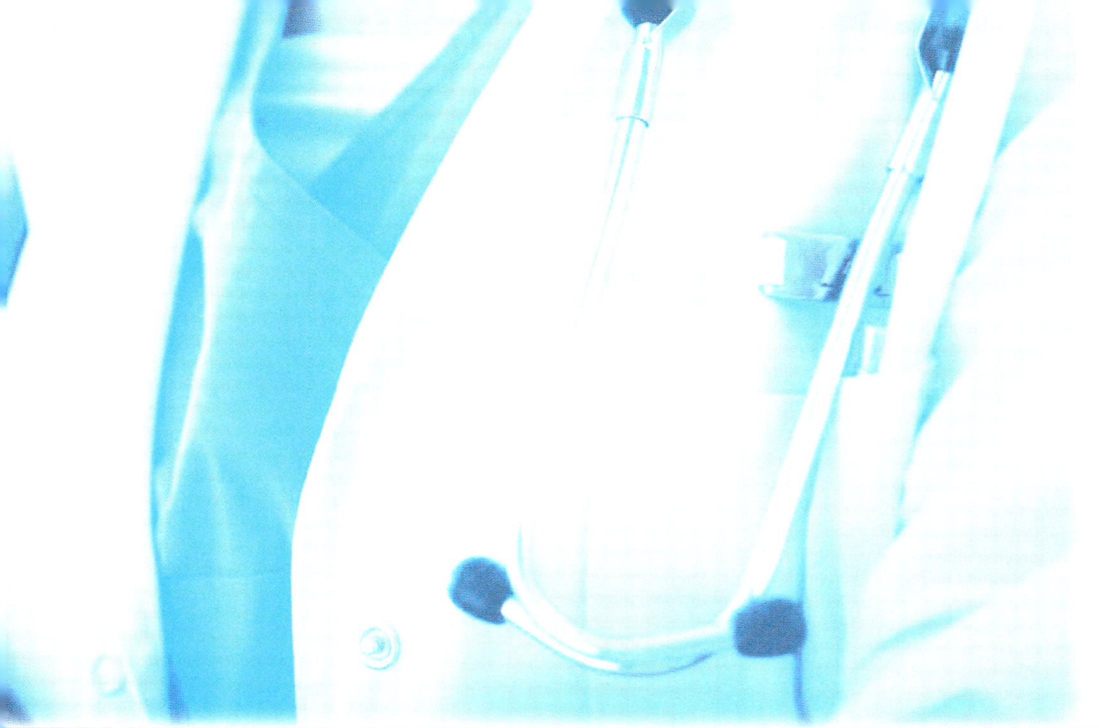

Unit 4

ORGANIZATIONAL BEHAVIOR AND HUMAN RELATIONS

Unit Outline

- Organizational Behavior
  - Definition
  - Concepts of Organizational Behavior
  - Elements/Factors Affecting Organizational Behavior
  - Approaches to Organizational Behavior
  - Organizational Behavior Models
  - Dependent and Independent Variables in Organizational Behavior
  - Challenges for Organizational Behavior
  - Communication
  - Transactional Analysis
  - Johari Window
  - Leadership
  - Motivation
  - Group Dynamics
- Human Relations
  - Public Relations
  - Union
  - Collective Bargaining

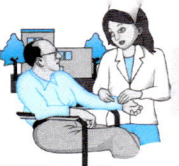

ORGANIZATIONAL BEHAVIOR

The management of organization is a challenging task. Global competition, increasing diversity, knowledge and information explosion and emphasis on total quality management makes an organization more challenging. To meet these challenges the administrator needs participation and cooperation from all employees in the organization. For effective management of organization an in-depth study of behavior of individuals within the work group is necessary.

Organizational behavior (OB) is valuable for examining the dynamics of relationship within small groups, both formal teams and informal groups. It also helps managers to examine the dynamics of relationship within a group and also to assess the behavior of employees. Organizational behavior is the study of both group and individual performances and activities within an organization. It examines the human behavior in the work environment and determines its impact on job structure, performance, communication, motivation, leadership, etc. It is the interdisciplinary field that includes sociology, psychology, communication and management.

DEFINITION

Organizational behavior is the field of study that investigates the impact that individuals, groups, organizational structure and behavior have within the organization for the purpose of applying such knowledge towards improvement of organizational effectiveness.

Organizational behavior is the study and application of knowledge about human behavior related to other elements of an organization such as structure, technology and social system. Organizational behavior is directly concerned with understanding, production and management of human behavior in organizations
—*Fred Luthans*

Organizational behavior is the study of application of knowledge about how people act within organization. It is human tool for human benefit and applies behavior of people in all types of organizations.
—*Keith Davis*

Organizational behavior is the field of study that investigates the impact that individuals, groups and structures have on behavior within the organizations for the purpose of applying such knowledge towards improving an organizations effectiveness
–*Stephens P Robbins*

Organization behavior is the systematic study of the action and attitudes that people exhibit within the organizations.

CONCEPTS OF ORGANIZATIONAL BEHAVIOR

- It is the field of study which investigates the impact that individuals, groups and structure have on behavior within the organization.
- It is the study and application of knowledge about how people act within the organization.
- It is the human tool for human benefit.
- It applies broadly to the behavior of the people in all types of organizations such as business, government, schools and service organization.
- It covers three dimensions of behavior in an organization: individuals, groups and structure.
- Organization behavior is the field of application and applies the knowledge gained about individuals and effect of structure of behavior in order to make organization more effective.
- Organization behavior covers the core topics of motivation, leadership, behavior and power.
- Organizational behavior is the study of human behavior in organizational settings, the interference between human behavior and organization and within the organization itself.

ELEMENTS/FACTORS AFFECTING ORGANIZATIONAL BEHAVIOR (FIG. 1)

- **People:** People are internal social systems. People are living, thinking, feeling beings who work in the organization to achieve objectives. This social system consists of individuals and groups. Each individual is unique. The administration has to deal with them and make them adapt to the environment. They form dynamic groups which may change and dissolve.
- **Structure:** Structure includes the forms of relationship of people in the organization, Organizational structure leads to division of work so that people can perform their duties to achieve the goals. Structure shapes employee's attitude and facilitates and motivates them to perform on higher level of performance.
- **Technology:** Technology provides the resources with which people can work and it affects the task that they perform. It allows doing work in better way.
- **Environment:** All organizations operate within the external and internal environment. Organization has to adapt in accordance with the changes of the environment for survival.

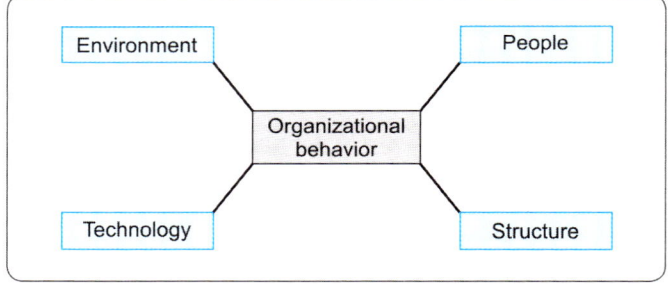

Figure 1: Elements affecting organizational behavior

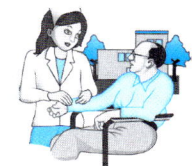

APPROACHES TO ORGANIZATIONAL BEHAVIOR

Different theoretical frame works will help to give a clearer perspective of OB. These approaches are as follows:

Behavioristic Approach

This approach is the outcome of the efforts by Pavlov and John B. Watson. They made an effort to establish the importance of observable behavior in learning. They tried to explore and understand behavior in terms of stimulus-response. The focus of the study was on the impact of the stimulus and a conclusion was drawn that learning took place when stimulus-response connection was established.

Cognitive Approach

The cognitive approach draws its inputs from various sources. Cognition takes place before the actual behavior, thereby forming an important input in an individual's thinking process or perception and processing of information. Cognition definitely plays an important role in determining behavior.

Social Learning Approach

Both behavioristic and cognitive approaches have been criticised as being deterministic. The cognitive theorists believe that the stimulus-response model gives a mechanical explanation of human behavior. The scientific approach used in the operant model has also immensely contributed to the study of human behavior.

The social learning approach is a behavioral approach. This approach goes by the belief that people are aware of their behavior and thus are engaged in purposive behavior. People are aware of their environment and try to modify and create the environment, which provides reinforcing variables.

Albert Bandura was of the opinion that the only way to define behavior was by explaining it in the form of a long lasting reciprocal interaction between behavioral, cognitive and environmental determinants. The person as well as the environmental situation cannot be treated as isolated independent units but are said to be in conjunction with the behavior itself and thus mutually interact to determine behavior.

ORGANIZATIONAL BEHAVIOR MODELS

Every organization develops a particular model in which behavior of the people takes place. This model is developed on the basis of management's assumptions about people and the vision of the management. Since these assumptions vary to a great extent, these result in the development of different organizational behavior models (OB models). In the field of OB, assumptions about people are on two extreme sides.

Two alternative approaches have been adopted for placing trust in people. One says "trust everyone unless there is a contrary evidence"; another says "do not trust anyone unless there is a contrary evidence". Naturally, interpersonal interactions take place differently under these two approaches.

Davis' OB Model

Davis has described four OB models which are as follows:
- Autocratic
- Custodial
- Supportive
- Collegial

Autocratic Model

In the autocratic model, managerial orientation is towards power. Managers see authority as the only means to get the things done, and employees are expected to follow orders. The result is high dependence on boss. This dependence is possible because employees live on the subsistence level. The organizational process is mostly formalized; the authority is delegated by right of command over people to whom it applies. The management decides what the best action for the employees is? The model is largely based on the 'Theory of X' assumptions of McGregor, where human beings are taken to find it inherently distasteful to work and try to avoid responsibility. A very strict and close supervision is required to obtain desirable performances from them. The autocratic model represents traditional thinking, which is based on the economic concept of man.

Custodial Model

In the custodial model, the managerial orientation is towards the use of money to pay for employee benefits. The model depends on the economic resources of the organization and its ability to pay for the benefits. While the employees hope to obtain security, at the same time they become highly dependent on the organization. An organizational dependence reduces personal dependence on boss. The employees are able to satisfy their security needs. Although employees working under a custodial model feel happy, their level of performance is not very high. Since employees are getting adequate rewards and organizational security, they feel happy. However, they are not given any authority to decide what benefits are best suited to the employees. Such an approach is quite common in many business organizations.

Supportive Model

The supportive model depends on managerial leadership rather than on the use of power or money. The aim of managers is to support employees in the achievement of results. The focus is primarily on participation and involvement of employees in managerial decision-making process. The supportive model is based on the assumption that human beings move to the maturity level and they expect the organizational climate which supports this.

Collegial Model

Collegial model is an extension of supportive model. The term 'collegial' refers to a body of people having common purpose. Collegial is based on the team concept in which each employee develops high degree of understanding towards others and shares common goals. Employees need little direction and control from management.

The Decision Making Model

Organizations are born with the purpose that more can be achieved by people working together in harmony and towards a stated goal. This is possible only if all resources - technology, expertise, information, finance and land are obtained for the stated goal/purpose. This involves taking decisions on activities which have to be determined, co-ordinated and controlled.

In an organization, decisions have to be taken at all levels. Irrespective of the level, there are certain fundamental aspects which have to be considered if the decision making process is to be effective and successful. The decision making model and process is given in the form of (a) Progression and (b) Process.

Various stages of decision making model are:

- **Defining the problem:** This is the first step in any process. Because only if the problem is defined, the likely effects and the outcome of the particular course(s) of action can be foreseen and understood.
- **Determination of the process:** This will to a great extent depend on the organizational culture, structure, environmental factors, working style and personality of persons involved in the decision making.
- **Time scale:** The time scale will depend on process determination and the quality and volume of information required and the time available to do this.
- **Gathering information:** Decision making process is based on the receipt of perfect information. Care needs to be exercised to ensure availability of quality information along with the means for understanding, evaluating and review of what has been gathered.
- **Identify the alternatives:** The result of the process is to identify the alternative courses of action.
- **Implementation:** The final course of action arrived at, will affect the future decisions. So the reasons for approving the final course of action are to be understood. It is necessary to understand that the implementation stage is a means by which opportunities and consequences of following the particular courses of action will be understood, assessed and evaluated.

There could be other factors affecting the decision making. These may be termed as:

1. Risk and uncertainty
2. Participation and consultation
3. Organizational adjustment
    - **Risk and uncertainty:** These two factors exist when insufficient information is available and the accuracy of its evaluation is in doubt. The element of risk and uncertainty in decision making can be avoided if a lot of emphasis is put on the quality and accuracy of the information gathered.
    - **Participation and consultation:** Participation and consultation will help generate understanding and acceptance of a courses of action. It also involves considering the legal aspects, government regulations and the interest of all persons concerned.
    - **Organizational adjustment:** The decision made usually involve adjustment/alteration on the part of the organization. Effective decisions are finally arrived at by combining the preferred and chosen direction, along with accommodating the means by which chosen decisions can be made successful.

Robbin OB Model

The three levels Robbin's OB Model are: individual level, group level and organization systems level.

DEPENDENT AND INDEPENDENT VARIABLES IN ORGANIZATIONAL BEHAVIOR

Dependent Variables

- *Productivity:* An organization is said to be productive if its output performance is effective as well as efficient. A business firm is said to be effective if it is able to achieve its market share goals and sales targets. Organizational efficiency will be measured by its high Return on investment (ROI); profit per rupee of sale and output per hour of labor. The dependent variables are:
- Absenteeism
- Turnover which could also be a reflection of the employee's perception of job satisfaction
- Job satisfaction
- Organizational citizenship

Independent Variables

Organizational behavior can be best understood if it is viewed as interlinking of the three levels of employee's behavior - individual, group and organization systems - level variables.

- **Individual level variables:** Each employee who joins an organization has certain characteristics which will influence his or her behavior at work. These characteristics are personal or biological such as age, gender, marital status, personality characteristics, an inherent emotional frame work, values and attitudes, basic ability levels, perception, learning, motivation and individual decision making. All the above variables are unique to each individual and definitely affects employee behavior and very often the management can do little to alter it.

- **Group level variables:** The behavior of people in groups is different from that of their individual behavior. It will be necessary to understand group dynamics - factors that influence people to exhibit certain patterns of behavior, group's acceptable standards of behavior, the communication pattern, leadership styles, power and politics, levels of conflicts in group etc.
- **Organization systems level variables:** Organizations are more than the sum of their individual member groups. The formal organization structure, specifically the design of the formal organization, work processes and jobs, the firm's HR policies and practices and work culture all have an impact on the dependent variables.

The model also refers to concepts of change and stress at the individual, group and organizational levels.

CHALLENGES FOR ORGANIZATIONAL BEHAVIOR

The relevance of understanding OB has tremendous significance in today's world, especially with constant changes and the uncertainty prevalent in the highly volatile environment in which organizations exist. This makes necessary for an organization to understand the changing employee profiles and behavioral patterns. Some of the changes affecting individuals and firms could be:
- The average age of any working Indian employee is growing younger and younger.
- Employees do not want to stick to the same organization throughout their lifetime.
- The average employee always seeks courses and programs which will lead to self development opportunities.
- Organizations have realised the need for downsizing and are offering Voluntary Retirement Scheme (VRS) to employees in order to become more proactive entities especially to match technological advances.
- In the post liberalisation age, the advent of the MNCs have made Indian companies wake up to adopt cutting edge strategies to meet and beat their foreign counterparts.

These changes have posed challenges for OB. One of the biggest challenges before organizations is how to attract, manage and nurture talented employees.

The challenges for use of organizational behavior include:
- Responding to globalization
  Now a days the entire world has turned in to a global village and employees in many parts of the world have advanced skills and knowledge and they struggle to produce quality outcomes.
- Managing workforce diversity
  Managing workforce diversity is one of the major challenges faced by management. Workforce diversity means the heterogeneity of employees in organizations in terms of their age, gender, culture, ethnicity, etc. Failure to manage workforce diversity may cause problems like conflict, turnover of employees, ineffective communication etc.
- Total quality management
  Now a days consumers are more conscious about quality care and consumer satisfaction is a big challenge. So managers have to observe the latest trends in management and advancements in technology and determine the right structure and process for organization to be competent.

COMMUNICATION

Communication is sending and receiving information. It is exchanging information by speaking, writing or using some other medium.

Communication has been derived from the Latin word 'communis' that means 'common'. Thus to communicate means to make common or to make known to share and includes verbal, non verbal and electronic means of human interaction. It is a meaningful exchange of information between two persons or group of people.

Definition

A process by which two or more people exchange ideas, facts, feelings, 'common understanding of meaning, intent and use of a message'.   –*Paul Leagens*

Communication refers to 'imparting, the conveying or the exchanging of ideas, knowledge, meanings among individuals through the medium of a sign of some kind', e.g. symbol.

Communication is any act by which one person gives or receives information from other person about that person's needs, desires, perception and knowledge.

Communication Process

Communication occurs as a sequence of process which begins with a sender who sends (encodes) the message and passes it to receiver. This is done through a channel. Communication is fruitful if and only if, the messages sent by the sender are interpreted with same meaning by the receiver. If any kind of disturbance blocks any step of communication, the message will be destroyed. Thus the managers must locate such barriers and take steps to get rid of them (Fig. 2).

Communication process, or *communications management* process, is a set of steps that are taken every time formal communications are undertaken in an organization. A communications process is undertaken as part of communications management and helps to ensure that stakeholders are kept regularly informed.

Types of Communication

- **Based on channels of communication,** communication can be classified as **verbal communication** and **non-verbal communication**.
  - **Verbal communication:** In verbal communication there is face to face communication. It can be either written or spoken from of communication.

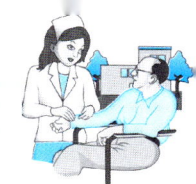

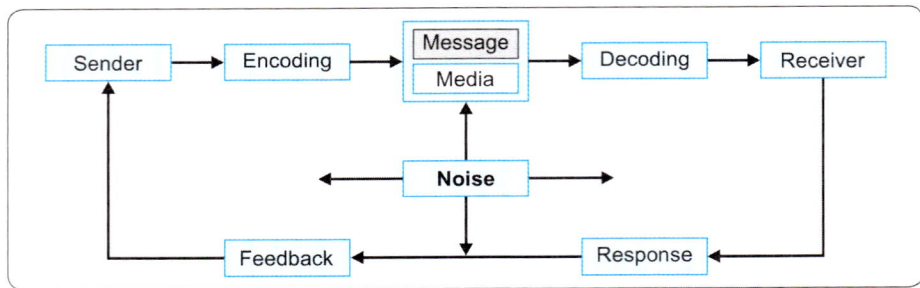

Figure 2: Process of communication

- **Non-verbal communication:** Nonverbal communication includes body languages, facial expression, gestures and physical appearance.
- Another type of communication is **Para verbal communication** that is with the use of tone, pitch and volume used during a verbal communication.
- **Based on style and purpose:** According to this, communication can be classified as formal and informal.
  - **Formal communication:** In formal communication, the style of communication is formal and it generally follows a well-defined hierarchical pattern. The communication in this form is formal and official. Official conferences and staff meetings are some examples of formal communication. Written memos, letters, circulars agreements and reports are some of the channels that facilitate formal communication.
  - **Informal communication:** Informal communication takes place in unstructured manner between co-workers, friends and family members. Informal communication takes place through informal talks, conversations etc. There is no hierarchy or guidance for informal communication.

Channels of Communication

- **Downward communication:** Downward communication moves from top to bottom from manager to subordinates. It includes, all written and oral communication from top level management to bottom level management and to employees. Example: manager to subordinates.
- **Upwards communication:** Upward communication moves from bottom to top level in the hierarchy. Here communication moves from employers to supervisors, supervisors to executives and so on.
  Example: Subordinates to management
- **Lateral or horizontal Communication:** In lateral communication, the communication is neither upward nor downwards. It progresses in a horizontal way. It occurs between two departments or person's at the same level of hierarchy. Example: Employee → Employer
  Manager → Manager

Barriers of Communication

There are several barriers in community which interrupt the flow of communication from sender to receiver. The main barriers of communication are:

- **Perceptual and language differences:** Language difference leads to incorrect or incoherent messages. The messages that are expressed poorly due to lack of clarity in communication, improper organization of ideas and poor expression are considered barriers.
- **Faulty transmission:** During the process of transmission also there are errors in communication. Here the purpose of message may not remain the same as it transmits from sender to receiver.
- **Environmental barriers:** Physical factors in the surroundings as noise, poor lighting, uncomfortable environment may affect communication. Noise is a factor which always disturbs communication other environmental barriers are—defect in the instruments or gadgets used for communication, disturbances in power, etc.
- **Employee–employer related factors:** It includes physical, psychological, linguistic, cultural factors and so on. The barriers include poor eye contact, poor emotional state, lack of clarity in conveying message, lack of consistency in communication, poor understanding of message etc.
- **Psychosocial factors**: There may be poor expression when the employees are fatigued and under severe stress. Stress, personal difficulties, worries, tension etc cause communication barriers.
- **Non-verbal communication barriers**: Some of the nonverbal communication barriers are eye rolling, deep and loud talking, failure to make eye contact, failing to pay attention or listening etc. are nonverbal barriers.
- **Verbal communication barriers:** They include asking closed ended questions, blaming client, constant interruption, making generalization, offering vague reassurance pointing finger while speaking etc. Paraverbal communication barriers include threatening or ordering taking rapidly.

TRANSACTIONAL ANALYSIS

Transactional analysis is a theory developed by Dr. Eric Berne in 1950. Transactional analysis is a very simple, early comprehensible method in understanding human behavior.

A 'transaction' is defined as an exchange between two people. The exchange is of thoughts and of feelings, expressed verbally in words or conveyed non-verbally in voice, variations and gestures. Study of such social transactions is known as Transactional Analysis. It is used to study and analyze interpersonal communication.

The objective of Transactional Analysis is to provide better understanding of how people relate to one another so that they may develop improved communication and human relationship.

Eric Berne also state that each person is made up of their alter ego statics.

- **Parent ego state:** Parent ego state is a set of feelings, thinking and behavior that we have copied from our parents and significant others. As we grow we receive ideas, beliefs, feelings and behaviors from our parents and caretakers. The characteristics of a person with parent ego states are judgmental, moralizing, overprotective and indispensable. Parent is our 'taught' concept of life. Adult is our 'thought' concept of life and child is our 'felt' concept of life.
- **Adult ego state:** Adult state is the ability to think and determine action for ourselves based on receive data. The adult ego has the capacity for understanding. People with adult ego state gather information carefully, analyze it, generate alternatives and make logical states.
- **Child ego state:** The child ego state is a set of behaviors, thoughts and feelings which are repaid from our own childhood. The important features of child ego are creativity, anxiety, depression, dependence, fear, joy, etc.

A transaction involves a stimulus and response

Types of Transactions

- Complementary or parallel transactions
- Crossed transaction
- Ulterior transactions

- **Complementary or parallel transactions:** Referes to the exchange of ideas in which the arrows are parallel. Here the conversation tends to flow back and forth in a consistent form

When transactions are complementary, communication will continue undisturbed (Fig. 3).

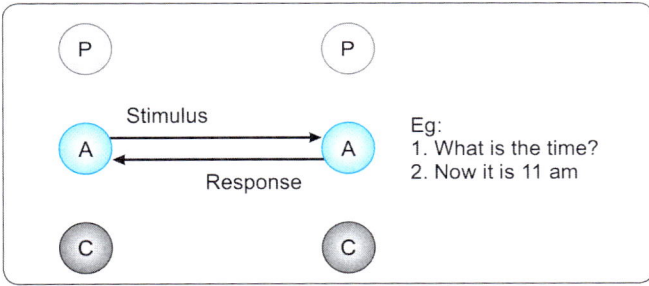

Figure 3: Adult to adult complementary transaction

- **Crossed transactions:** If the response is not from response R to stimuli (S), but from any other ego state, the two lines will cross each other. The transaction is then called crossed transaction. It is an unexpected response (Fig. 4).

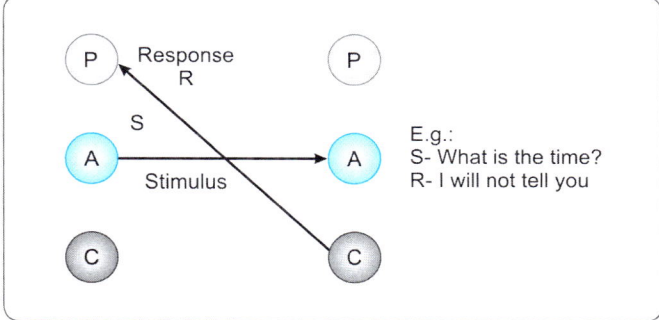

Figure 4: Adult to adult, parent to child crossed transaction

- **Ulterior transactions:** Interactions, responses, actions which are different from those explicitly stated (Fig. 5).

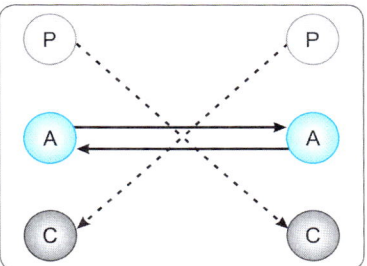

Figure 5: Ulterior transactions

Transactional Analysis – Life Positions (Fig. 6)

The important concept of transactional analysis is life positions. Life positions are basic beliefs about oneself and about others in general. Basically there are four life positions.

I am OK, you are OK

It appears to be an ideal life position. People with this type of life positions have confidence in themselves as well as trust and confidence in others. This behavior is respectful, supportive and collaborative.

I am OK you are not OK

This is a distrustful psychological positions. This is the attitude of those people, who think that whatever they do is correct. There is arrogance, lack of trust, tendency to blame everyone, feel annoyed, non–cooperative and unfriendly.

I am not OK you are OK

This is a common position for those people who feel powerless when they compare themselves to others. The person is insecure and depressed.

I am no OK, you are not OK

People in this position tend to feel bad about them and see the whole world is miserable. They do not trust others. Person is indifferent and neglect. They have no confidence in themselves.

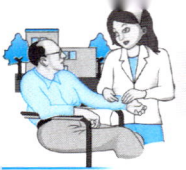

	You are okay with me		
I am not okay with me	I am not OK You are OK Own down position Get away from helpless	I am OK You are OK Healthy position Get on with happy	I am okay with me
	I am not OK You are not OK Hopeless position Get nowhere with hopeless	I am OK You are not OK You are not OK One – up position Get rid of angry	
	You are not OK with me		

Figure 6: Life positions of transactions

Transactional Analysis–Strokes

Strokes are the acts of an individual to get recognition. People need strokes for their sense of survival and well being on the job. Lack of stroking can have negative consequences both on physiological and psychological wellbeing of a person. The three types of strokes are:

- **Positive strokes:** The stroke one feel good is a positive stroke. Recognition, compliment, praise, approval and rewards are examples of positive stroke.
- **Negative strokes:** A stroke one feel or not good is a negative stroke. eg: criticism, degrading, punishment, ridicule. Negative strokes hurt physically and psychologically.
- **Mixed stroke:** A stroke may be mixed type also

Games Analysis

When people fail to get enough strokes at work they try a variety of things. One of the most important thing is that they play psychological games. They provide satisfaction to the players. Game players fall into one of these basic categories.

Persecutors → Those people make unrealistic rules, implement those rules in crucial ways.

Victim → These people do the things to put others down, use them and to hurt them.

Rescuer → these people help others to keep others dependent on them.

Benefits/Utility of Transactional Analysis

- Improved interpersonal communication
- Understanding ego state
- Motivation
- Organizational development
- Source of positive energy
- Useful at work and management of organization
- Demonstrated successful in organization

Transactional analysis is a good method for understanding interpersonal behavior. It offers a model of personality and dynamics of self and its relationship to others that makes possible a clear and meaningful discussion of behavior.

	Information known to others	Information not known to others
Information known to others	1 Open self (Public area)	2 Blind self (Blind area)
Information not known to others	3 Hidden self (Private area)	4 Unknown self (Dark area)

Figure 7: Johari window

JOHARI WINDOW

A johari window is a communication model developed by American psychologist Joseph Luft and Harry Ingham. This model can be used to improve relationship between groups and it became a widely accepted tool for understanding and training self-awareness, interpersonal relations, team development etc.

The above Figure 7 indicates that there are four parts(self) in all of us that has been indicated by four quadrants.

- **Open self (Public area):** It indicates information about self is known to oneself and also to others .The information relates to feelings ,motivation and behavior of an individual, knowledge skill etc which he is willing to share with those whom he comes in conduct. The individual behaves in a straight forward manner and is sharing. In the organizational setting, because of the openness of the individuals the chances of conflict are reduced to minimum.
- **Blind self (Blind area):** The information is not known to self but known to others who interact with you, know more about you. This area is known as blind area. It is important that an individual should reduce blind area to the maximum by interacting with people more intimately and by asking questions about self. By seeking feedback from others the individual aims to reduce this area and increase open area that is self-awareness. So managers should help an individual to reduce their blind area by giving feedback. Therefore individual should reduce conflict situations to a great extent in interpersonal behavior
- **Hidden self (Private area):** Self knows information but others do not know it. There are certain aspects , which are private , such type of area is called hidden area, and it include sensitiveness, fears, secrets, hidden agenda, etc. Individual therefore does not want to share it with subordinates and wants to keep hidden. By sharing these feelings with others we can reduce hidden areas and it enables better understanding co-operation, trust and team working effectiveness
- **Unknown self (Dark area):** It is characterized by facts unknown to the self and to others. There is nothing much that can be done about it. It should be an endeavour to improve upon one self by obtaining feedback from others about self. Individuals should carry out improvement and perceive oneself correctly so that one perceives each person in the right manner. Managers can provide opportunity to employees to try new things to discovers

unknown abilities. So manager should all ways try to reduce blind area and increase open areas by proper feedback.

LEADERSHIP

Leadership is the ability of a manager to induce subordinates to work with confidence and zeal. It can be an important modification of behavior of people working in an organization.

A leader is a person who delegates or influences others to act so as to carry out the objectives of an organization. Health care organizations too need effective leaders to manage changing health care environment.

Leadership is stated as the "process of social influence in which one person can enlist the aid and support of others in the accomplishment of a common task.

Definition

- "Leadership is the art of motivating a group of people to act towards achieving a common goal".
- "Leadership is the quality of behavior of individuals whereby they guide people or their activities in organizing efforts" —*Chester Barnard*
- "Leadership is a process of giving purpose (meaningful direction) to collective effort, and causing willing effort to be expended to achieve purpose." —*Jacobs and Jaques*
- "Leadership is the process of influencing the activities of an individual or a group in efforts toward goal achievement in a given situation." —*Hersey and Blanchard*
- "Leadership is the ability to influence other people" —*Lansdale*
- "Leadership is influence—nothing more, nothing less" —*John C Maxwell*

Characteristics of Leadership

- Leadership is a continuous process of behavior and it is not one shot activity.
- Leader tries to influence the behavior of individuals around him/her to achieve common goals.
- Leadership gives an experience of help to followers to attain common goals.
- Leadership is exercised in a particular situation, at a given point of time, and under a specific set of circumstances.
- Leadership may be seen in terms of relationship between a leader and his followers, which arises out of their working for common goals.

Importance of Leadership

- **Motivating employees:** Motivation is necessary for work performance. Higher the motivation, better would be the performance. A good leader motivates the employees for high performance by exercising his leadership.
- **Creating confidence:** A good leader creates confidence among his followers by directing them, giving suggestions and getting good results.
- **Building morale:** Morale is the attitude of employees towards the organization, management and voluntary cooperation to offer their abilities to the organization. High morale leads to high productivity and organizational stability.

Theories of Leadership

Trait Theory

Trait is defined as *a relatively enduring quality of an individual.* The trait approach seeks to determine 'what makes a successful leader' from the leader's own personal characteristics. Research on leadership traits suggests that some factors differentiate leaders from non-leaders. The most important traits are a high level of personal drive, desire to lead, personal integrity, and self-confidence. Cognitive (analytical) ability, business knowledge, charisma, creativity and flexibility are also desired. The various traits can be classified into innate and acquirable traits, on the basis of their source.

Innate Qualities

Innate qualities are those which are possessed by various individuals since their birth. These qualities are natural and often known as God-gifted. The individuals cannot acquire these qualities. Major innate qualities in a successful leader are:

- *Physical features:* Physical features of a man are determined by heredity factors. Heredity is the transmission of the qualities from ancestor to descendent. Physical characteristics and rate of maturation determines the personality formation which is an important factor in determining leadership success.
- *Intelligence:* For leadership, higher level of intelligence is required. Intelligence is generally expressed in terms of mental ability. Intelligence, to a very great extent, is a natural quality in the individuals because it is directly related to the brain.

Acquirable Qualities

Acquirable qualities of leadership are those which can be acquired and enhanced through various processes. Many of these traits can be increased through training programs. Following are the major qualities essential for leadership:

- **Emotional stability:** A leader should have high level of emotional stability. He should be free from bias, consistent in action and refrain from anger. He should be well adjusted and must believe that he can meet most situations successfully.
- **Human relations:** A successful leader should have adequate knowledge of human relations. An important part of a leader's job is to develop people and get their voluntary cooperation for achieving work. He should have intimate knowledge of how human beings behave and how they react to various situations.
- **Empathy:** Empathy relates to observing the things or situations from other's points of view. The ability to look at things objectively and understanding them from others' point of view is an important aspect of successful leadership. Empathy requires respect for the rights, beliefs, values and feelings of others.

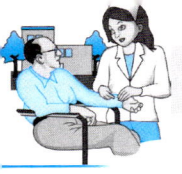

- **Objectivity:** Objectivity implies that what a leader does should be based on relevant facts and information. He should make an objective diagnosis and implement the action required.
- **Motivating skills:** A leader should be self-motivated and have the requisite quality to motivate his followers. There is an inner drive in people for motivation to work. The leader can play an active role in stimulating the inner drives of his followers.
- **Technical skills:** The ability to plan, organise, delegate, analyse, seek advice, make decisions, control and win cooperation requires the use of important abilities which constitute technical competence of leadership.
- **Communicative skills:** *A* successful leader knows to communicate effectively. A leader uses communication skilfully for persuasive, informative and stimulating purposes.
- **Social skills:** *A* successful leader has social skills. He understands people and knows their strengths and weaknesses. He has ability to work with people so that he gains their confidence and loyalty.

Behavioral Theory

According to this theory, a leader behaves according to the role expectations of the group. Strong leadership is the result of effective role behavior. To operate effectively, group needs someone to perform two major functions:
- Task related or problem solving functions and
- Group maintenance or social functions.

Assumptions

- Leaders can be made, rather than are born.
- Successful leadership is based in definable, learnable behavior.

Behavioral theories of leadership do not seek inborn traits or capabilities. Rather, they look at *what leaders actually do*. This leadership theory focuses on the actions of leaders, not on mental qualities or internal states.

This theory failed to explain why a particular leadership behavior is effective in one situation, but fails in another situation. Thus, situational variables are not considered.

McGregor Theory

Douglas McGregor categorized leadership style into two brand categories in his management theories, i.e. theory X and theory Y, having two different beliefs and assumptions about subordinates (Table 1).

McGregor (1906-1964) postulated that managers tend to make two different assumptions about human nature.

> **Box: 1**
>
> **Theory X**
> - The average human being has an inherent dislike of work and will avoid it if he or she can.
> - Because of this human characteristic, most people must be coerced, controlled, directed, and threatened with punishment to get them to put forth adequate effort toward the achievement of organizational objectives.
> - The average human being prefers to be directed, wishes to avoid responsibility, has relatively little ambition, and wants security above all.
>
> **Theory Y**
> - The expenditure of physical and mental effort in work is as natural as play or rest.
> - External control and threat of punishment are not the only means for bringing about effort toward organizational objectives. People will exercise self-direction and self-control in the service of objectives to which they are committed.
> - Commitment to objectives is a function of the rewards associated with their achievement.
> - The average human being learns, under proper conditions, not only to accept responsibility but to seek it.
> - The capacity to exercise a relatively high degree of imagination. Ingenuity, and creativity in the solution of organizational problems is widely, not narrowly, distributed in the population.
> - Under the conditions of modern industrial life, the intellectual potentialities of the average human being are only partially utilized.

An effective leader needs to examine carefully his own ideas about the motivation and behavior of subordinates and others, as well as situation, before adapting any particular leadership.

Table 1: McGregor theory

Basis of distinction	Theory X	Theory Y
1	2	3
View about the human behviour	It represents a negative or pessimistic view of human behavior	It represents a positive or optimistic view of human behavior
Liking for work	This theory assumes that people dislike work and will try to avoid work, if possible	This theory assumes that people regard work as natural as play or rest.
Direction	It also assumes that people seek direction from superior	It assumes that people will exercise self-control if they are committed to the objectives
Responsibility	It assumes that people avoid responsibility	It assumes that people seek and acept responsibility

Contd...

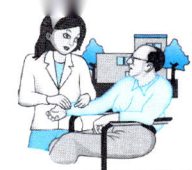

Basis of distinction	Theory X	Theory Y
1	2	3
Creativity and change	It assumes that people lack creativity and resist change	It assumes that people are creative by nature and ready to accept change.
Focus on needs	It focuses on lower-level needs i.e. physiological and safety needs	If focuses on higher-level needs i.e. social esteem and self-actualisation needs
Style of leadership	It represents autocratic leadership	It represents democratic leadership
Role of incentives	It emphasises the role of financial incentive in motivation	It emphasises the role of non-financial incentives in motivation
Role of job factors or job	It assumes key role of job factors in motivation	It assumes key role of job itself in motivation
Nature	It is a traditional theory of motivation	It is a modern theory of motivation
Applicability	It is more applicable to illiterate or unskilled and lower-level employees	It is more applicable to skilled employees occupying higher positions

Contingency Theory

Contingency theories propose that for any given situation there is a best way to manage. Contingency theories go beyond situational approaches, which observe that all factors must be considered when leadership decisions are to be made. Contingency theories attempt to isolate the key factors that must be considered and to indicate how to manage when those key factors are present.

The continuum of Leadership Behavior

The model put forward by Robert Tannenbaum and Warren H. Schmidt framed leadership in terms of choices managers may make regarding subordinates' participation in decision making (Fig. 8).

The actions shown at the left side of the continuum are relatively authoritarian; those at the right side are relatively participative (Fig. 8). The manager's choices depend on three factors:

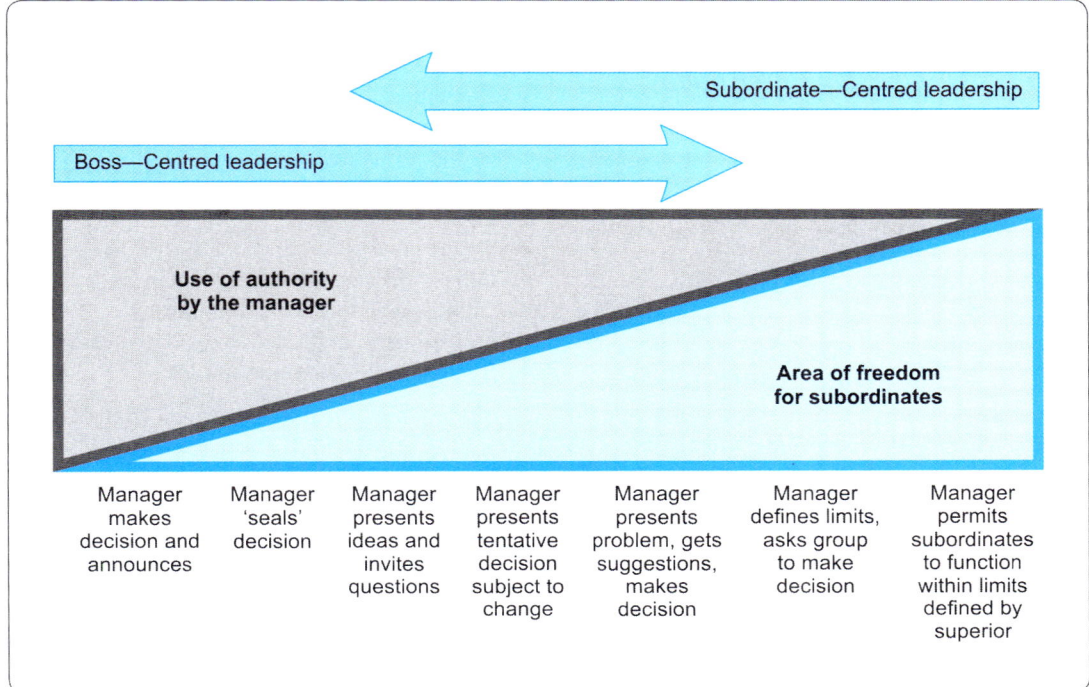

Figure 8: Continuum of leadership behavior

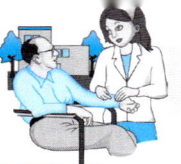

- **Forces in the manager:** The manager's value system, confidence in subordinates, leadership inclinations, and feelings of security in an uncertain situation.
- **Forces in the subordinate:** Expectations, need for independence, readiness to assume decision-making responsibility, tolerance for ambiguity in task definition, interest in the problem, ability to understand and identify with the goals of the organization, and knowledge and experience to deal with the problem.
- **Forces in the situation:** Type of organization, effectiveness of the group, the problem itself (the task) and time pressure.

Path Goal Theory (Situational Leadership)

The path-goal theory of leadership was developed to describe the way that leaders encourage and support their followers in achieving the goals they have set by making the path that they should take, clear and easy.

In particular, leaders:
- Clarify the path so subordinates know which way to go
- Remove roadblocks that are stopping them going there
- Increasing the rewards along the route

Leaders can take a strong or limited approach in these:
- In clarifying the path, they may be directive or give vague hints.
- In removing roadblocks, they may clear the path or help the follower to move the bigger blocks.
- In increasing rewards, they may give occasional encouragement or pave the way with gold.

This variation in approach will depend on the situation, including the follower's capability and motivation, as well as the difficulty of the job and other contextual factors.

Great Man Theory of Leadership/Charismatic Leadership Theory

The great man theory of leadership states that some people are born with the necessary attributes that set them apart from others and that these traits are responsible for their assuming positions of power and authority. This is also known as Charisma. *Charisma* is a Greek word, meaning 'gift'.

A leader is a hero who accomplishes goals against all odds for his followers. The theory implies that those in power deserve to be there because of their special endowment. Furthermore, the theory contends that these traits remain stable over time and across different groups. Thus, it suggests that all great leaders share these characteristic regardless of when and where they lived or the precise role in the history they fulfilled.

Limitation is, firstly, if we assume that there are certain inborn qualities of a great leader, it implies that nothing can be done to develop leaders in the organizations. But, through various training program, leaders can be developed in the organizations. Whereas, a charismatic leader may fail in a changed situation.

Leadership Styles

Leadership styles are the patterns of behavior which a leader adopts in influencing the behavior of his followers. Different leadership styles are either based on the behavioral approach or situation approach of leadership. Important theories/models prescribing leadership styles are given below:

Based on behavioral approach
- Power orientation
- Leadership as a continuum
- Employee-production orientation
- Likert's management system
- Managerial grid
- Tri-dimensional grid

Based on situational approach
- Fiedler's contingency model
- Hursey and Blanchard's situational model
- Path-goal model

Leadership Styles Based on Behavioral Approach

Lewin's Leadership Styles

Kurt Lewin and colleagues did leadership decision experiments in 1939 and identified three different styles of leadership, in particular around decision-making.

Autocratic/authoritarian style

In this style of leadership, a leader has complete command and hold over his employees/team. The team cannot put forward their views even if they are best for the team's or organizational interests. They cannot criticize or question the leader's way of getting things done. The leader himself gets the things done.

The advantage of this style is that it leads to speedy decision-making and greater productivity under leader's supervision.

The drawbacks of this leadership style are that it leads to greater employee absenteeism and turnover. This leadership style works only when the leader is the best in performing or when the job is monotonous, unskilled and routine in nature or where the project is short-term and risky.

In short,
- Strong control is maintained over the group
- Others are motivated by coercion
- Communication flows downwards
- Decision and making does not involves others
- Emphasis on difference and status

Democratic/ participative leadership style

In democratic leadership, the workers in the organization take a participative role in the decision making process. In this style of leadership every employee is given opportunity to participate in decision making.

The leaders invite and encourage the team members to play an important role in decision-making process, though the ultimate decision-making power rests with the leader. The leader guides the employees on what to perform and how to perform, while the employees communicate to the leader their experience and the suggestions if any.

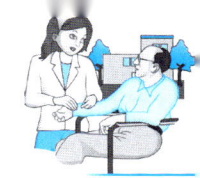

The advantages of this leadership style are that it leads to satisfied, motivated and more skilled employees. It leads to an optimistic work environment and also encourages creativity. The only drawback is time-consuming.

In short,
- Less control is maintained
- Economic and ego awards are used to motivate
- Others are directive through suggestions and guidance
- Communication flows up to down
- Decision making involves others
- Emphasise in 'We' rather than 'I' and 'You'
- Criticism is constructive

Laissez-Faire

The Laissez-Faire style is to minimize the leader's involvement in decision-making, and hence allowing people to make their own decisions, although they may still be responsible for the outcome.

Here, the leader totally trusts their employees/team to perform the job themselves. He just concentrates on the intellectual/rational aspect of his work and does not focus on the management aspect of his work. The team/employees are welcomed to share their views and provide suggestions which are best for organizational interests. This leadership style works only when the employees are skilled, loyal, experienced and intellectual.

In short,
- The manager is permissive with little or no control
- Motivates by support when requested by the group or individual
- Little or no direction is provided
- Communication between members of group and upwards and downwards
- Decision making is dispersed throughout the group
- Emphasis on the group
- Criticism is not given

Table 2: Comparison of different leadership styles

Variables	Autocratic	Democratic	Laissez faire
Control and direction	Strong control, directed with commands	Less control, directed with suggestions, guidance	No control, no direction, permissive
Motivation	Coercion	Economic/ego awards	Support when requested by individual/group
Emphasis	Difference in status (I and You)	We (group cohesion)	Group
Communication	Downward	Up and down	Upward downward grape wine
Decision making	Does not involve others	Involves group	Disperses throughout
Criticism	Punitive	Constructive	Does not criticize

Contd…

Leadership as a Continuum

There are a variety of styles of leadership behaviors between two extremes of automatic and free rein. Tannenbaum and Schmidt have depicted a broad range of styles on a continuum moving from authoritarian leadership behavior at one end to free rein behavior at the other end.

Each type of action represents the degree of authority used by a leader and the degree of freedom which a subordinate enjoys in relationship to his superior. The point along with the continuum at which, a manager adopts his behavior depends upon three aspects:

- Forces in the manager such as the manager's value system, his confidence in subordinates, his own leadership inclinations, and his feeling of security in an uncertain situation.
- Forces in subordinates such as a need for independence, readiness to assume responsibility for decision-making, level of tolerance for ambiguity, understanding and identifying organizational goals, interest in problems and the knowledge and experience to deal with the problems.
- Forces in the situation such as type of organization, group effectiveness, the problem itself and the pressure of time.

Employee-Production Orientation

Studies have shown about employee orientation and production orientation. The employee orientation stresses the relationship aspects of employees' jobs. It emphasises that every individual is important and takes interest in every one, accepting their individuality and personal needs. Production orientation emphasises production and technical aspects of jobs and employees are taken as tools for accomplishing the jobs.

The leadership studies initiated by the Bureau of Research at Ohio State University identified two dimensions of leader behavior: Initiating structure and considerations. **'Initiating structure'** refers to the leader's behavior in delineating the relationship between himself and members of the work group. **'Consideration'** refers to behavior indicative of friendship, mutual trust, respect, and warmth in the relationship between the leader and the members of his staff. Leadership behavior can be plotted on two separate axes.

The four quadrants show various combinations of initiating structures and considerations. In each quadrant, there is a relative mixture of initiating structure and consideration and a manager can adopt any one style (Fig. 9).

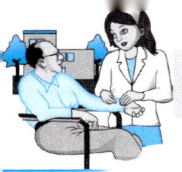

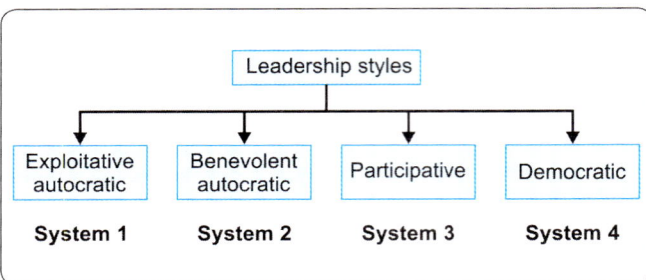

Figure 9: Leadership quadrants

Figure 10: Likert's leadership styles

Likert's Management System

Rensis Likert and his associates have studied the patterns and styles of managers and developed certain concepts about leadership behavior. He has given a continuum of four systems of management. Likert has taken seven variables of different management systems. These variables include leadership, motivation, communication, interaction influence, decision making process, goal setting and control process (Fig. 10). Likert's four systems of management in terms of leadership styles may be referred to as:

- Exploitative autocratic (System 1)
- Benevolent autocratic (System 2)
- Participative (System 3)
- Democratic (System 4). High producing departments are marked by System 4 (democratic).

He states that leadership and other processes of the organization must be such as to ensure a maximum probability that, in all interactions and in all relationships within the organization, each member will view the experience as supportive and the one which builds and maintains sense of his personal worth and importance.

Likert has also isolated three variables which are representative of his total concept of System. These are: (i) the use of supportive relationships by managers; (ii) the use of group decision-making and group methods of supervision; and (iii) his high performance goals.

Leadership Styles Based on Situational Approach

Fiedler's Contingency Model

The appropriateness of leadership styles depends on their matching with situational requirements. Leadership effectiveness is situational. Fiedler along with his associates made an attempt to identify the situational variables and their relationship with appropriateness of leadership styles. Fiedler's model consists of three elements: leadership styles, situational variables, and their inter-relationship (Fig. 11).

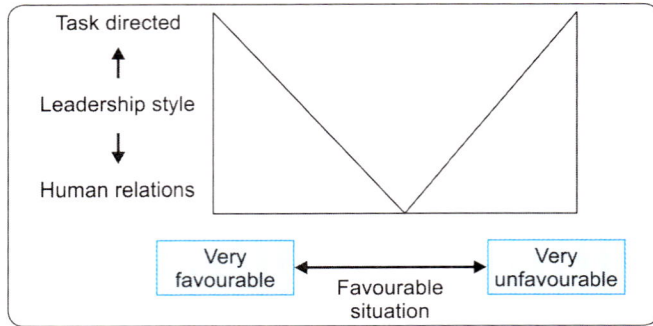

Figure 11: Fiedler model of leadership

Leadership Styles

Fiedler has identified leadership styles on two dimensions: task-directed and human relations oriented. **Task-directed** style is primarily concerned with the achievement of task performance. **Human relations** style is concerned with achieving good inter-personal relations and achieving a position of personal prominence.

Situational variables: Fiedler has identified three critical dimensions of situation which affect a leader's most effective style. These are leader's position power, task structure and leader-member relations.

Leaders position power: This is determined by the degree to which a leader derives power from the position held by him in the organization which enables him to influence the behavior of others

Task structure: Task structure refers to the degree to which the task requirements are clearly defined in terms of task objectives, processes and relationship with other tasks.

Leader-member relations: It is the degree that tells about follower's confidence, trust and respect in the leader.

All these situational variables taken together may define the situation to be favourable or unfavourable (Fig. 12).

A very favourable situation is one (cell 1) where leader-member relations are good, task is highly structured, and the leader has enormous position power to influence his subordinates. At the other extreme, a very unfavourable situation is one (cell 8) where leader-member relations are poor, task is highly unstructured, and leader's position power is weak. Between these two extremes, the degree of favourableness/unfavourableness varies.

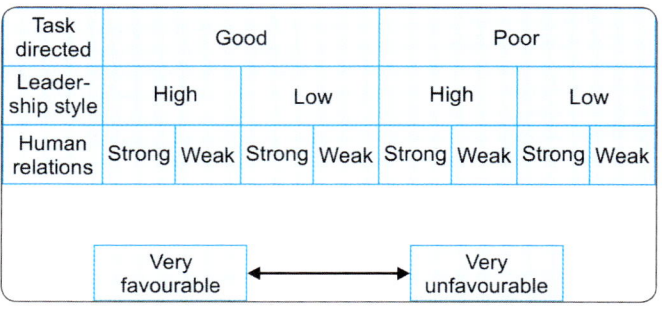

Figure 12: Favourableness/unfavourableness of situation

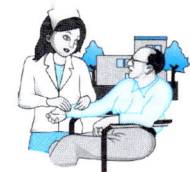

Task and relationship oriented		
High	High relationship and low risk	High relationship and high risk
Low	Low relationship and low task	Low relationship and high task
	Low	High
	Task orientation	

Figure 13: Leadership behavior styles

Fiedler feels that the effectiveness of leadership style depends on the situation. Appropriateness of leadership styles in different situations is given below:

Task-directed and human relations oriented styles tend to be effective in different situations:

Task-directed leadership styles tends to be better in group situations that are either very favourable or very unfavourable to the leader.

Human relations oriented leadership styles tends to be good in group situations that are intermediate in favourableness.

Hursey-Blanchard's Situational Model

Hursey and Blanchard feel that the leader has to match his leadership style according to the needs of maturity of subordinates which moves in stages and has a cycle. This theory is also known as life-cycle theory of leadership. There are two basic considerations in this model: leadership style and maturity of subordinates.

Leadership styles (Fig. 13)

Leadership styles may be classified into four categories based on the combination of two considerations: relationship behavior and task behavior. Relationship behaviors are determined by socio-emotional support provided by the leader.

Subordinates maturity

Maturity means ability and willingness of the people for directing their own behavior. All persons tend to be more or less mature in relation to a specific task, function, or objective that a leader is attempting to accomplish through their efforts. When both components of maturity—ability and willingness—are combined, there can be four combinations:
1. Low ability and low willingness—low maturity
2. Low ability and high willingness—low to moderate maturity
3. High ability and low willingness—Moderate to high maturity
4. High ability and high willingness—high maturity

Path-goal Model of Leadership

Robert House and others have developed a path-goal model of leadership. Path-goal model of leadership is basically a combination of situational leadership and Vroom's expectancy theory of motivation.

According to this model, the main function of a leader is to clarify and set goals with subordinates, to help them to find the best path for achieving the goals, and to remove the obstacles to their performance and need satisfaction. In providing this path-goal process, the leader adopts different leadership styles based on the situations. Thus, the combination of these two —leadership styles and situations—helps the employees to achieve goals.

Leadership Skills

To be an effective leader, the nurses need the primary leadership skills that are as follows:
- Skills of personal behavior
  - Be sensitive to feelings of group.
  - Identify ourself with the needs of the group
  - Considers others suggestions
  - Helps other feel important and needed
  - Abstain from agrument
- Skills of communication: A nurse should:
  - Listen attentively
  - Make sure that policies are made clear to all
  - Maintain good interpersonal relations and open communication in the group
- Skills of organization: The effective leader helps the group to:
  - Develop long and short range objectives
  - Share opportunities and responsibilities
  - Plan, act, follow-up and evaluate
- Skills of self-examination: A nurse must be:
  - Aware of personal motivations
  - Aware of the group members
  - Helpful to the group to be aware of their attitudes and values

Effective Leadership in Nursing

For leadership to be effective in nursing, the nurse leader must possess certain qualities and apply The certain techniques in health care setting as follows:

Qualities of Nurse Leaders

- Self-awareness
- Personal qualities like integrity, honesty, ability to cooperate, ability to attract, motivate, etc.
- Initiative qualities like willing to help and assist, along with self-confidence,
- Technical qualities like mastery over subject, expertise to work
- Teaching abilities
- Administrative abilities
- Intellectual skills
- Enthusiasm
- Emotional stability
- Quality of building human relations

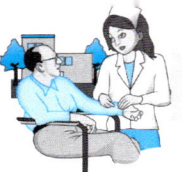

Techniques

- Planning and organizing the work schedule according to the availability of resources
- Assigning work to subordinates should be defined with clear cut objectives
- Proper teaching and guidance to subordinates
- Good communication
- Democratic supervision
- Evaluation of performance

Box: 2

What is Emotional Intelligence (EQ)?

For most people, emotional intelligence (EQ) is more important than one's intelligence quotient (IQ) in attaining success in their lives and careers. As individuals, our success and the success of the profession, today depend on our ability to read other people's signals and react appropriately to them.

Therefore, each one of us must develop the mature emotional intelligence skills required to better understand, empathize and negotiate with other people — particularly as the economy has become more global. Otherwise, success will elude us from our lives and careers.

"Your EQ is the level of your ability to understand other people, what motivates them and how to work cooperatively with them," says Howard Gardner, the influential Harvard theorist. Five major categories of emotional intelligence skills are recognized by researchers in this area.

MOTIVATION

Motivation is defined as a driving force within individuals by which they attempt to achieve some goals to fulfill some needs or expectation.

The word motivation is coined from the Latin word 'movere' means 'to move'. Motivation is the internal drive that activates behavior and gives its direction.

Motivation is psychological drive that directs a person toward an objective. Motivation is an important factor which leads to employee's satisfaction, effective cooperation and thereby leads to stability of employees in an organization. There will be better organizational relations.

Motivation is defined as the willingness to exert high level of efforts toward organizational goals, conditioned by efforts and ability to satisfy some individual needs—**Stephen P Robbins**

Need/Importance of Motivation

Motivation is important for an organization as it:
- Improves level of efficiency of employers which will result in increase in productivity, reducing cost of operation and improving overall efficiency.
- It leads to achievement of goals
- It builds friendly relationship as motivation is an important factor which brings employee's satisfaction.
- Also helps employees to realize organizational goals and achieve objectives
- Give positive view
- Creates a power of change
- Helps to build self-esteem
- Helps to improve level of efficiency
- Gives job satisfaction and opportunity of self-development to an employee
- Makes employees more quality oriented
- Makes workers become more productive.

Types of Motivation

- **Positive motivation:** Positive motivation induces people to work in the best possible manner and improves their performance. Rewards and better facilities are provided in positive motivation for better performance. Rewards may be financial or nonfinancial. For example: promotion, recognition, allowances etc.
- **Negative motivation:** Aims at controlling the positive efforts of the work and seeks to create a sense of fear in the worker, and due to this he has to suffer for lack of good performance. If a worker fails in achieving the desired results, he should be punished. For example: demotion, transfer, penalties etc.
- **Intrinsic motivation:** Intrinsic motivation renders to motivation that comes from inside of an individual. The motivation comes from the pleasure one gets from the tasks itself or from the sense of satisfaction in completing or even working on a task.

  Managers are interested to increase intrinsic motivation. The ideal employee may be one who is self-motivated and does not require constant supervision. Supervisors may increase intrinsic motivation by allowing employee to have greater autonomy and encouraging his creativity.
- **Extrinsic motivation:** In extrinsic motivation the individual's motivation stimuli are coming from outside of a person, i.e., our desire to perform a task is controlled by an outside source, for example, discounts, bonus etc.

Theories of Motivation

The term motivation theory is concerned with the processes that describe why and how human behavior is activated and directed.

Classification of motivational theories

Motivational theories can be classified into two.
1. Content theories or Need Theories
2. Process theories

Content theories focus on what motivates people and Process theories focus on how people's needs influence their behavior.

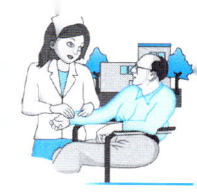

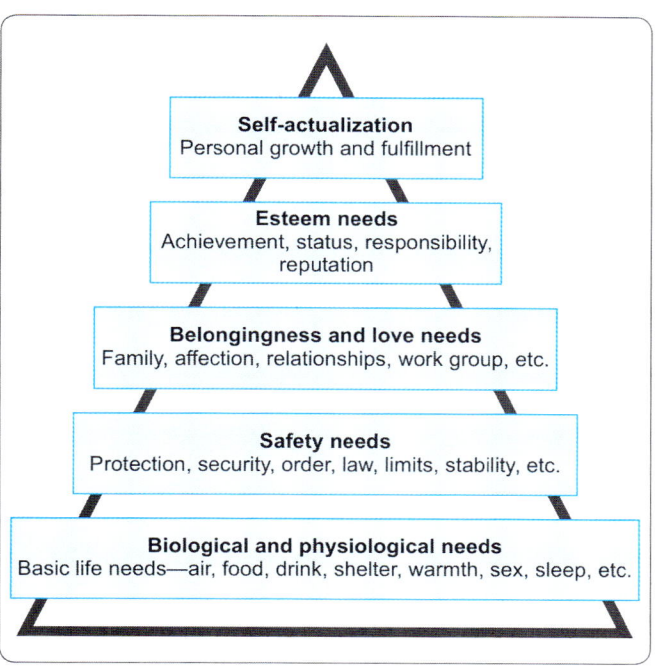

Figure 14: Maslow's hierarchy of needs

Content theories or Need Theories
- Maslow's Need Hierarchy Theory
- Herzberg Two Factor Theory
- David McClelland's Theory of Needs
- Alderfer's ERG Theory
- Theory X and Theory Y

Abraham Maslow's Need Hierarchy Theory

One of the most popular theories of motivation is the hierarchy of needs theory put forth by psychologist Abraham Maslow. Maslow saw human needs in the form of a hierarchy, ascending from the lowest to the highest, and he concluded that when one set of needs is satisfied, people will go for the next needs. He classified the human needs into five (Fig. 14):
1. Physiological needs
2. Safety needs
3. Social needs
4. Esteem needs
5. Self-actualization needs

Physiological needs

Physiological needs are those needs which are required to sustain life, such as:
- Air
- Water
- Nourishment
- Sleep

According to Maslow's theory, if physiological needs are not satisfied then one's motivation will arise from the search to satisfy them.

Safety needs

Once physiological needs are met, the attention turns to safety and security in order to be free from the threat of physical and emotional harm and they are:
- Living in a safe area
- Medical insurance
- Job security
- Financial reserves

If a person feels that he is insecure, he will not give much attention to higher needs.

Social needs

Once a person has met the lower level physiological and safety needs, higher level needs become important, the first of which are social needs. Social needs are those related to interaction with other people and may include:
- Need for friends
- Need for belonging
- Need to give and receive love

Esteem needs

It is fourth stage in Mashlow's hierarchy of needs. Esteem needs refer to the need for respect, self-esteem and self-confidence. Esteeem needs are basis for the human desire to be accepted and valued by others.

Some of the esteem needs are:
- Self-respect
- Achievement
- Attention
- Recognition
- Reputation

Maslow later refined his model to include a level between esteem needs and self-actualization: The need for knowledge and aesthetics.

Self-actualization needs

Maslow regards this as the highest need in his hierarchy. It is the quest of reaching one's full potential as a person. Self-actualized people tend to have needs such as truth, justice, wisdom, meaning, etc.

According to Maslow only a small percentage of people reaches the level of self-actualization

Implications for management

Maslow's theory has some important implications for management. This model helps the managers to understand and deal with issues of employee's motivation at work place. Managers who understand the need patterns of their staff can help the employees to meet the different work activities and some of the implications.
- **Physiological needs:** Provide lunch periods, rest breaks, and wages that are sufficient to purchase the essentials of life.
- **Safety needs:** Provide a safe working environment, retirement benefits, and job security.
- **Social needs:** Create a sense of community via team-based projects and social events.

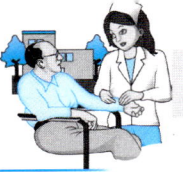

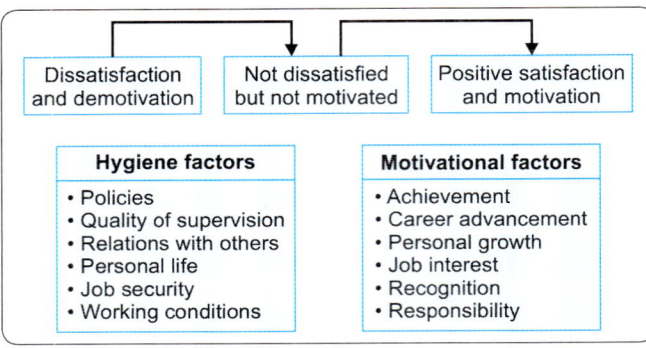

Figure 15: Herzberg's two-factor theory

- **Esteem needs:** Recognize achievements to make employees feel appreciated and valued. Offer job titles that convey the importance of the position.
- **Self-actualization:** Provide employees a challenge and the opportunity to reach their full career potential.

Frederick Herzberg's Motivation-hygiene Theory or Herzberg's Two-Factor Theory (Fig. 15)

Herzberg stated that there are certain satisfiers and dissatisfiers for employees at work. The intrinsic factors (satisfieds) are related to job satisfaction and extrinsic factors (dissatisfiers) are associated with dissatisfaction. Removing dissatisfying characteristics from a job does not necessarily make the job satisfying. According to Herzbersg, there are two factors which can satisfy or dissatisfy an employee. They are:

Hygiene factors → These can demotivate when not present, for example: Security, status, relationship with subordinates, personal life, salary, work conditions, relationship with supervisor and administration.

Motivational factors → These will motivate when present, for example, growth prospects, job advancement, responsibility, challenges, recognition and achievements.

Herzberg states that presence of certain factors like security, status, relationship with subordinates, personal life, salary, work conditions, relationship with supervisor and administration in the organization does not lead to motivation. However, their absence leads to dissatisfaction. These are called hygiene factors (or) dissatisfiers.

Similarly the absence of certain factors like growth prospectus, job advancement, responsibility, challenges, recognition and achievement causes no dissatisfaction, but their presence has motivational impact. These are called motivational factors or satisfiers.

Implications

In order to motivate employees the manager must ensure to provide the hygiene factors and then motivating the motivating factors. So if we want to motivate employees on their jobs, it is suggested to give much importance on those job content factors such as opportunities for personal growth, recognition, responsibility and achievement. These are the factors of intrinsic motivation.

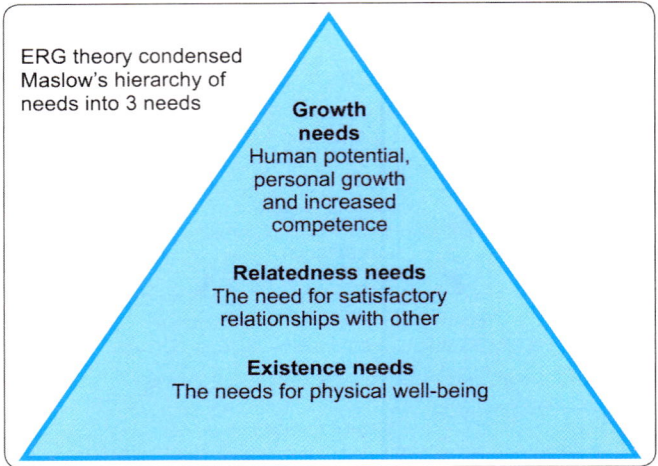

Figure 16: ERG theory

Herzberg model sensitizes that managers should utilize the skills, abilities and talents of workers.

Clayton Alderfer's ERG Theory (Fig. 16)

According to Clayton there are 3 groups of core needs.
1. **The existence needs:** These are concerned mainly with providing basic material existence.
2. **The relatedness needs:** The individuals' need to maintain interpersonal relationship with other members in the group.
3. **The growth needs:** The individual's desire to grow and develop personally.

Implications

Alderfer has proposed two sets of views on individual's aspirations and fulfillment. One is satisfaction – progression and other is frustration – regression.

Satisfaction: Progression views that once an individual's basic needs are satisfied, he/she will progress to the next level to satisfy the succeeding higher level to have them satisfied. He proposed another view of individual's aspirations and fulfillment. If people eventually become frustrated in trying to satisfy their needs at one level, their next lower level will re-emerge and they will regress to the lower level to satisfy more basic needs. This is called as frustration - regression. This theory provides the manager with the opportunity of directing employee behavior in a constructive manner even though higher order needs are temporarily frustrated.

The major conclusions of this theory are:
- In an individual, more than one need may be operative at the same time.
- If a higher need goes unsatisfied, then the desire to satisfy a lower need will be strong.

McClelland's Theory of Needs

David McClelland in his theory mentions three types of motivating needs.

1. Need for power
2. Need for affiliation
3. Need for achievement

Need for power

Basically people having high need for power are inclined toward influence and control. They like to be at the center and are good speakers. They are demanding in nature, forceful in manners and ambitious in life. They can be motivated to perform if they are given key positions or power positions.

Need for affiliation

In the second category are the people who are social in nature. They try to affiliate themselves with individuals and groups. They are driven by love and faith. They like to build a friendly environment around themselves. Social recognition and affiliation with others provides them motivation.

Need for achievement

People in the third area are driven by the challenge of success and the fear of failure. Their need for achievement is moderate and they set for themselves moderately difficult tasks. They are analytical in nature and take calculated risks. Such people are motivated to perform when they see at least some chances of success.

McClelland's Theory of Need Implications

David McClelland proposed that there are three needs which are major motives in work life. They are: need for achievement, needs for power and needs for affiliation.

Need for achievement is a drive to excel, to achieve in relation to a set of standards and to strive to succeed. People with this need have a desire to do something efficiently. They are motivated and prefer the challenges of working at a problem and accept personal responsibility for success or failure.

Need for power is the need to make others behave in a way that they would not have behaved otherwise.

Further McCelland proposed that there are two types of powers—personal power and institutional power. Persons with high need for power would naturally turn on by holding positions of authority. They like to take charge and control of situations.

People high in need for affiliation perform better in their job when they are given supportive feedback. Thus friendly supervisors can influence individuals with high need for affiliation and motivate the workers harder.

"Theory X and Theory Y" of Douglas McGregor

McGregor states that people inside the organization can be managed in two ways. The first is basically negative, which falls under the category X and the other is basically positive, which falls under the category Y.

Assumptions of theory X

- Employees inherently do not like work and whenever possible, will attempt to avoid it.
- Because employees dislike work, they have to be forced, coerced or threatened with punishment to achieve goals.
- Employees avoid responsibilities and do not work till formal directions are issued.
- Most workers place a greater importance on security over all other factors and display little ambition.

Assumptions of theory Y

- Physical and mental effort at work is as natural as rest or play.
- People do exercise self-control and self-direction if they are committed to those goals.
- Average human beings are willing to take responsibility and exercise imagination, ingenuity and creativity in solving the problems of the organization.

Theory X tends to be "authoritarian" in nature. In contrast organizations with theory Y can be described as "participative", where the aims of the organization and of the individuals in it are integrated. Individuals can achieve their own goals best by directing their efforts toward the success of the organization.

Process Theories of Motivation

The following are the process theories of motivation:
- Vroom's Expectancy Theory
- Adam's Equity Theory
- Reinforcement Theory
- Goal Setting Theory
- Cognitive Evaluation Theory

Vroom's Expectation Theory

The Vroom's theory says that the strength of a tendency to act in a specific way depends on:
- The strength of an expectation that the act will be followed by a given outcome
- The attractiveness of that outcome to the individual
- To make this simple.

    Motivation = Valence x Expectancy.

    Valence means the strength of an individual's preference to a particular outcome.

    Expectancy means the probability that a particular action will lead to the outcome.

The theory focuses on three things:
- Efforts and performance relationship
- Performance and reward relationship
- Rewards and personal goal relationship

Adam's Equity Theory

As per the equity theory of J. Stacey Adams, people are motivated by their beliefs about the reward structure as being fair or unfair, relative to the inputs. People have a tendency to compare the outcomes and inputs with different individuals and then they will be motivated based on the comparison.

Accordingly if people feel that they are not equally rewarded, they either reduce the quantity or quality of work or move to some other organization. However, if people perceive that they are rewarded higher, they may be motivated to work harder.

Reinforcement Theory

BF Skinner, who propounded the reinforcement theory, holds that by designing the environment properly, workers can be motivated. He also states that work environment should be made suitable to the individuals and that punishment actually leads to frustration and demotivation.

Goal Setting Theory of Edwin Locke

The goal setting theory states that when the goals to be achieved are set at higher standards then employees are motivated to perform better and they put in maximum effort. It revolves around the concept of "Self-Efficacy" i.e. individual's belief that he/she is capable of performing a hard task.

Cognitive Evaluation Theory

As per this theory a shift from external rewards to internal rewards results into motivation. It believes that even after the stoppage of external stimulus, internal stimulus survives. It relates to the pay structure in organization.

Instead of providing external factors like pay, incentives and promotion, the internal factors like interests, drives, responsibility should be provided. The cognition is to be such that even when external motivators are not there, the internal motivation continues. However, practically extrinsic rewards are given much more importance.

Process of Motivation or Basic Motivation Model

An individual may have many needs. These needs may be classified into primary needs and secondary needs. Primary needs are known as physiological, biological and basic needs. These needs are common to all human beings. Some of these needs are food, sex, sleep etc.

Secondary needs are natural but are learned by an individual through his experience and interaction. They are learned or derived needs, for example, need for power, status, achievement etc.

These needs are the driving force that accelerates individuals into specific actions that are directed toward the achievement of goals. These goals may be general or specific. If a person achieves his goals (Fig. 14), he will be getting satisfaction. Otherwise, he will get dissatisfaction. As a result he has to change either his expectations or goals.

Motivational Factors

There are two types of factors/incentives: Monetory factors and nonmonetory factors.

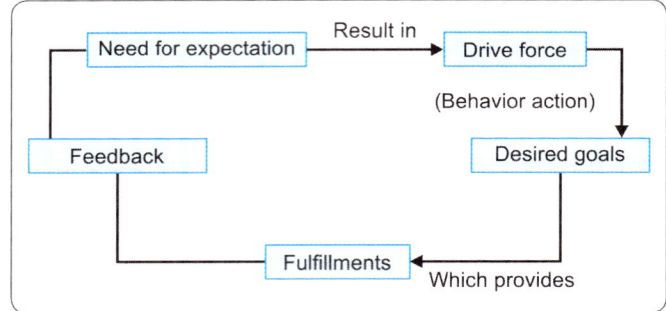

Figure 17: Factors of motivation

Monetory Factors

Providing reward to employee in terms of money, wages and bonus schemes. Reasonable wages must be paid to employees because salaries are one of the most important motivational factors. Bonus, i.e., extra payment to employees over and above salary must be paid to employees which motivates them to do. The organization may also provide additional incentives as medical allowances, educational allowances, etc.

Nonmonetory Factors

- **Recognition:** It is an incentive which satisfies the ego needs of the employees.
- **Security of job:** Security provides motivation.
- **Job enrichment:** Increases responsibility and increasing nature of work is a motivation.
- **Promotion opportunities:** It is a motivation and an employee feels satisfied.
- **Participation in planning activities:** Invites employees to give suggestions.
- Stature or job title give an employee feeling of pride as they feels elected by higher designation.
- Appreciation and recognition
- Provision of better working condition motivates employees, e.g. proper physical layout, proper sanitation.
- Workers participation in planning motivates them.
- Healthy relation within the organization also motivates employees.
- Experienced and intelligent superiors also motivate workers.

Other factors of motivation are:
- In-service education
- Proper placement
- Proper performance feedback
- Proper welfare facilities

Strategies for Employee Motivation For Nurse Manager

- The nurse managers should understand the dynamics of employee motivation theories.
- Consider employees as individuals and be available for them.

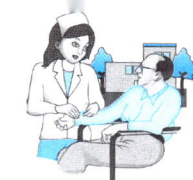

- Initiate communication and be a good listener.
- Involve them to set challenging but realistic goals for the welfare and care of patients.
- Create clear work objectives for workers, so that best available care be given to patients and their family.
- Create incentives by paying high laden pay scales (more output = more pay) and incentives.
- Include all nurses in planning process
- Provide workers with resources, freedom and authority to meet expectations
- Initiate cooperation and team works
- Give special honor or rewards to top performers
- Be fair and consistent
- Give workers lots of feedback about the way they are performing
- Give credit to everyone that contributes
- Assign tasks that require their skills and talents
- Provide opportunities for professional development of nurses so that they can update with changing technology
- Provide opportunities for social interaction with employees

GROUP DYNAMICS

Administration is an intellectual, social, dynamic and continuous process. It is a team effort for the achievement of goal of an organization that is combined effort of a group of people working together as a team to achive targets. For effective management, the administrator should have adequate knowledge regarding group behavior and group psychology.

Kurt Lewin, a social psychologist from USA was the founder of the term 'group dynamics'. Group dynamics refer to the study of human behavior in a group. It is a branch of social psychology which studies problems involving the structure of a group. A group is a social unit which consists of a number of individuals who stand in definite status and role relationship to one another which possess a set of values or norms of its own, regulating the behavior of individual members at least in matters of consequence to the group. —*Sheriff and Sheriff*

Group is also defined as two or more people who interact regularly to accomplish a common goal. Individuals in a group have a tendency to follow their own ideas and they create a feeling of unity, purpose and mutual understanding.

Group dynamics is the study of groups and group process, the personal interrelationships among members of the group. Group dynamics refers to the complex forces that are acting upon every group throughout its existence which cause it to behave the way it does. It deals with the interactions and forces between group members in a social institution.

—*Stephen Robbins*

Group dynamics is a system of behavior and psychological process occurring within a social group or social groups. Group dynamics helps to identify and analyze the social process that impact group development.

A group may be defined as a number of individuals who join together to achieve a goal. People always join groups to achieve goals that cannot be achieved by them alone.

—*Jonson and Jonson 2006*

Stephen Robbins defines a group as two or more individuals interacting and interdependent, who have come together to achieve particular objectives.

Qualities of a Group

The qualities of a group are:
- A definite membership
- Ability to act in a unitary manner
- Group consciousness, group members should have collective perception of a decision.
- The group members have same goal
- In group, there are interdependence between members to achieve goals
- In groups, there are interactions between members

In every organization, groups are very important to accomplish goals and coordinate interdependent efforts. Individuals in a group have a tendency to follow their own ideas and they create a feeling of unity, purpose, mutual understanding etc.

Types of Groups

CH Cooley on the basis of forms of relationship among the group members classified groups into primary group and secondary group.

Primary Group

Primary group is composed of people who are emotionally close and who know one another. In primary group people will have face to face, close cooperative relationship. The group members will have intimate contact with each other. Group members will provide love, security, belongingness, tolerance, mutual concerns etc. For example, family, neighborhood.

Secondary Group

Secondary groups are groups that are constituted for some specific aims. They are relatively casual and impersonal in their relationship. Relationship in them is usually competitive rather than mutually helpful. —*H. Landis*

After achieving the goal, the members will not maintain required relationship within the group, **e.g.** occupational associations.

The groups can also be classified as below:
- **Formal groups:** Formal groups are formulated with structural associations to accomplish specific goals of an organization. Formal groups are permanent in nature and members have to follow organizational mission, policy, rules and regulations, e.g., trade unions.
- **Informal groups:** Informal groups refer to aggregate of personal contact and interactions, e.g., friendship group. The members of the group relate to each other for

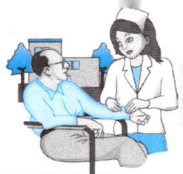

the purpose of mutual benefit and achievements. In an organization, informal groups are formed by employees in an organization at the workplace while working together, e.g., example: teachers, friendship groups in recreation club etc.

- **Task groups:** Task groups are groups composed of people who work together to perform a task. Task groups are specifically created to solve the problem or to perform a task.
- **Social group:** Special groups refer to a group formulated to accomplish a definite purpose, e.g., political group.
- **Command group:** Formed by subordinates reports directly to a particular manager. It is determined by formal organizational charts.

Group Development

Dr Bruce Tuckman in 1965 formulated a group development model which described 4 stages of group development as forming, storming, norming and performing. He added the 5th stage of group development—adjourning in 1970's. The five stage model includes:

1. **Forming:** It is the stage when groups first come together. During this stage the group members come to know one another and build rapport and are enthusiastic to know about the group. There is uncertainty about group's purpose, structure and relationships. This stage is marked by uncertainty and confusion. The managers have a major role at this stage.
2. **Storming:** During this stage the members accept the existence of the group. This is a conflicting stage. In this stage, the employees come to know each other's position and level. When complete, there will be a relatively clear hierarchy of leadership within the group.
3. **Norming:** In this stage there is relationship between members of the groups, i.e., there is group cohesiveness. At this stage the group members become clear about their roles and responsibilities. This stage is complete when the group structure solidifies and the group has assimilated a common set of expectations of what defines correct member behavior.
4. **Performing:** During this stage of development, the group becomes fully functional and accepted and the group moves toward performing stage. The group members work independently. Team is self-directing in development of plans and strategy to meet their goals and carry out work. The leader at this stage becomes a facilitator and helps the team. Through effective team work, the group completes the assigned tasks.
5. **Adjourning:** The fifth stage of group development is adjourning stage. When the groups are temporary in nature or if they have limited tasks to do, they go through this stage. At this stage, the group prepares for its dismissal. For permanent groups performing is the last stage.

Sometimes groups do not always proceed from one stage to the next as several stages go on simultaneously that is when groups are forming and performing. The administrators should be with the group members during all the stages of development and organization should provide the rules and regulations, information and resources needed for the group to perform.

There are group development models like Bass and Ryterband's model (1979), Poole's multiple- sequence model, systematizing the Person group relation theory on group development etc.

Factors Affecting Group Behavior

Factors affecting group behavior are: group member resources, group structure, group process and group tasks.

- **Group member resources:** Group member resources include knowledge, skill and attitude of members in the group and effective utilization of the same for the achievement of organization.
- **Group structure:** Group structure is the layout of the group. It includes group roles, group behavior, group status, group achievements etc. Group structure include:
  - **Formal leadership:** All groups in each organization have an administrator or manager as leader and the role of leader is very important for the attainment of objective.
  - **Group roles:** Roles are set of expected behavior patterns of employees occupying various positions in a social unit. In a group the members are expected to act diverse roles set to individuals.
  - **Role identity:** Role identity is certain attitude and actual behavior that is consistent with a role.
  - **Role perception:** Role perception is the group member's view to decide how they are supposed to act in a given situation and they get these perceptions from the stimuli around them as books, friends etc.
  - **Role expectation:** Role expectation is how others in the group expect each member must act in a group.
  - **Role conflict:** Role conflict occurs when an individual is confronted by divergent role expectation. Role conflict increases internal tension, fluctuations and dissatisfaction.
  - Group roles are of work roles, maintenance roles and blocking roles. Work roles are task oriented activities to achieve the goals. The specific work roles are: initiator, informer, clarifier, summarizer etc.
  - **Maintenance roles:** Maintenance roles are social and emotional activities that help members maintain their involvement in the group. The maintenance roles are harmonizer, encourager, and compromiser. Blocking roles are activities that disrupt the group. It does not always have a negative effect.
- **Group norms:** Norms are acceptable standards of behaviors. Group norms are standards set by the group that every member has to follow. All groups have norms and

for each group norms are unique. Norms are formulated to facilitate group survival. The norms reflect the level of commitment, motivation and performance of the group.

Group norms are rules or guidelines of accepted behavior which are established by a group and used to monitor the behavior of its members. —*Micheal Argyle*

Group norms are important in an organization as they regulate the activities or roles of members in the group to achieve the objectives and facilitate survival of the group. The norms may be of different types like performance norms which determine the level of performance; the norms of equality that dictate equal treatment of all the members; social responsibility norms, and behavior norms which include norms that standardize the behavior of employees in the group.

- **Group cohesiveness:** Cohesiveness is the degree to which members are attracted to each other and are motivated to stay in the group. Cohesiveness refers to the degree and strength of interpersonal attraction among members of the group. The more the members are attracted to the group, the greater will be group cohesiveness. Cohesiveness is a very important group attribute. The positive consequences of group cohesiveness are increased participation of employees in group affairs and activities, achievement of goals of the organization, high productivity, increased communication and interpersonal relations etc.

Attributes of cohesive group are:
- The members in the group shares the goals of the group
- The individuals in the group have some common interests.
- The group members maintain good interpersonal relations.
- The group functions to attain the goals
- The number of members in the group is relatively small

Activities that increases cohesiveness are:
- Makes the group small
- Encourages agreement with group goals
- Increases time the members spend together
- Increases group status
- Stimulates competition with other groups
- Gives reward to the group, not to individual members
- Increases interaction among members.

Relation between group cohesiveness, performance norms and productivity is depicted below in Figure 18.

- **Group roles:** Group roles are work roles, maintenance roles and blocking roles. Work roles are task oriented activities to achieve the goals. The specific work roles are initiator, informer, clarifier and summarizer.

Performance norms		Cohesiveness	
		High	Low
	High	High productivity	Moderate productivity
	Low	Low productivity	Moderate to low productivity

Figure 18: Relation between group cohesiveness, performance norms and productivity

Maintenance roles are—Social emotional activities that help members maintain their involvement in the group. The maintenance roles are harmonizer, encourager, compromiser etc. Blocking roles are activities that disrupt the group.

Role conflicts arise when there is ambiguity which leads to frustration and dissatisfaction.

- **Status:** Group status is the socially defined position given to each member of the group by others. Group structure status includes group norms, culture, status, equity. Group members get high status or low status in the group based on their authority and performance.
- **Group size:** The size of the group has a great impact on the behavior of the group. The groups with smaller number of employees are found to be faster in accomplishing the tasks or goals. It is found to be difficult for the large group to identify with one another and experience cohesion. Social loafing is a tendency for employees to put fewer efforts when working collectively in a group than working individually.
- **Group composition:** Group activities usually require knowledge and skill. These knowledge and ability of group members may influence the outcome or achievement of objectives of the group. The groups in which the individuals have diverse abilities are found to me more creative.
- **Group process:** Group process includes decision making by a group. Group generates more information; knowledge and it develop alternatives and formulate solutions. Group process also includes leadership communication, conflict management and interpersonal relations.

Group Decision Making Techniques

The group decision making is a participating process where the individuals in the group work together to analyze a situation and find out solutions. There are several techniques for group decision making. Group decision making methods/techniques are:
- Brain storming
- Nominal group technique (NGT)
- Delphi Technique
- Didactic Interactions
- Interacting groups
- Electronic meeting or computer assisted group meeting
- **Brain storming:** Brain storming is a group technique by which efforts are made to find out solution for a specific problem or decision making by gathering ideas spontaneously contributed by the members in the group.

During brain storming, the group members sit together around a table and the group leader introduces the situation clearly to the group. The members are encouraged to give suggestions regarding the idea. Criticisms are not allowed. All the alternate suggestions are recorded, discussed and analyzed to formulate solutions.

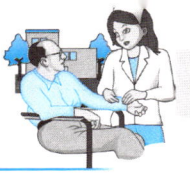

- **Nominal group technique (NGT):** This technique was developed by Andre Delbecq and Andrew Van de Ven at the University of Wisconsin. The organizer explains the purpose and asks individuals to write down their ideas without any discussion or communication. The individual members silently list their ideas. Each member is allowed to share their ideas they have generated before the group. The group then discusses the idea and each group member independently rank orders the ideas. The idea with the highest aggregate ranking determines the final decision. NGT is a structured group decision making process in which members are requested to prepare a comprehensive list of their ideas in writing. This method helps to provide more information and alternatives to a situation.
- **Delphi technique:** Delphi technique was developed by Norman Dalkey and Olaf Helmer. In Delphi technique, a group of 15-20 experts are selected. Here also there is no face to face interaction. All group members are given a structured questionnaire with questions relevant to decision making. The experts complete and return the questionnaire after completing. The organizer summarize the options of the experts and again sends back to the experts seeking their response to the results and askes to review the results. The process is repeated several times until an agreement among experts is obtained.
- **Didactic interactions:** These type of interactions are used when the type of problem is such that it result in a 'yes' or 'no' solution. There may be two groups, one favoring 'yes' and other favoring 'no'. Both the groups discuss their views and find out strengths and weaknesses and finally result in mutual acceptance of facts or solutions.
- **Interacting group:** In this group method, the members meet face to face and rely on both verbal and nonverbal interaction to communicate with each other. Interacting groups often censor themselves and pressurise individual members toward conformity of opinion.
- **Electronic meetings:** In this method, of decision making, the members in the group interact with the help of computers through connected computer terminals. The projector screen is used to show the individual suggestions. The group members sit around and issues are presented to participants and they type their responses on to their computer screens. These comments are displayed on a projection screen in the room. This method of meeting are significantly faster and cheaper.

Groups are integral part of modern organization. Group dynamics is concerned with interaction of the group members in a social situation or in an organization. Group dynamics is essential and helps to find out how the relationships are maintained in an organization. It helps to recognize the formation of group and how group should be organized etc.

HUMAN RELATIONS

Human relation is an area of management practice which is concerned with the integration of people into a work situation in a way that motivate them to work productively, cooperatively with economic, psychological and social satisfaction.

—*Keith davis*

Human relations are the relations between human beings that are affected by many other factors and helps in the accomplishment of goals of an organization. Human relation in nursing refer to the relationship of nurses with colleagues and other department personal and of nurses with patients. It is interdepartmental, intradepartmental and interpersonal relationship.

The nurse assumes the role of a professional helper. In such relationships, helping relationships are the foundations of clinical nursing practice. In nurse-patient helping relationship, nurse often encourage patients to share personal stories, which are called narrative interactions.

PUBLIC RELATIONS

Public relation activities are now considered as one of the important functions of hospital, Nowadays patients are becoming better informed and they become more active participants in decisions regarding treatment processes. Moreover a large number of new hospitals are entering in the field of health care and there is increased competitions among them. The consumers are becoming more selective and they are using health related information to make informed choices. Public relation helps to develop image of the organization.

Public relation is a management function that identifies, establishes and maintains mutually beneficial relationships between an organization and the various publics to whom its success or failure depends.

"Public relation practice is a planned and sustained effort to establish and maintain good will and mutual understanding between an organization and the public".

(Institute of Public Relation – Gt. Britain)

Publics are group of people, internal or external that an organization communicates with and it includes employees working in the orgaization and communities (people neighboring to the organization who must be treated with friendship and support), mass media, Government (Health organization whether it is in private sector or public sector must work closely with government policy) and consumer of health care services.

—*Baron (2004)*

"Public relations are the deliberate, planned and sustained efforts to establish and maintain mutual understanding between an organization and its publics."

—*Institute of Public Relations, USA*

"Public relations are a combination of philosophy, sociology, economics, language, psychology, journalism, communication and other knowledges into a system of human understanding."

—*Herbert M Baus*

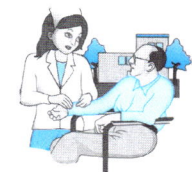

Need of Public Relation

It has been estimated that 80% of the problems confronting management have public relations implications. Management has to foresee the impact of policy decisions on the opinion of the public in accordance with follwing:
- Increased governmental activities
- Population explosion creating communication problems
- Increased educational standards resulting in rise in expectations
- Progress in communication techniques.

Public Relation Activities in Hospital

- **Counselling:** Counselling includes providing advice policies, relationship and publicity.
- **Advertisement:** Giving publicity through newspapers, health magazines, news letters, online chat groups, posters etc.
- **Media relation:** For publicity works with mass media. Media relation includes press conferences through which information can be given through face to face communication and through press release.
- **Public participation:** Organization can plan activities that give benefits to the public and can conduct activities which facilitate interactions between organization and the public.
- **Employee communication:** Employees should be properly directed and satisfied employee is an effective and credible person.
- **Community relations:** Organize activities with the neighboring community that benefits both to the community and the organization.

Tools and Technique of Public Relation

- Working with individuals/groups
- Advertisement
- Direct method of communication
- Community relations
- Government relations
- Media relations

For in house people in the organization use internal media like:
- **Journals:** It is an effective tool through which organization can communicate with the employees. Journals are periodic publications through which effective communication can be maintained between organization and employees.
- **Bulletin board:** Organization can publish important notices, orders, events etc. for the employees in bulletin board.
- **Annual reports and accounts:** Annual reports, budget for the fiscal years, accounts etc. are also used as communication tool.

For external media the organization can use tools like:
- **Newspapers:** Newspapers have a predominant influence in our society, so through new papers, information can reach to public.
- **Television:** Television is a most influential mass media communication to public.
- **Radio:** Radio is a best media for publicity as it reaches to people especially in rural village.
- **Films:** These are powerful media of communication, education and marketing.

Other publicity methods include direct methods like, using leaflets etc.

Each and every employee in an organization must have the responsibility of gaining confidence of public by performing services in efficient and effective way.

The measures to get public confidence in a health care institution, or measures to adopt for good public relation include.
- High quality health care services.
- Reception/enquiry that promptly respond to enquiries.
- Cleanliness and good surroundings.
- Outpatient department, reception and casualty must be equipped with adequate staff.
- Hospital information booklet with adequate information to patients relatives.
- All areas of hospital should be marked clearly with sign boards.
- Adequate space for waiting area and parking facilities.
- Employees should be qualified and neatly dressed with name labels.
- Complaint and suggestions should be welcomed.

Responsibilities of Public Relation Department in a Hospital

- Employees should be properly informed about organizations objectives, policies and goals.
- Establish enquiry/information desk to give information of patient enquiries.
- Special consideration must be given to physical appearance and environmental hygiene of the hospital. The interior of hospital must be decorated from the point of being esthetic and relaxing.
- Employees must be informed of organizations programs and activities and kept updated with latest changes.
- Organize and implement programs that are supporting to the community as giving aids/donations to local organizations
- Organize in-service education programs to improve professional knowledge and skills of employees.
- Prepare posters and brochures and educational literature with annual reports.
- Produce staff magazines.
- Establish web page for hospitals.
- Conduct opinion surveys and research activities.

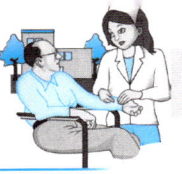

UNION

An organization of workers joined to protect their common interests and improve their working conditions is known as union.

Union may be referred to a trade union which is an organization of workers that have banded together, often for the purpose of getting better working conditions or pay.

A trade union or labor union is an organization of workers that have banded together to achieve common goals such as better working conditions. The trade union, through its leadership, bargains with the employer on behalf of union members (rank and file members) and negotiates labor contracts (collective bargaining) with employers. This may include the negotiation of wages, work rules, complaint procedures, rules governing hiring, firing and promotion of workers, benefits, workplace safety and policies. The agreements negotiated by the union leaders are binding on the rank and file members and the employer and in some cases on other nonmember workers. Activities of trade unions include:

- Provision of benefits to members
- Collective bargaining
- Industrial action
- Political activity

The Indian Trade Unions Act 1926

- Union is that they must work to protect and promote the interests of the workers and the conditions of their employment.
- To secure better wages and living conditions for their members.
- To acquire the control of the industry by the workers.
- To provide the workers self-confidence and a feeling of identity in the organization.
- To imbibe sincerity and discipline in the workers.
- To makeup welfare measures for improving morale of the workers.

COLLECTIVE BARGAINING

It is a process in which the employer representative and worker representative negotiate condition of employment as wages, hours of work and other benefits. The term collective is used in collective bargaining because both the employer and the employee put a collective effort to establish mutually agreeable conditions related to employment.

Nurses have the right to negotiate the condition of their employment either as individuals or collectively in all practice settings.

Collective bargaining is the process used by the representatives of an employer and the certified representatives of a group of the employees to negotiate and sign an agreement covering terms of employment.

Objectives of Collective Bargaining

To establish mutually agreeable terms and conditions for employment in an organization:
- To maintain employer employee relations
- To establish agreement on wages, hours of work and other benefits.

Collective Bargaining Process

The process of collective bargaining includes negotiation between representatives of management and employees union. The process involves:

Prebargaining Stage

This phase consists of selection of negotiation team and examination of the situation. During this stage, both sides are engaged in gathering data to be used in the negotiations. Managements analyze trends and create projections of what it can offer to the union. Union professionals survey the nurses in the bargaining unit to see what issues are of high priority, moderate priority and low priority. Both sides also examine recently negotiated local and regional contacts in other organizations for use as benchmarks in the current negotiations.

Negotiation teams are also established at this point. Each team will have members processing "on-the-floor" expertise, for example: staff nurses for labor, first- and second-level supervisors. Most negotiations are carried out between one organization and one union. The courts have broken the subject areas into three categories—mandatory, prohibited and permissive.

- Mandatory bargaining subjects are major issues that affect a nurse's work life. Examples are wages, hours and layoff procedures.
- Prohibited bargaining subjects involve language that would violate other laws. Examples of prohibited bargaining issues are—pay differentials based on race or requiring employers to only hire workers who already are members of the union.
- Permissive bargaining subjects are any topics that are neither excluded nor prohibited, such as color options for uniforms.

Discussion Phase

In the discussion phase they decide on the time and venue for discussion and decide on the ground rules. This phase involves active discussion of problems and issues between both parties with active listening and decision making. Possible alternatives are to solve issues and problems are discussed.

Bargaining Phase

After the exchange of demands made at the initial bargaining meetings, both sides get down to real negotiations. Formal mediation often becomes necessary at this point, with the

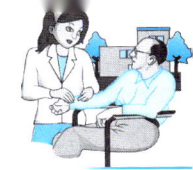

mediator serving as a neutral third party counselor working to bring both sides closer to an agreement. Formal draft of agreement are prepared and both parties should sign on it and take steps to implement it immediately.

Bargaining Outcomes

Collective bargaining outcomes typically follow one of the two avenues. The first and much more desired route is a settlement. An alternative to settlement is an impasse. An impasse means both sides have bargained to a point where each side refuses to offer anymore concessions to the other side. At this juncture, the union can call for a strike. If the impasse cannot be resolved in ten days the union is free to go out.

- **Strike activity among registered nurses:** Strikes have been a relatively uncommon event in the history of health care collective bargaining. It appears that the worst majority of all bargaining outcomes are settlements, not walkouts.
- **Alternative to strike:** The strike is considered as most significant weapon, other job actions and alternative avenues of dispute resolution.
- **Interest arbitration:** When labor and management reaches an impasse, they may decide to submit their case to an arbitrator for resolution. An arbitrator is a neutral third party, jointly selected by both sides to resolve the dispute.
- **Strikeouts:** A strikeout is a temporary one or two days strike used to show management how important the nurses are for the successful functioning of a facility.
- **Mass resignations:** Similar to strikeouts, this is the tactic used to pressurise to give management concessions of some sorts when other job actions are not possible or desirable.
- **Donated time:** This alternative is a ploy to bring public sentiments to hear on a health care facility. Under this scheme, nurses would continue to work their normal shifts but refuse to accept payment for their services.

Merits of collective bargaining are:

- Collective bargaining provides employees an opportunity to discuss professional issues.
- Helps to establish working relationship between employees representatives and employers.
- Enhance employees motivation.

Demerits of collective bargaining are:

- If bargaining process is not managed properly it may end in strike or lockout.
- The decisions of bargaining process may be influenced by power and politics.

Issues Leading to Collective Bargaining

- Absence of procedures for reporting unsafe or poor patient care.
- Short staffing and improper skills mix to compliment patient acuity.
- Floating without orientation and training.
- Use of temporary personnel and unlicensed assistive personnel.
- Resistance of employers to accept joint decision making.
- Adversarial relationships between nurses and management and exploitation of nurses by management.
- Lack of respect for employees.
- Lack of autonomy, that is, incursion by management into the scope of practice.
- Lack of promotional opportunities.
- Lack of professional practice committees.
- Lack of staff development and continuing education opportunities.
- Lack of child care and elder care.
- Lack of involvement.
- Poor differentials for shift work, education, and experience.
- Low wages and limited benefits.
- No pension portability.
- Lack of employee assistance programs.
- Poor on-call arrangement and lack of flexible schedules.
- Overwork, mandatory overtime and shift rotation.
- Low morale.
- Performance of non-nursing duties.
- Poor management and poor communication.
- Being able to take sufficient breaks.
- Having and implementing fair policies and practices for discipline and dismissal.
- Assurance that patient classification systems have practicing nurse inputs.
- Fair and consistent standards, policies and practices.
- Adequate health insurance.
- Assurance that competence and qualification are considered with seniority.
- Vacancy posting so, that all nurses have an opportunity.
- Lack of a system to apply peer review.
- Lack of career ladders.

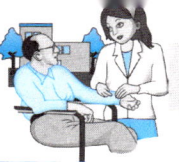

Suggested Reading

- Marquis BL, Huston CJ. Leadership Roles and Management Functions in Nursing Theory and Application 2nd ed; Lippincott. Pp. 53-71
- Swansburg RC. Management and Leadership for Nurse Managers. Boston Jones and Bartlett Publishers. Pp. 27-45
- Basvanthappa BT. Nursing Administration. Jaypee Brothers Medical Publishers Pvt. Ltd.: New Delhi, 2000.
- Bryson A, Wilkinson D. Collective Bargaining and Workplace Performance: An Investigation using the Workplace Employee Relations Survey 1998. Crown Copyright 2001 available from URL:http:/www. dti. gov. uk/er/EMAR
- Lalit Bhasin. Labor and Employment Laws of India. Available from URL: http://www. mondaq. com/ 08/24/2007
- Labor and Employment Laws of India. Ministry of Labor and Employment Government of India.
- Trade Unions Act. Available from URL: res://ieframe. dll/dnserror. htm#http://www. exportersindia. com/india/
- Lalitha K. Mental Health and Psychiatric Nursing. (1st ed). Gajanana Book Publishers and Distributors. Bangalore; 2006.
- Shives LR. Basic Concepts of Psychiatric Mental Health Nursing (7th ed). Lippincott Williams and Wilkins.
- Mohr WK. Psychiatric Mental Health Nursing (6th ed). Lippincott Williams and Wilkins. Philadelphia.
- KP Neeraja;(2009), "Essentials of Mental Health and Psychiatric Nursing" Jaypee Brothers Medical Publishers Pvt. Ltd. New Delhi; Pp. 39-43. http. /www. googles. com
- Benjamin J Sadock, Virginia A Sadock, Menas S Gregory. Comprehensive Textbook of Psychiatry, 8th edition.
- Stuart W Gail, Laraia T Michele. Principles of Psychiatry Nursing, 8th edition, Mosby Publication, Pp. 140-168.
- Handbook on Decision Making. Lakshmi C. Jain. Vol 4.
- Susan J Penner. Introduction to Health Care Economics and Finance Management. Lippincott Williams and Wilkins. Pp. 61-87.
- Katherine W Vestal. Nursing Management Concepts and Issues. JB Lippincott Company. Pp. 15-47.
- Steven A Finkler. Budgeting Concepts for Nurse Managers. Grune and Stratton Inc. Pp. 89-95.
- Mary Lucita. Nursing: Practice and Public Health Administration. Current Concepts and Trends. BI Churchill Livingstone. New Delhi. Pp. 173-186.
- Nursing Service Administration CM Francis, Mario C de Souza. Hospital Administration. Jaypee Brothers Medical Publishers (P) Ltd. New Delhi.
- Janice Rider Ellis, Celia Hartley. Managing and Coordinating Nursing Care, 5th ed. Lippincott Williams and Wilkins. Pp. 69-810.
- RC Goyal. Handbook of Hospital Personnel Management, 2nd ed. Pp. 69-81.

Assess Yourself

LONG ANSWERS

1. Define leadership and list out the qualities of leader. Discuss the various leadership styles.
2. Define communication. Write in detail about channels of communication and communication systems used in hospitals.
3. What is group? Describe various types of group and explain in detail about group dynamics.
4. What is meant by public relation? Which are the tools of public relation in context of nursing.

SHORT NOTES

1. Job description
2. Methods of patient assignment
3. Duties and responsibilities of a head nurse
4. Four ethical concepts relating to nursing
5. Four factors affecting ward management
6. Role of head nurse in material management
7. Material management
8. Quality assurance
9. Nursing audit
10. Performance appraisal
11. Inventory control

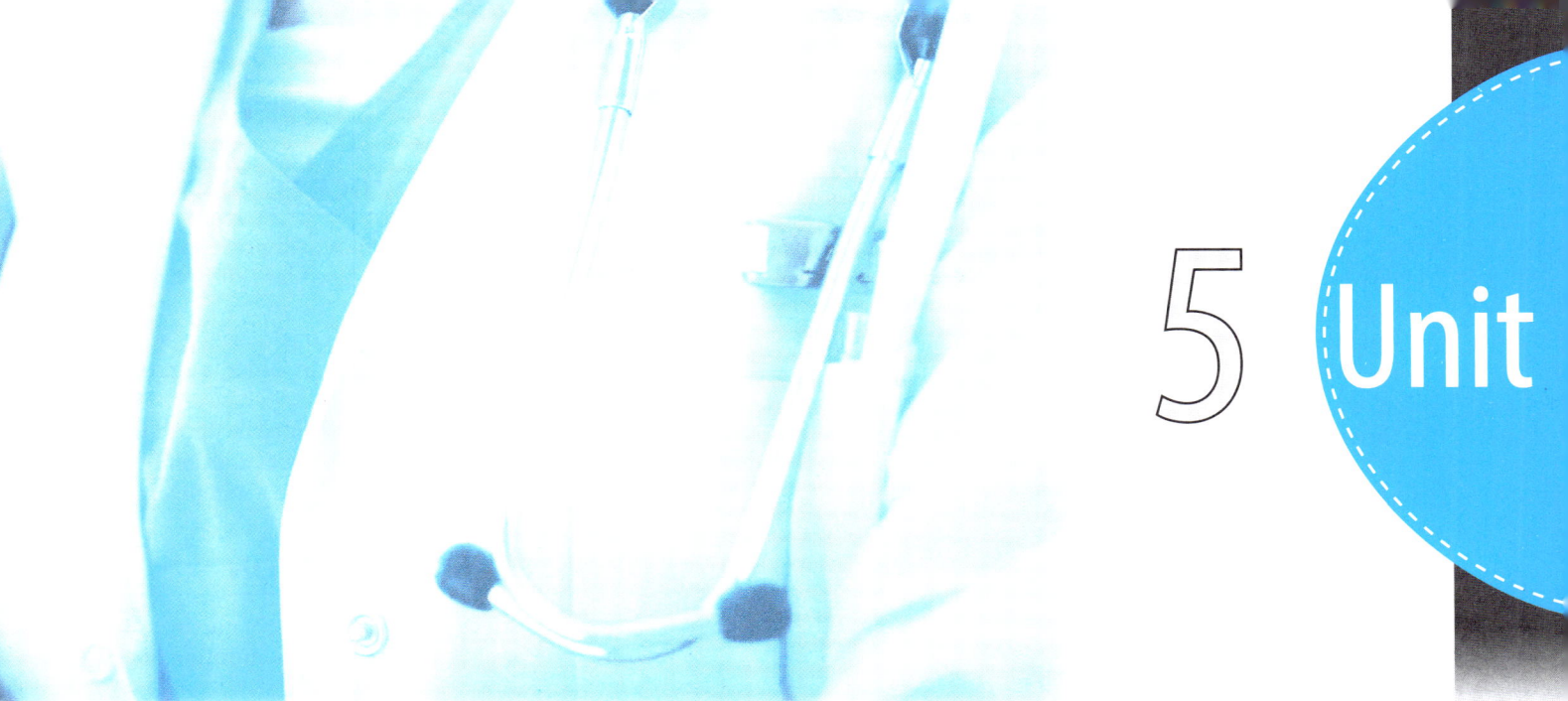

Unit 5

IN-SERVICE EDUCATION

Unit Outline

- Staff Development
- Types of Staff Development Program
- In-service Education
  - Definition of In-service Education
  - Objectives of In-service Education
  - Aims of In-service Education
  - Concept of In-service Education
  - Scope of In-service Education
  - Components/Organization/Types of In-service Education
  - Approaches/Types of In-service Education
  - Factors Affecting In-service Education
  - Characteristics of a Good In-service Education Program
  - Principles for Developing an In-service Education Program
  - Problems of In-service Education Program
  - Benefits of In-service Education Program
  - Planning of In-service Educational Program
  - Steps in Developing In-service Program
  - Conditions for Success of In-service Program
  - Methods of In-service Educational Program
  - Evaluation of In-service Program
  - Sample In-service Education Plan
  - Conclusion
- Adult Learning
  - Principles of Adult Learning
  - Knowles' 5 Assumptions of Adult Learners
  - Knowles' 4 Principles of Andragogy
  - Characteristics of Adult Learners
  - Adult Learning Cycle
  - Factors Affecting Adult Learning
- Standards of Staff Development Program According to American Nurses Association

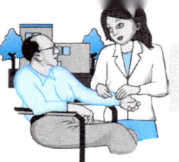

STAFF DEVELOPMENT

Staff development includes all training and education endeavors undertaken by employer to improve knowledge, skill and attitude of employees. It is a process consisting of orientation, in-service education and continuing education for the people promoting the development of personnel within an employment setting, consistent with goals and responsibilities of the employment (American Nurses Association).

TYPES OF STAFF DEVELOPMENT PROGRAM

- Induction training
- Job orientation
- In-service education
- Continuing education

In-service training in nursing is seen as a necessary component to help the professional nurse to keep up-to-date on the most recent developments in nursing and to be able to manage the demands of nursing practice. When the nurses are enriched with 'In-service education', their capabilities or work output is balanced by what is expected from them.

Among these we are discussing here, in-service education.

IN-SERVICE EDUCATION

DEFINITION OF IN-SERVICE EDUCATION

- In-service education is a continued training that the organization provided to its employees to increase the knowledge, skill and competency of employees in a specific area of work.
- In-service education is defined as a continued program of education provided by the employing authority, with the purpose of developing the competencies of personnel in their functions appropriate to the position they hold, or to which they will be appointed in the service.
- In-service education is a planned learning experience provided by the employer for employees.
- In-service education is a planned instructional or training program provided by an employing agency in the employment setting and designed to increase competence in a specific area.
- **In-service education:** In-service education is a planned continuous education for people already employed by a health authority. —*Blackwell*
- In-service education is an ongoing on-the-job instruction that is given to enhance the worker's performance in their present job.

OBJECTIVES OF IN-SERVICE EDUCATION

The objective of in-service education is to improve the quality of nursing care by updating knowledge and skills of nurses. In-service education aims to develop the ability for efficient working and the capacity for continuous learning so that nurses can quickly adapt to changes in order to produce effective services.

It will help nurses to get acquainted with modern technologies, to recognize their own resources and abilities, to broaden the outlook and increase professional competencies.

AIMS OF IN-SERVICE EDUCATION

- To update the knowledge, skill and ability of nurses.
- To improve creative ability of nurses for acquisition of new knowledge.
- To eliminate deficiencies in practice.
- Improvement of professional practice and development of the person as an individual and a responsible citizen.
- To develop interest and job satisfaction of nurses.
- It helps to develop confidence through acquisition of up-to-date knowledge.
- It reduces turnover and absenteeism in nursing.
- It helps to maintain high standards in nursing.

CONCEPT OF IN-SERVICE EDUCATION (FIG. 1)

Concepts of in-service education can be defined as the relevant activities or courses by which professional knowledge skills and competence of participation is increased.

SCOPE OF IN-SERVICE EDUCATION

- Maintenance of familiarity with new knowledge and subject matter.
- Increased skill in providing care.
- Improved attitudes and skills.

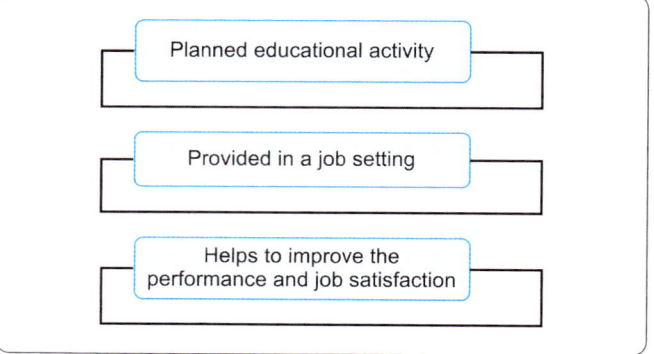

Figure 1: Concepts of in-service education

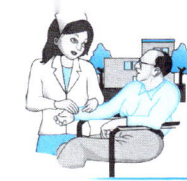

- Greater skill in utilizing community resources and in working with adults.
- Development and refinement of common values and goals.

COMPONENTS/ORGANIZATION/TYPES OF IN-SERVICE EDUCATION

- Orientation program
- Skill training program
- Leadership and management development
- Continuing education

Orientation Program

Orientation is a process of acquainting a newly joined employee to the policies, rules and regulations and practices of the organization. Orientation is given to employees during first 2 or 3 days of employment.

Once employees are selected in an organization, first step is to give them orientation and training. Orientation is the process of acquainting a new staff with the existing work environment so that he/she can relate quickly to his/her new surroundings.

Why Orientation?

- It helps the employee to adjust himself to new situations
- It helps them to familiarize with the philosophy, objectives, organizational pattern, policies and practices of organization.
- It helps to improve the performance of employees and having a feeling of being part of organization.
- It helps in socializing new employees.
- Improve employees morale and increase productivity.

Components of Orientation

- **Centralized orientation:**
  - General orientation
  - Orientation to hospital
  - Orientation to nursing
- **Decentralized orientation:**
  - Orientation to nursing unit
  - Orientation to nursing team

Orientation programs cover general orientation; which is about the organization, its physical layout, philosophy, objectives and support services. Orientation is given on personnel in the organization like director, administrators, nurse educators, doctors, co-workers, subordinates and services available. Orient about personnel policies, rules and regulations, leave policy, legal issues, records and reports and channels of communication. In nursing department, responsibilities are explained by giving job description, and task responsibilities.

Advantages

- Adjust to work situation
- Be strongly motivated to learn
- Able to function effectively
- Feel wanted and needed by coworkers and supervisors

Skill Training Program

Skill training may be a manual or technical skill of doing for people or skill in dealing and working well with people. It provides the nursing staff with the skills and attitude required for job and to keep them abreast of changing methods and new techniques. Often it is the continuation of the orientation program. It is designed to provide training to new and older staff. Presentation of skill can be through **Objective Structured Clinical Examination** (OSCE) or **Objective Structured Practical Examination** (OSPE).

Types of skills include psychomotor skill, cognitive skill, teaching skill, affective skill, communication skill, supervisory skill etc.

Benefits of Skill Training

It gives an opportunity to the nurses to improve and reinforce their level of preparation, it also fills any gap in their knowledge by making them aware of changing methods and new technology.

Training Principles

- The trainee must be motivated to learn.
- Learning must be reinforced.
- Materials must be meaningful and communicated.
- Multiple senses learning should be applied.
- The material taught must be transferred to the job situation.
- Feedback is must to achieve required and appropriate learning.

Leadership and Management Development

- To improve the managerial abilities of persons at every management level as well as potential managers to produce the greatest degree of organizational progress.
- By establishing agreement among top level and middle level managers like proper authority, responsibility and accountability for managers at every level.
- Need can be identified by incident reports, turnover rates, patient audits and quality control reports.

Objectives of Leadership and Management Development

- Decentralize leadership management competency and spread this among personnel.
- Permit increased delegation of authority.
- Promote good morals among administrative personnel which in turn influence staff morale.
- Aid in reducing costly turnover in top positions.

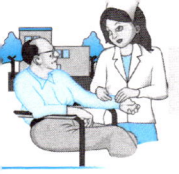

Continuing Education

By continuing education we mean any extension of opportunities for study or training to any person and adult following completion of their full time course. It is a planned activity directed toward meeting the learning need of nurse following basic nursing education, exclusive of full time formal post-basic education.

Continuing education is all the learning activities that occur after an individual has completed his basic education.

—*Cooper*

It is the education that builds on previous education

—*Shanon*

It is a method of staff development in which the employees are given opportunities to learn new knowledge and skill or review and add to new knowledge already gained.

Continuing education is a formal, organized, educational program designed to promote the knowledge, skills and professional attitude of nurses. Continuing education includes the experience after initial training which helps employees to maintain and improve existing knowledge.

Needs for Continuing Education

- It develop employee by updating their knowledge.
- It helps employee to respond effectively to the challenge of current social changes.
- It helps to improve the health care, economic and educational opportunities.
- It helps to improve the new health patterns of health care.
- It enables a worker to provide excellent service.
- It ensures professional development.
- It aids in carrier advancement.
- Specific skills to practice nursing are developed.
- 73% of hospital nurses cited shift work as the major barrier to their continuing education. Shift work is a necessary inconvenience for nurses because of the care that the patients require on a 24 hour basis.
- The cost was cited by 50% of nurses as a deterrent to continuing education.
- 18% of the nurses reported having to travel up to one hour by public transportation to be able to participate in continuing educational activities, (Ofosu, 1993).
- Difference between in-service education and continuing education is depicted below in Table 1.

Table 1: Difference between in-service education and continuing education

Features	In-service education	Continuing education
Responsibility	Employing agency	Individual
Basic concept	Improve worker performance	Self-directed learning
Venue	Employment setting	Not limited to area of employment
Utility value	In areas of employment	In areas of employment and all aspects of living
Work performance	Improved in area of work	Improved in general

Extramural Education

It is a community-based continuing education directed toward meeting job related learning needs of the nurse and other personnel. These are exclusive of full time formal study at a degree/training institution, e.g. conferences, workshops, seminars, etc.

APPROACHES/TYPES OF IN-SERVICE EDUCATION

- Centralized approach
- Decentralized approach
- Coordinated approach
- **Centralized in-service education:** In centralized approach a separate nursing department will take the responsibility for improvement of knowledge and skills.
- **Decentralized approach:** The employees are expected to keep administration informed of their activities and they are expected to develop and direct their own learning experiences. It is planned by employees in a unit giving care to patients with similar conditions.
- **Coordinated approach:** In coordinated approach the central administration of nursing personnel is responsible for a broad program which is of importance to all nursing personnel.

FACTORS AFFECTING IN-SERVICE EDUCATION

- **Cost of health care:** Conduct of in-service education needs additional expenses to the organization, The additional should be taken into consideration even though in-service education program increases quality of nursing care.
- **Manpower:** In-service education needs qualified, competent personnel, which means an increase in human resources component.
- **Standards:** It is very important to maintain highest standards of nursing practice.
- **Organization of nursing department:** Planned approaches are regular and for this concern in-service education is affected as it includes staff availability, workload etc. Well organized approaches are important.

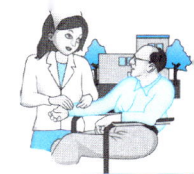

- **Changes in nursing practice:** There are frequent changes in 'in-service education' programs to meet the standards in practice.

CHARACTERISTICS OF A GOOD IN-SERVICE EDUCATION PROGRAM

- It is based on real and specific problems of patients or health care workers.
- It involves all personnel in planning.
- Participation and cooperation should be ensured.
- All activities are evaluated continuously to get feedback

PRINCIPLES FOR DEVELOPING AN IN-SERVICE EDUCATION PROGRAM

- Continuity should be ensured while planning in-service education program.
- Scientific approach should be adopted.
- Move from simple to complex situations.
- Flexibility
- Clear planning is needed. Success of an in-service education depends on effective planning.
- Adopt step-by-step approach

PROBLEMS OF IN-SERVICE EDUCATION PROGRAM

- Inappropriate methodology
- Inadequate training of trainers
- Lack of confidence of trainers
- Inadequate evaluation methods
- Lack of motivation
- Lack of interest
- Lack of management support
- Lack of proper follow-up
- Lack of time
- Inadequate resources
- Lack of clarity about organization of the program

BENEFITS OF IN-SERVICE EDUCATION PROGRAM

For Employee

- It keeps the employees enthusiasm in their learning.
- It develops interest among the staff members to learn new things.
- Develops a sense of responsibility for being knowledgeable and competent.
- Helps in decision making process through improvement in knowledge and skills.
- Helps the nurses to manage and become aware of new technologies and practice.
- Develops leadership skills, motivation and better attitude.
- Aids in achieving self-confidence.
- It helps the employees to update their knowledge and skills and improve quality care.
- Helps the employees to improve the professional practice.
- Helps the employees to keep abreast with the changing techniques and use of sophisticated tools and equipments.
- Helps employees to learn new techniques and to maintain old competencies.
- Equip the nurses with knowledge of current research and development.

For the Organization

- It will keep the nursing staff enthusiastic in their learning.
- It will help in developing interest and job satisfaction amongst the staff.
- Develops sense of responsibility.
- Creates an appropriate environment for growth and communication.
- It helps the nurses to make appropriate decision as well as effective problem solving techniques.
- Helps them to adjust according to change adopted in the field of nursing.
- Helps in developing leadership skills, motivation and better attitude.
- Helps in developing self-confidence and self-development.
- Makes the organization a better place to work.

PLANNING OF IN-SERVICE EDUCATIONAL PROGRAM

- Study staff needs through use of suggestion box/survey/questionnaire.
- Establish goals compatible with mission of the organization
- Formulate program objectives.
- Determine the course of action required to meet the objectives.
- Assess available resources (physical, financial, others).
- Formulate committees.
- Secure staff assistance.
- Plan for evaluation of the results of the program.

STEPS IN DEVELOPING IN-SERVICE PROGRAM

- **Assessment:** Participant resources, community and professional needs.
- **Planning:** Objectives, participant, method, content.
- **Implementation:** Participant's program recording.
- **Evaluation:** Participant's program follow-up.

The different steps in organizing program are:

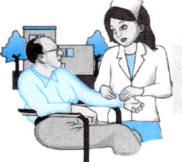

Need Assessment

The primary step-in-service education is determination of educational needs of nurses. For analyzing needs the nurse administrator can contact the employees personally, use survey questionnaires, analyze records and reports or through evaluation and performance appraisal, analysis of quality of service, etc. After analyzing the needs set priorities. Develop goals and objectives of in-service program and formulate criteria for evaluation. Plan the learning activities and course of action required to meet the objectives.

Design and Planning

The administrator has to plan and decide the training method. The different training method that can be used are workshops, conferences, seminars, etc. The organizer has to develop learning objectives and program schedule. Fix time and venue of ISE program in consultation with management. Find out resource persons who are competent enough to fulfil the educational objective. The venue should have all the physical facilities, transportation facilities and facilities to meet the basic needs. Develop resource material. Arrange all teaching-learning activities for the conduct of ISE.

Implementation

Implementation involves conduct of actual teaching-learning session. Ensure that all planned session are implemented properly to achieve the goal of ISE. Ongoing evaluation is also necessary.

Evaluation

Evaluation is an essential part of ISE. It is necessary to identify the extent to which the objectives are achieved and need for improvement. It can be done by establishment of evaluation criteria, pretest and post- test before and after completion of the program. After conducting evaluation, analyze information collected and identify the deficiencies.

CONDITIONS FOR SUCCESS OF IN-SERVICE PROGRAM

- Must be planned and systematic
- Must be based on organizational philosophy
- Must be realistic with approval and support of administration
- Have attendance and participation of personnel concerned
- Proper arrangement for welfare measures

How to Promote Participation

- Develop awareness
- Involve staff in all activities
- Use motivation, not manipulation
- Reward system—Positive reinforcement by holding appraisal programs.

Preparation of report

- Date and duration of in-service education program.
- Coordinator and resource persons.
- Purpose of the topic.
- Group of individuals with qualification and number of individuals in the group.
- Plan of in-service education program.
- Evaluation report related to change in knowledge, attitude and skill based on the program.
- Brief summary of all this should be recorded and submitted to a higher authority.

METHODS OF IN-SERVICE EDUCATIONAL PROGRAM

- Demonstrations
- Conference
- Class room observations
- Committee
- Field trip
- Role playing
- Panel discussions
- Workshops

EVALUATION OF IN-SERVICE PROGRAM

Evaluation is the process of determining the degree of achieving the predetermined objectives.

Evaluation Methods

- Questionnaires
- Interviews
- Observation of behavior in in-service program

SAMPLE IN-SERVICE EDUCATION PLAN

It is planned to organize an in-service education program as per following schedule:

Date	
Duration	60 minutes
Setting	Lecture hall, maternity ward
Participants	Staff nurses
Teaching methodology	Lecture and discussion
Presented by	Ms Judith, clinical nurse specialist

Topic

Role of nurses in prevention of HIV/AIDS and in providing comprehensive care to the positive mothers.

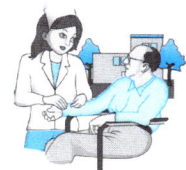

Objectives

At the end of the session, participants will be able to:
- Apply knowledge of HIV/AIDS, its prevention and comprehensive care.
- Recognize the role of nurses as a team member toward HIV care.
- Provide care to the HIV positive patients with confidence.
- Apply or utilize various HIV prevention interventions.
- Follow infection control and standard precautions in prevention of HIV.
- Utilize knowledge in providing patient education and counseling.
- Plan comprehensive care and will be confident in decision making in providing care.
- Guide mothers related to prevention of parent child transmission of HIV/AIDS.

Sample Topics for in-service Education in Hospital

- Drug calculation
- Fluid electrolyte imbalance
- Anaphylaxis
- Records, reports and team nursing
- Phlebitis assessment
- Basics in ECG
- Pediatric Nursing- assessment, I/V calculation, dehydration assessment
- Management of emergency conditions I
- (ACS, poisoning, hypoglycemia)
- Burns training
- Equipment handling
- Biomedical waste management
- Safe injection and infusion practices
- Documentation
- Physical assessment and scales in assessment
- BLS/ACLS
- Blood transfusion
- Dengue fever - management
- IV essentials
- Management of a patient on ventilator—Hands on training
- Breastfeeding- BFHI, techniques
- Critical care nursing through OSCE evaluation
- Prevention of bedsore—Implementing Braden scale
- Aseptic practises, reconstitution of medication and safe patient handling techniques
- Nutritional management of critically ill patients
- Advances in management of diabetes mellitus

Contd…

- Insulin administration
- Temperature, pulse, respiration, BP and respiratory assessment for novice nurses
- Hand washing, waste management and aseptic practices
- Ventilator associated pneumonia
- Patient instruction training on common conditions
- Closed suction system - session for ICU staffs

CONCLUSION

The main purpose of in-service education program is to provide educational activities for all nurses employed by the health care agency directed towards change in behavior related to role expectations, which build upon the individuals varied education and experimental basis. In-service education program must be concerned with the growth and development of personnel from their initial contact with the health care agency until the termination of services.

ADULT LEARNING

The term andragogy was coined in 19th century. Andragogy refers to education of adults. Knowles is referred to as the father of adult learning. Knowles defines andragogy as the art and science of helping adults to learn. He explained that education of adult is a process of self-directed inquiry. Participants prefer to decide for themselves what they want to learn and enter into learning process with a task centered orientation. He also described adult learners are persons who perform best when asked to use their experience and apply new knowledge to solve problems.

The European Commission defines adult learning as all forms of learning undertaken by adults after having left initial education and training.

PRINCIPLES OF ADULT LEARNING

- **Adult learners are self-directed:** Self-directed adult learners actively participate in teaching and learning process.
- **Life experience:** Adult learners have life experiences, like work related experiences, previous education etc., which enhance their abilities to guide their education.
- **Adults need learning to be relevant and practical:** Adults are practical oriented and the learning must be applicable to their work.
- **Adults have their own learning styles:** Each individual adult has different learning style and each individual should be given preference.
- **Goal oriented:** For adult learning, select an educational program that is organized and has clearly defined objectives.
- In adult learning, learners actively participate in learning process and pace with their own learning.

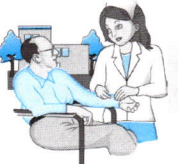

- Adult learners need an environment that enables them to assume responsibilities.

Adult learners need to determine their own goals and needs and work collaboratively to achieve goals. So create a relaxed, psychologically safe climate with an environment of trust and mutual respect. Teacher should acts as a facilitator, guide and or a coach. Give respect to learner's idea. Introduce them to new opportunities and experience. Guide learners in developing learning strategies and to identify resources. Introduce them to new opportunities and experiences.

KNOWLES' 5 ASSUMPTIONS OF ADULT LEARNERS

1. **Self-concept:** As a person matures, his/her self-concept moves from one of being a dependent personality toward one of being a self-directed human being.
2. **Adult learner experience:** As a person matures, he/she accumulates a growing reservoir of experience that becomes an increasing resource for learning.
3. **Readiness to learn:** As a person matures, his/her readiness to learn becomes oriented increasingly to the developmental tasks of his/her social roles.
4. **Orientation to learning:** As a person matures, his/her time perspective changes from one of postponed application of knowledge to immediacy of application, and accordingly his/her orientation toward learning shifts from one of the subject-centeredness to one of problem centeredness.
5. **Motivation to learn:** As a person matures the motivation to learn is internal.

KNOWLES' 4 PRINCIPLES OF ANDRAGOGY

Malcolm knowles is the father of adult learning. In 1984, Knowles suggested 4 principles that are applied to adult learning:
1. Adults need to be involved in the planning and evaluation of their instruction.
2. Experience (including mistakes) provides the basis for the learning activities.
3. Adults are most interested in learning subjects that have immediate relevance and impact to their job or personal life.
4. Adult learning is problem-centered rather than content-oriented.

CHARACTERISTICS OF ADULT LEARNERS

- Adult learners are self-directed.
- Life experiences enhances the abilities of adult learners and guide their education.
- Adult learners work collaboratively to achieve goals.
- Adult learners have work related experience.

Characterstics of adult learners according to Jackson and Caffarella (1994)
- Adult learners have life experience that serve as rich sources for learning.
- Adults have their own learning style.
- Adults are more likely to prefer being actively involved in the learning process.
- Adults are supportive to each other in learning process.
- Adults have individual responsibilities and life situation that provide a context for learning.

ADULT LEARNING CYCLE

- **Phase 1:** Experiencing (Doing)
- **Phase 2:** Processing (Reflecting)
- **Phase 3:** Generalizing (Deriving meaning)
- **Phase 4:** Applying (Taking action)

FACTORS AFFECTING ADULT LEARNING

Hands-on

Adults want to involved in training process. They would rather "do" or perform than simply sit and watch. Even a demonstration will not be as effective as doing it oneself. Although providing hands-on experiences takes more time and preparation, the results are well worth in effectiveness and increased implementation.

Active Involvement

Adults can tune out during a training session. Sitting passively opens the door to day-dreaming or worrying about outside responsibilities. Many adults have few opportunities to talk with others about their work-related concerns or experiences and will desire such interactions.

Performance Feedback

Most adults need reassurance that their attempts are not inconsistent with expectations. Coaching helps to keep them motivated and wanting to learn. Feedback through comments from the instructor and support through recognition of their efforts and performance are essential to effective training.

Movement

Adults will need opportunities to move around either through instructor-planned activities or through their choices. Adults become conditioned to frequent changes. Change the type of activity often and schedule activities and breaks to allow movement.

Repetition and Reinforcement

Adults need opportunities to repeat tasks or to have ideas repeated to reinforce learning and skills. Practice is important in their learning, but it should not consist of boring drill. Provide reinforcement by incorporating the same information or skill in different ways through a variety of activities.

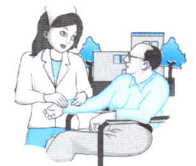

STANDARDS OF STAFF DEVELOPMENT PROGRAM ACCORDING TO AMERICAN NURSES ASSOCIATION

Standard I: Organization and Administration
The nursing service department and the nursing staff development unit, philosophy purpose and goals and address the staff development needs of nursing personnel.

Standard II: Human Resources
Qualified administrative, educational and support personnel are provided to meet the learning and developmental needs by nursing service personnel.

Standard III: Learner
Nursing staff development educators assist nursing personnel in identifying their learning needs and planning-learning activities to meet those needs.

Standard IV: Program Planning
Provides the unit systematically, plan and evaluate the overall nursing staff development program in response to health care needs.

Standard V: Educational Design
Educational offering and learning experiences are designed through the use of educational process.

Standard VI. Material Resources and Facilities
Material resources and facilities are adequate to achieve the goals and implement the function of overall nursing staff development unit.

Standard VII: Records and Report
The nursing staff development unit establishes and maintains record keeping system.

Standard VIII: Evaluation
Evaluation is an integral ongoing and systematic process which include measure in the impact of learning.

Standard IX: Consultation
The nursing staff development educators use the consultation process to facilitate and enhance the achievement of individual, departmental and organizational goals.

Standard X: Climate
The nursing staff development educators foster a climate which promote open communication, learning and professional growth.

Standard XI: Systematic Enquiring
Encourage systematic enquiring and application of the result into nursing practice.

Suggested Reading

- Knowles, MS. Informal Adult Education. Guide for educators based on the writer's experience as a program organizer in the YMCA. New York: Association Press; 1950.
- Knowles, MS. (1962). A History of the Adult Education Movement in the USA, New York: Krieger. A revised edition was published in 1977.
- Sharan B Merriam, Ralph G Brockett. The Profession and Practice of Adult Education: An Introduction. Jossey-Bass; p. 7. 2007.
- "Adult Education". The Canadian Encyclopedia, Retrieved 19 October, 2014.
- Lisa M Baumgartner, Sharan B Merriam, et al. Learning in Adulthood: A Comprehensive Guide (3rd ed.). San Francisco: Jossey-Bass; 2007. p. 7. ISBN 978-0-7879-7588-3.
- Spencer, Bruce. The Purposes of Adult Education: A Short Introduction (2nd ed.). Toronto: Thompson Educational Publishing pp. 9–10. ISBN 9781550771619.
- Tomey AM. Guide to Nursing Management and Leadership. 5th Ed. St. Louis; Mosby.
- Barrett Jean. Ward Management and Teaching. 2nd Ed. New Delhi; The English Book Store.
- Gillies DN. Nursing Management. A System Approach. Tokyo; WB Saunders Company.

Assess Yourself

LONG ANSWERS

1. Define in-service education program. Nature, scope and components of in-service education program. Write down the principles of good in-service education program.
2. Define adult learning. Write the types and principles of learning.
3. Define staff development program. Explain the role of nurse manager in organizing a staff development program.

SHORT NOTES

1. In-service education
2. Principles of adult learning

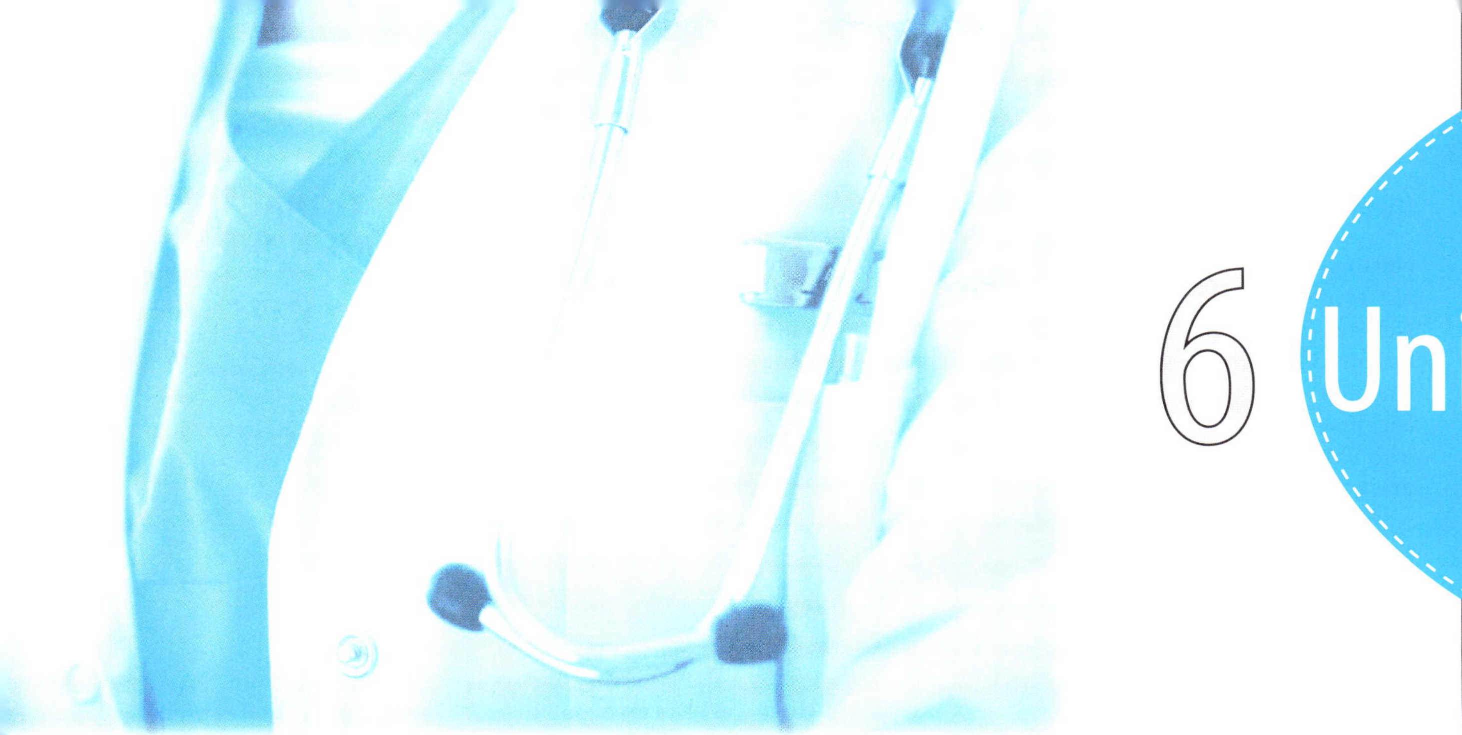

Unit 6

Management of Nursing Educational Institutions

Unit Outline

- Introduction
- Organization of Nursing Educational Institutions
- Essentials of Educational Institutions as per INC Norms
- Guidelines and Minimum Requirements to Establish School of Nursing
- Minimum Requirement to Establish General Nursing and Midwifery Program
- Teaching Faculty—Qualifications and Experience in School of Nursing
- Budget
- Affiliation
- Distribution of Beds
- Staffing
- Admission Terms and Conditions
- Health Services
- Institutional Records
- Transcript
- Credit System
- Guidelines and Minimum Requirements to Establish BSc (N) College of Nursing
- Recognition, Affiliation and Accreditation
- Management of Faculty
- Job Description of Faculty College of Nursing
- Staff Welfare
- Staff Development Program
- Administration of Students
- Discipline in Educational Institutions
- Administration of Curriculum

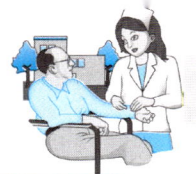

INTRODUCTION

Nursing education is a professional education to prepare nurses to provide quality nursing service to humanity. Nursing education is dominated by theories, models and systems that are generally adopted and applied with little attention to bridging the gap between nursing education and practice. History of modern nursing education began with Florence Nightingale. Her theoretical model for nursing practice emphasized discipline, good character and a nursing service hierarchy and a strong ability to follow protocol and procedures. Nursing education has the challenging mandate of preparing a generation of practitioners who are knowledgeable and equipped with values and critical thinking abilities required in an emerging and ever changing health care systems.

The aim of nursing education is to prepare nursing workforce to provide quality service to people in all settings. The quality of nursing education depends on the organizational framework within which it operates. Nursing education institutions are organizations which provide scientific knowledge and skill and prepare nursing students to assume the responsibilities of a professional nurse. Organization pattern of a nursing educational institution is influenced by the institutions vision, mission, philosophy, objectives, number of educational programs, students etc.

The statement of philosophy is the foundation on which the objectives of the program will be determined and the policies are framed. The points to be considered while formulating philosophy are the responsibilities of nurse to the society, belief regarding the role of nurse educators toward the students, belief regarding contribution of the hospital and community to the students, belief regarding professional status of nursing etc.

ORGANIZATION OF NURSING EDUCATIONAL INSTITUTIONS

Steps in the organization of nursing educational administration:
- Formulation of board of management
- Formulation of philosophy of nursing education institutions.
- Preparing infrastructure and other facilities.
- Selection, recruitment and appointment of faculty.
- Inspection and obtaining permission from India Nursing Council (INC), State Government and concerned university.
- Development of curriculum.
- Selection of student.
- Periodic credentialing and accreditation of the educational institution.
- Maintenance of records and registers.

ESSENTIALS OF EDUCATIONAL INSTITUTIONS AS PER INC NORMS

INC is a statutory body that regulates nursing education in the country through examination, certification and maintaining its standards for uniform syllabus at each level of nursing education.

The different levels of nursing education in India today are:
- Auxilliary Nursing and Midwifery (ANM) or Multi-purpose Health Workers Male and Females
- General Nursing and Midwifery (GNM)
- Basic Bachelor of Nursing (BSc Nursing)
- Post Basic Bachelor of Nursing (PBBSc Nursing)
- Post Basic Diploma in Specialty Nursing
- Masters in Nursing (MSc Nursing)
- Masters in Philosophy in Nursing (M. Phil)
- Doctorate in Philosophy in Nursing (PhD)
- Post Doctoral Fellowship in Nursing

GUIDELINES AND MINIMUM REQUIREMENTS TO ESTABLISH SCHOOL OF NURSING

- Any organization under: (i) Central Government/State Government/Local body (ii) Registered Private or Public Trust (iii) Missionary or any other organization registered under Society Registration Act (iv) Company incorporated under section 25 of Company's Act are eligible to establish General Nursing and Midwifery School of Nursing.
- Any organization having 100 bedded Parent (Own) hospital is eligible to establish General Nursing Course.
- Above organization shall obtain the Essentiality Certificate (EC)/No Objection Certificate (NOC) for the General Nursing and Midwifery program from the respective State Government. The institution name along with Trust Deed/Society address shall be mentioned in NOC/EC.
- An application form to establish nursing program is available on the website viz., www.indiannursingcouncil.org, which can be downloaded. Duly filled in application form with the requisite documents mentioned in the form shall be submitted before the last date as per the calendar of events of that year.
- The INC on receipt of the proposal from the Institution to start nursing program, will undertake the **first inspection** to assess suitability with regard to physical infrastructure, clinical facility and teaching faculty in order to give permission to start the program.
- After the receipt of the permission to start the nursing program from INC, the institution shall obtain the approval from the State Nursing Council and Examination Board.
- Institution will admit the students only after taking approval of State Nursing Council and Examination Board.

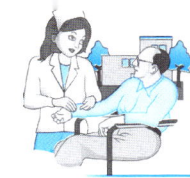

- The INC will conduct inspection every year till the first batch completes the program and permission will be given year by year till the first batch completes.

Note:
- If, no admission are made for two consecutive academic years then it shall be considered as closed for the said program.
- If the institution wants to restart the program they have to submit the first inspection fees within 5 years, i.e., from the year they did not have admissions.

MINIMUM REQUIREMENT TO ESTABLISH GENERAL NURSING AND MIDWIFERY PROGRAM

Teaching Block

The School of Nursing should have a separate building/teaching block. For a School with an annual admission capacity of **40–60** students, the constructed area of the school should be **23720** square feet.

The School of Nursing can be in a rented/leased building for first two years. After two years institute shall have own building in an institutional area. Otherwise ₹50,000 penalty has to be paid for every year for 3 years. During the penalty period institute shall be able to construct own building. If the institution is not able to have their own building, permission/suitability will be withdrawn however institution will be given chance to submit the proposal toward first inspection with the latest guidelines.

Adequate hostel/residential accommodation for students and staff should be available in addition to the above mentioned built up area of the nursing school respectively. The details of the constructed area are given below in Table 1 for admission capacity of **40-60** students:

Table 1: Area of teaching block

S.No.	Teaching block area	Figures in sq feet
1	Lecture Hall 4 × 1080	4320
2	**Laboratories**	
	• Nursing foundation lab	1500
	• CHN	900
	• Nutrition	900
	• OBG and Pediatrics lab	900
	• Preclinical science lab	900
	• Computer lab	1500
3	Multipurpose hall	3000
4	Common room (male and female)	1100
5	Staff room	1000
6	Principal room	300

Contd…

S.No.	Teaching block area	Figures in sq feet
7	Vice-principal room	200
8	Library	2400
9	AV aids room	600
10	One room for each head of departments	800 each
11	Faculty room	2400
12	Provisions for toilets	1000
	Total	**23720 Sq feet**

Table 2: Area of hostel block

S. No.	Hostel block area	Figures in sq feet
1.	Single room Double room	24000
2.	Sanitary one latrine and one bath room (for 5 students)	500
3.	Visitor room	500
4.	Reading room	250
5.	Store	500
6.	Recreation room	500
7.	Dining hall	3000
8.	Kitchen and store	1500
	Total	**30750 Sq feet**

Grand Total (Total requirement for the nursing program): 23720 (Teaching Block) + 30750 (Hostel block) = **54470 Sq feet.**

Hostel Block

Hostel provision is mandatory and shall also be owned by the institute within the period of two years (Table 2.)

Physical Facilities

- Nursing educational institution should be in Institutional area only and not in residential area.
- If the institute has non-nursing program in the same building, nursing program should have separate teaching block.
- Shift-wise management with other educational institutions will not be accepted.
- Separate teaching block shall be available if it is in hospital premises.
- Proportionately the size of the built-up area will increase according to the number of students admitted.
- School and college of nursing can share laboratories, if they are in same campus under same name and under same trust, that is the institution is one but offering different nursing programs. However, they should have equipments and articles proportionate to the strength of admission and the class rooms should be available as per the requirement stipulated by INC of each program.

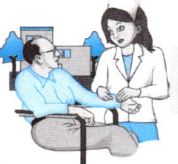

Class Rooms

There should be at least four classrooms with the capacity of accommodating the number of students admitted in each class. The rooms should be well ventilated with proper lighting system. There should be built in Black/Green/White Boards. Also there should be a desk or a big table and a chair for the teacher. Adequate number of racks/cupboards for keeping teaching aids are also needed.

Laboratories

There should be at least six laboratories as listed below:
1. Nursing Practice Laboratory
2. Community Health Nursing Practice Laboratory
3. Nutrition Laboratory
4. Computer Laboratory
5. OBG and Pediatric Laboratory
6. Pre-clinical Sciences Laboratory

Nursing Practice Laboratory

There should be demonstration beds with dummy and mannequins in proportion to the number of students practicing a nursing procedure at a given point of time (the desired ratio being 1 bed: 6 practicing students).

It should be fully equipped with built-in-cupboards and racks. Wash-basins with running water supply, electric fitting, adequate furniture like table, chairs, stools, patient lockers footsteps etc. Sufficient necessary inventory articles should be there i.e. at least 10–12 sets of all items needed for the practice of nursing procedure by the students.

Community Practice Laboratory

It should have all required articles needed for practicing nursing procedures in a community set-up.

Nutrition Laboratory

It should have facilities for imparting basic knowledge of various methods of cooking for the healthy as well as for the sick. The furnishing and equipment should include work-tables, cooking cutlery, trays, plates, dietetic, scales, cooking utensils, microwave, racks/shelves, refrigerator, pressure cookers, mixer and cupboards for storage of food items. The food items shall be purchased for the conduct of practical classes as and when required. Sets of crockery and cutlery for preparation, napkins for serving and display of food also should be there.

Computer Laboratory

It can be shared with other departments.

OBG and Pediatric Laboratory

Laboratory should have equipment and articles as mentioned in laboratory equipment and articles.

Pre-clinical Science Laboratory

It is the laboratory of biochemistry, anatomy and microbiology. The laboratory articles mentioned in the laboratory equipment and articles shall be available.

Auditorium

Auditorium should be spacious enough to accommodate at least double the sanctioned/actual strength of students, so that it can be utilized for hosting functions of the college, educational conferences/workshops, CNEs examinations etc. It should have proper stage with green room facilities. It should be well-ventilated and have proper lighting system. There should be arrangements for the use of all kinds of basic and advanced audio-visual aids or **multipurpose** hall—it should have multipurpose hall, if there is no auditorium in the school.

Library

There should be a separate library in the school. It should be easily accessible to the teaching faculty and the students, during school hours and extended hours also. It should have comfortable seating arrangements for half of the total strength of the students and teachers in the school. There should be separate budget for the library. The library committee should meet regularly for keeping the library updated with current books, journals and other literature. Internet facility should be provided in the library. The library should have proper lighting facilities and it should be well-ventilated. It should have a cabin for librarian with intercom phone facility. There should be sufficient number of cupboards, books shelves and racks with glass doors for proper and safe storage of books, magazines, journals, newspapers and other literature. There should be provision for catalogue-cabinets, racks for students bags etc., book display racks, bulletin boards and stationery items like index cards, borrowers cards, labels and registers. Current books, magazines, journals, newspaper and other literature should be available in the library.

A minimum of 500 of different subject titled nursing books (all new editions), in the multiple of editions, 3 kinds of nursing journals, 3 kinds of magazines, 2 kinds of newspapers and other kinds of current health related literature should be available in the library.

Office Requirements

Principal's Office

There should be a separate office for the principal with attached toilet and provision for visitor's room. Independent telephone facility is a must for the principal's office with intercom facility connected/linked to the hospital and hostel.

Office for Vice-Principal

There should be a separate office for the vice-principal with attached toilet and provision for visitor's room. Independent telephone facility is a must for vice-principal's office with intercom facility connected/linked to the hospital and hostel.

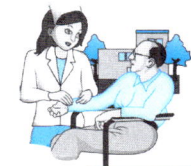

Office for Faculty Members

There should be adequate number of office rooms in proportion to the number of teaching faculty. One office room should accommodate **2** teachers only. Separate toilet facility should be provided for the teaching faculty with hand washing facility. There should be a separate toilet for male teachers.

One separate office room for the office staff should be provided with adequate toilet facility. This office should be spacious enough to accommodate the entire office staff with separate cabin for each official.

Each office room should be adequately furnished with items like tables, chairs, cupboards, built-in racks and shelves, filing cabinets and book cases. Also, there should be provision for equipment like photocopier, computers and telephone.

Common Rooms

A minimum of **3** common rooms should be provided. One for the teaching faculty, one for the student and one for the office staff. Sufficient space with adequate seating arrangements, cupboards, lockers, cabinets, built-in-shelves and racks should be provided in all the common rooms. Toilet and hand washing facilities should be made available in each room.

Record Room

There should be a separate record room with steel racks, built-in shelves and racks, cupboards and filing cabinets for proper storage of records and other important papers/documents belonging to the college.

Store Room

A separate store room should be provided to accommodate the equipment and other inventory articles which are required in the laboratories of the college. This room should have the facilities for proper and safe storage of these articles and equipment like cupboards, built-in-shelves, racks, cabinets, furniture items like tables and chairs. This room should be properly lighted and well-ventilated.

Room for Audio-Visual Aids

This room should be provided for the proper and safe storage of all the audio-visual aids. The school should possess all kind of basic as well as advanced training aids like chalkboards, overhead projectors, slide and film-strip projector, models, specimen, charts and posters, TV and VCR, Photostat machine, tape recorder and computers, LCD, laptop.

Other Facilities

Safe drinking water and adequate sanitary/toilet facilities should be available for both men and women separately in the school. Toilet facility to the students should be there along with hand washing facility.

Garage

Garage should accommodate **50** seather vehicles.

Fire Extinguisher

Adequate provision for extinguishing fire should be available as per the local byelaws.

Playground

Playground should be spacious for outdoor sports like volleyball, football, badminton and for athletics.

Hostel Facilities

There should be a separate hostel for the male and female students. It should have the following facilities:

Hostel Room

It should be ideal for 2 students. The furniture provided should include a cot, a table, a chair, a book rack, a cupboard or almirah for each student.

Toilet and Bathroom

Toilet and bathroom facilities should be provided on each floor of the students hostel at the ratio of one toilet and one bathroom for 2-6 students. Geysers in bathroom and wash basins should also be provided.

Recreation

There should be facilities for indoor and outdoor games. There should be provision for TV, radio and video cassette player.

Visitor's Room

There should be a visitor's room in the hostel with comfortable seating, lighting and toilet facilities.

Kitchen and Dining Hall

There should be a hygienic kitchen and dining hall to seat at least 80% of the total student's strength at one time with adequate tables, chairs, water coolers, refrigerators and heating facilities. Hand washing facilities must be provided.

Pantry

One pantry on each floor should be provided. It should have water cooler and heating arrangements.

Washing and Ironing Room

Facility for drying and ironing clothes should be provided in each floor.

Sick Room

A sick room should have a comfortable bed, linen, furniture and attached toilet. Minimum of 5 beds should be provided.

Room for Night Duty Nurses

Should be in a quiet area.

Guest Room

A guest room should be made available with toilet facility.

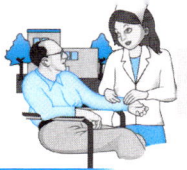

Warden's Room

Warden should be provided with a separate office room besides her residential accommodation. Intercom facility with school and hospital shall be provided.

Telephone Facility

This facility accessible to students in emergency situation shall be made available.

Canteen

There should be provision for a canteen for the students, their guests, and all other staff members.

Transport

School should have separate transport facility under the control of the principal. Twenty five and fifty seater bus is preferable.

Crèche

There should be a crèche in the college campus.

Staff for the Hostel

- Warden (Female)-3: Qualification—BSc Home Science or Diploma in Housekeeping/Catering. Minimum three wardens must be there in every hostel for morning, evening and night shifts. If number of students are more than 150, one more warden/Asst. Warden/House keeper for every additional 50 students.
- Cook-1: (For every 20 students for each shift).
- Kitchen and dining room helper-1: (For every 20 students for each shift).
- Sweeper-3
- Gardener-2
- Security Guard/Chowkidar-3

General Points

- Notice/Circular for prohibition of ragging shall be available on:
  - Notice Boards
  - Admission Brochure/Prospectus
- Display posters/charts on prohibition of ragging in common places.
- **Constitute:**
  - Antiragging committee with name, designation and telephone no.
  - Antiragging squad
- Complaint boxes placed at places accessible to students

The Principal should be the administrative head of the school. He/she should hold qualification as laid down by INC. The principal should be the controlling authority for the budget of the school and also be the drawing and disbursing officer. The Principal and Vice-Principal should be gazetted officers in government schools and of equal status (though non-gazetted) in non-government schools.

Ratio of female and male nursing teachers in school program is for every 7 female nursing teacher there shall be 3 male nursing teacher i.e. 7:3 female to male nursing teacher ratio. [i.e., maximum of 30% will be male] it does not direct that female teachers are to be replaced by male.

TEACHING FACULTY—QUALIFICATIONS AND EXPERIENCE IN SCHOOL OF NURSING

Teaching Faculty

- Principal: MSc nursing with 3 years of teaching experience or BSc nursing (Basic)/Post Basic with 5 years of teaching experience.(1)
- Vice-Principal: MSc nursing or BSc nursing (Basic)/Post Basic with 3 years of teaching experience.(1)
- Tutor: MSc. Nursing or BSc Nursing (Basic/Post Basic) or Diploma in Nursing Education and Administration with 2 years of professional experience.(10)
- **Total 12 Faculty = 1 Principal + 1 Vice-principal + 10 Tutor**
- Teacher student ratio should be 1:10 on sanctioned strength of students.
- One of the tutors need to stay at the community health field by rotation.
- The salary structure of the teaching faculty in private schools of nursing should not be less than what is admissible in the schools of the nursing under State/Central Government.
- Nursing service personnel should actively participate in instruction, supervision, guidance and evaluation of student in the clinical and field/community practice areas.
- The teaching faculty of the school of nursing should work in close coordination with nursing service personnel.
- The teaching faculty of the school and the nursing service personnel should be deputed to attend short-term educational courses/workshops/conferences etc. to update their knowledge.
- It is mandatory for school authorities to treat teaching faulty of the school of nursing on duty when nominated/selected for the purpose of examination or inspection or inspection by the Council.
- All nursing faculty including principal shall spend at least four hours each day in the clinical area for clinical teaching and/or supervision of care by the students.
- 50% of the non-nursing subjects should be taught by the nursing teachers.
- However, it will be supplemented by the guest faculty who are doctors/PG. Qualification in the requisite subject as per INC norms. Nursing teachers who are involved in non-nursing subjects shall be examiners for the program.

External Lecturers

Besides the regular teaching faculty in the school of nursing, there should be provision for external lectures for teaching the students. They should possess the desired qualification in the respective subjects which are to be taught. Remuneration of these external lecturers is to be paid as per the institute/government policy. The external lecturers may comprise nursing experts medical faculty and scientists, general educationist including teaching experts in english, computer education, physical education/yoga, psychologists, sociologists, hospital dieticians, nursing service personnel like nursing superintendent, ward-in-charge or ward sister, health economist/statistician etc. working in or outside the institution.

School Management Committee

Following members should constitute the Board of Management of the school.

Principal—Chairperson
Vice-Principal—Member
Tutor—Member
Chief Nursing Officer/Nursing Superintendent—Member
Representative of Medical Superintendent—Member
Administrative Staff for School of Nursing—Member

Additional Staff for School of Nursing

Stenographer/Personal Assistant
Senior Clerk cum Cashier/Accountant
Junior Clerk cum Typist
Librarian -1
Laboratory Attendant -1
Chowkidar/Watchman -2
Driver One/each vehicle
Cleaner One/each vehicle
Peon - 3
Sweeper/Safai Karmachari - 2
Machine (Duplicating/Xerox) Operator -1

BUDGET

In the overall budget of the institution, there should be provision for school budget under a separate head. Principal of the school of nursing should be the drawing and disbursing officer.

School of nursing should have a **100** bedded Parent (Own Hospital) for 40-60 annual intake in each program:

- **Distribution of beds** in different areas

Medical	– 30
Surgical	– 30
Obstetrics and gynecology	– 30
Pediatrics	– 20
Ortho	– 10

- The size of the Hospital/Nursing Home for affiliation:
  - Should not be less than **100** beds apart from having own hospital.
  - Maximum 3 hospital can be attached with 100 beds each.

- Bed occupancy of the hospital should be minimum **75%**.
- **Other specialties/facilities** for clinical experience required are as follows:
  - Major OT
  - Minor OT
  - Dental
  - Eye/ENT
  - Burns and plastic
  - Neonatology with mursery
  - Communicable disease
  - Community health nursing
  - Cardiology
  - Oncology
  - Neurology/neurosurgery
  - Nephrology
  - ICU/ICCU
- There should be a variety of patients of all age groups in all the clinical areas where the students are posted for obtaining the requisite learning experiences.
- **Affiliation of psychiatric hospital** should be of minimum 30-50 beds.
- The nursing staffing norms in the affiliated hospital should be as per the INC norms.
- Affiliated hospitals should be in the radius of 15-30 km.
- **1:3 student patient ratio** to be maintained.
- For tribal and hilly area the maximum distance is 50 km for affiliated hospital.

AFFILIATION

If all the required learning experience are not available in the parent hospital, the students should be sent to affiliated hospital/agencies/Institutions where it is available.

Criteria for Affiliation

The types of experience for which a nursing school can affiliate are:
- Community health nursing
- Communicable diseases
- Mental Health (psychiatric) nursing
- Specialties like cardiology, neurology, oncology nephrology etc.

The physical facilities like staffing and equipment of the affiliated hospitals should be of the same standard as required in the parent hospital.

The staff of the selected hospital should be prepared to recognize student status and their educational program.

DISTRIBUTION OF BEDS

At least one third of the total number of beds should be for medical patients and one-third for surgical patients. The number of beds for male patients should not be less than 1/6th

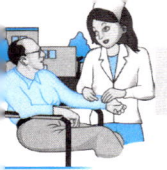

of the total number of beds, i.e. at least 40 beds. There should be minimum of 750 deliveries per year (for annual admission capacity of 20 students). Provision should be made for clinics in health and family welfare and for preventive medicine.

STAFFING

• For 500 beds and above chief nursing officer (CNO)	Qualification as for Principal, SON
• Nursing Superintendent (NS)	Qualification as for Principal, SON
• Deputy Nursing Superintendent (DNS)	Qualification as for vice-principal SON
• Assistant Nursing Superintendent (ANS) and for every additional 50 beds one more	Qualification as for vice-principal SON

Norms recommended by experts committee on health manpower production and management (resolution of fourth conference of central council of health and family welfare, on nursing, 1995)

Categories requirements
- Nursing superintendent 1:200 beds
- Deputy nursing superintendent 1:300 beds
- Departmental nursing supervisors 7:1000
- Ward nursing supervisors/sisters 8:200+30% leave reserve
- Staff nurse for wards 1:3 (of 1:9 each Shift) +30% leave reserve
- For OPD, blood bank, X-ray - 1:100 OPD patients diabetic clinic CSR etc. (1 bed: 5 OPD patients) + 30% leave reserve.
- For intensive care unit (ICU) 1; 1 per shift+ 30% leave
- For specialized departments 8:200 + 30% leave reserve and clinic such as OT, labor room.

Justification
- Needs may vary from one hospital to another, depending on its size and service rendered, more staff than anticipated will be required.
- Special attention is needed for supervision of patient care in the evening and night shifts.
- 30% leave reserve posts are mandatory.

Other points to be considered
- The staff of the parent hospital should be strictly as per the criteria laid down by INC in terms of doctors, nurses and paramedical staff.
- Wards/Area/OPDs/OTs/Clinical departments etc. must have adequate coverage of the staff in all the shifts to ensure that students are only for attending clinical experience in these areas and not utilized for service purposes.
- Continuing/in-service education program must be attended by all staff nurses to keep themselves abreast with latest technologies and sophistication used in day to day patient care in these areas.

Community Health Nursing Field Practice Area

The students should be sent for community health nursing experience in urban as well as rural field area. Institute can be attached to primary health centre. A well setup field teaching center should be provided with facilities for accommodation of at least 10-15 students and one staff member at a time. Peon, cook and chowkidar should be available at health centre. Each school of Nursing should have its own transport facilities.

ADMISSION TERMS AND CONDITIONS

- Minimum education eligibility criteria for admission **to GNM**: 10+2 with 40% marks from any recognized board. However science is preferable
  Candidates are also eligible from State Open School recognized by State Government and National Institute of Open School (NIOS) recognized by Central Government.
  Registered ANM
  10+2 vocational ANM course from the school recognized by INC
  10+2 Health care Science – Vocational stream from a recognized CBSE board/State/Centre
  For Foreign Nationals
  The entry qualification equivalency i.e., 12th standard will be obtained by Association of Indian Universities, New Delhi. Institution, State Nursing Council will be responsible to ensure that the qualification and eligibility will be equivalent to what has been prescribed as above.
- **Reservation**
  - **For disabled candidates:** 3% disability reservation to be considered with a disability of locomotor to the tune of 40% to 50% of the lower extremity and other eligibility criteria with regard to age and qualification will be same as prescribed for each nursing program.
    Note: A committee to be formed consisting of medical officer authorized by medical board of state government and a nursing expert in the panel which may decide whether the candidates have the disability of locomotor of 40–50%.
  - 5% seats are reserved for SC/ST candidates
  - Any other quotas as per the State Government under the reservation policy
    Note: Quotas shall be applicable within the sanctioned number of the seats sanctioned and not above it.
- Admission of students will be once in a year.
- Students should be medically fit.
- Minimum age for admission is 17 years (as on 31st December of that year). The upper age limit is 35 years. For ANM/for LHV, there is no age bar.

Admission/Selection Committee

This committee should comprise of:
- Principal Chairperson

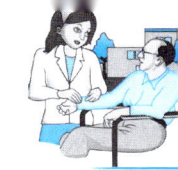

- Vice-Principal
- Senior Tutor
- Chief Nursing Officer or Nursing Superintendent

Admission Strength

More than 60 students can be sanctioned (maximum 100) if the institution has a parent-medical college or parent hospital having more than 300 beds.

HEALTH SERVICES

There should be provisions for the following health services for the students.
- An annual medical examination
- Vaccination against tetanus, hepatitis B or any other communicable disease as considered necessary
- Free medical care during illness
- A complete health record should be kept in respect of each individual student. The question of continuing the training of a student, with long-term chronic illness, will be decided by the individual school.

INSTITUTIONAL RECORDS

Following are the minimum records which needs to be/should be maintained in the school:
- **For students:**
  - Admission record
  - Health record
  - Class attendance record
  - Clinical and field experience record
  - Internal assessment record for both theory and practical
  - Mark lists (State Council/Board Results)
  - Record of extracurricular activities of student (both in the school as well as outside)
  - Leave record
  - Practical record books – Procedure book and Midwifery record book to be maintained as prescribed by INC
- **For each academic year, for each class/batch**
  - Course contents record (for each subjects)
  - The record of the academic performance
  - Rotation plans for each academic year
  - Record of committee meetings
  - Record of the stock of the school
  - Affiliation record
  - Grant-in-aid record (if the school is receiving grant-in-aid from any source like State Government etc.)
  - **Cumulative record:** Record of educational programs organized for teaching faculty and student, both in the school as well as outside.

Annual reports (Record of the achievement of the school prepared annually.

School of nursing should possess detailed and up-to-date record of each activity carried out in the school.

TRANSCRIPT

Transcript is an official copy of student's academic record. It records all courses successfully and unsuccessfully completed and all courses that were withdrawn after the registration deadline. It comes from the Latin Word, 'Transcriptum' that means things copied.

Transcript is defined as certified document that includes your full name, course and the date of enrollment. It details the module marks, clinical hours and curriculum information for each academic year and confirms the final award classification. It is a record of a student's performance and history at a particular academic institution.

Uses of Transcript
- Provide evidence
- Used for advanced education
- Used for employment
- Used for immigration

CREDIT SYSTEM

A credit system is a systematic way of describing an educational program by attaching credits to its component.

Objectives
- Giving opportunity to student who are diligent and having high capacity to finish their studies in the possible shortest time.
- Giving opportunity to students in general for being able to follow educational activity that best suit their interest, talent and capacity.
- Improving student capacity evaluation system.

GUIDELINES AND MINIMUM REQUIREMENTS TO ESTABLISH BSc (N) COLLEGE OF NURSING

Guidelines for Establishment of New BSc (N) College of Nursing

- Any organization under: (i) Central Government/State Government/Local body (ii) Registered Private or Public Trust (iii) Missionary or any other organization registered under Society Registration Act (iv) Company incorporated under section 25 of Company's Act are eligible to establish BSc (N) College of Nursing.
- Any organization having 100 bedded Parent (Own) hospital is eligible to establish BSc (N) Course.
- Above organization shall obtain the Essentiality Certificate (EC)/No Objection Certificate (NOC) for the BSc (N) program from the respective State Government. The

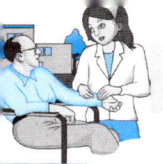

institution name along with Trust Deed/Society address shall be mentioned in NOC/EC.

- An application form to establish Nursing program is available on the website viz., www.indiannursingcouncil.org, which shall be downloaded. Duly filled in application form with the requisite documents mentioned in the form shall be submitted before the last date as per the calendar of events of that year.
- The INC on receipt of the proposal from the Institution to start nursing program, will undertake the **first inspection** to assess suitability with regard to physical infrastructure, clinical facility and teaching faculty in order to give permission to start the program.
- After the receipt of the permission to start the nursing program from INC, the institution shall obtain the approval from the State Nursing Council and University.
- Before admission of the students institute will submit the renewal/validity form as per the calendar of events every year.
- Institution will admit the students only after taking approval of INC, State Nursing Council and University.
- Seats sanctioned by INC shall be final. i.e. admission shall not exceed the sanctioned strength of Indian Nursing Council.
- Upgradation is not an additional BSc (N) program, but is the conversion from School of Nursing into College of Nursing.

Note: If any School of Nursing wants to convert to College of Nursing, essentiality Certificate for BSc (N) course is not essential, as they already possess essentiality certificate for School of Nursing. However, the private institutions has to produce document with regard to resolution of the management for conversion of School of Nursing into College of Nursing and INC norms will be followed. The School of Nursing should have been recognized by INC.

Minimum Requirement to Establish BSc (N) Program

Physical Facilities

Building

The college of nursing should have a separate building. The college of nursing should be near to its parent hospital having space for expansion in an institutional area. For a college with an annual admission capacity of **40-60** students, the constructed area of the college should be **23,720** square feet.

Adequate hostel/residential accommodation for students and staff should be available in addition to the above mentioned built up area of the nursing college respectively. The details of the constructed area is given below for admission capacity of **40-60** students Table 3:

Table 3: Area of teaching block

S. No.	Teaching Block	Area (Figures in Sq feet)
1	• Lecture hall	4 × 1080 = 4320
2	• Nursing foundation lab	1500
	• CHN	900
	• Nutrition	900
	• OBG and pediatrics lab	900
	• Preclinical science lab	900
	• Computer Lab	1500
3	• Multipurpose hall	3000
4	• Common room (Male and female)	1100
5	• Staff room	1000
6	• Principal room	300
7	• Vice principal room	200
8	• Library	2400
9	• A-V aids room	600
10	• One room for each head of departments	800
11	• Faculty room	2400
12	• Provisions for toilets	1000
Total		**23720 Sq feet**

- Nursing educational institution should be in Institutional area only and not in residential area.
- If the institute has non-nursing program in the same building, Nursing program should have separate teaching block.
- Shift-wise management with other educational institutions will not be accepted.
- Separate teaching block shall be available if it is in hospital premises.
- Proportionately the size of the built-up area will increase according to the number of students admitted.
- School and College of nursing can share laboratories if they are in same campus under same name and under same trust, that is the institution is one but offering different nursing programs. However, they should have equipment and articles proportionate to the strength of admission, and the class rooms should be available as per the requirement stipulated by INC of each program.

Class Rooms

There should be at least four classrooms with the capacity of accommodating the number of students admitted in each class. The rooms should be well-ventilated with proper lighting system. There should be built in black/green/white boards. Also there should be a desk, table and a chair for the teacher and racks/cupboards for keeping teaching aids.

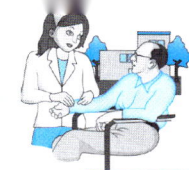

Departments

College should have following departments
- Fundamentals of nursing including nutrition
- Medical surgical nursing
- Community health nursing
- Obstetric and gynecological nursing
- Child health nursing
- Mental health nursing

Laboratories

There should be at least seven laboratories as listed below:
- Nursing foundations and medical surgical
- Community health nursing
- OBG and pediatrics
- Nutrition
- Computer lab with 10 computers
- Preclinical science labs. (Biochemistry, microbiology, biophysics, anatomy and physiology)

Auditorium

Auditorium should be spacious enough to accommodate at least double the sanctioned/actual strength of students, so that it can be utilized for hosting functions of the college, educational conferences/workshops, examinations etc. It should have proper stage with green room facilities. It should be well-ventilated and have proper lighting system. There should be arrangements for the use of all kinds of basic and advanced audio-visual aids.

Multipurpose Hall

College of Nursing should have multipurpose hall, if there is no auditorium.

Library

There should be a separate library for the college. The size of the library should be minimum **2400 square feet**. It should be easily accessible to the teaching faculty and the students. Library should have seating arrangements for at least **60** students for reading and having good lighting and ventilation and space for stocking and displaying of books and journals. The library should have at least **3000 books**. In a new college of nursing the total number of books should be proportionately divided on yearly basis in four years. At least 10 sets of books in each subject to facilitate for the students to refer the books. There should be at least 15 journals of which one-third shall be foreign journals and subscribed on continuous basis. There should be sufficient number of cupboards, book shelves and racks with glass doors for proper and safe storage of books, magazines, journals, newspapers and other literature.

In the library there should be provision for:
- Staff reading room for **10** persons.
- Rooms for librarian and other staff with intercom phone facility
- Video and cassette/CD room (desirable)
- Internet facility.

Offices Requirements

- ***Principal's office:*** There should be a separate office for the Principal with attached toilet and provision for visitor's room. Independent telephone facility is a must for the Principal's office with intercom facility connected/linked to the hospital and hostel and a computer with internet facility. The size of the office should be **300** sq. ft.
- ***Office for vice-principal :*** There should be a separate office for the Vice-Principal with attached toilet and provision for visitor's room. Independent telephone facility is a must for vice-principal's office with intercom facility connected/linked to the hospital and hostel and a computer with internet facility. The size of the office should be **200** sq. ft.
- ***Office for faculty members:*** There should be adequate number of office rooms in proportion to the number of teaching faculty. One office room should accommodate **2** teachers only. Separate toilet facility should be provided for the teaching faculty with hand washing facility. There should be a separate toilet for male teachers. The size of the room should be **200 sq. ft**. Separate chambers for heads of the department should be there.
- One separate office room for the office staff should be provided with adequate toilet facility. This office should be spacious enough to accommodate the entire office staff with separate cabin for each official. Each office room should be adequately furnished with items like tables, chairs, cupboards, built-in racks and shelves, filing cabinets and book cases. Also there should be provision for typewriters, computers and telephone.

Common Rooms

A minimum of **3** common rooms should be provided. One for the teaching faculty, one for the student and one for the office staff. Sufficient space with adequate seating arrangements, cupboards, lockers, cabinets, built-in-shelves and racks should be provided in all the common rooms. Toilet and hand washing facilities should be made available in each room.

Record Room

There should be a separate record room with steel racks, built-in-shelves and racks, cupboards and filing cabinets for proper storage of records and other important papers/documents belonging to the college.

Store Room

A separate store room should be provided to accommodate the equipments and other inventory articles which are required in the laboratories of the college. This room should have the facilities for proper and safe storage of these articles and equipments like cupboards, built-in-shelves, racks, cabinets, furniture items like tables and chairs. This room should be properly lighted and well-ventilated.

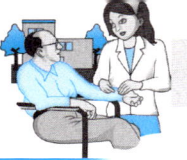

Room for Audio-Visual Aids

This room should be provided for the proper and safe storage of size **600** sq. ft. for all the audio-visual aids.

Other Facilities

Safe drinking water and adequate sanitary/toilet facilities should be available for both men and women separately in the college in each floor common toilets for teachers (separate for male and female) i.e. **4** toilets with wash basins. Common toilets for students (separate for male and female) **12** with wash basins for **60** students.

Garage

Garage should accommodate **60** seater vehicles.

Fire Extinguisher

Adequate provision for extinguishing fire should be available as per the local byelaws.

Playground

Playground should be spacious for outdoor sports like volleyball, football, badminton and for athletics.

Hostel Facilities (Table 4)

There should be a separate hostel for the male and female students. It should have the following facilities:

- **Hostel room:** It should be ideal for 2 students with the minimum 100 sq. ft. carpet area. The furniture provided should include a cot, a table, a chair, a book rack, a cupboard and a cloth rack for each student.
- **Toilet and bathroom:** Toilet and bathroom facilities should be provided on each floor of the student's hostel at the rate of one toilet and one bathroom for 2-6 students. Geysers in bathroom and wash basins should also be provided.
- **Recreation:** There should be facilities for indoor and outdoor games. There should be provision for TV, radio and video cassette player.

Table 4: Hostel Block (60 Students)

S. No.	Hostel block	Area (Figures in sq feet)
1.	Single room/double room	24000
2	Sanitary	One latrine and one bath room (for 5 students) - 500
3	Visitor room	500
4	Reading room	250
5	Store	500
6	Recreation room	500
7	Dining hall	3000
8	Kitchen and store	1500
	Total	30750 Sq feet

Grand Total : 23720 + 30750 = 54470 Sq feet.

- **Visitor's room:** There should be a visitor room in the hostel with comfortable seating, lighting and toilet facilities.
- **Kitchen and dining hall:** There should be a hygienic kitchen and dining hall to seat at least 80% of the total students strength at one time with adequate tables, chairs, water coolers, refrigerators and heating facilities. Hand washing facilities must be provided.
- **Pantry:** One pantry on each floor should be provided. It should have water cooler and heating arrangements.
- **Washing and ironing room:** Facility for drying and ironing clothes should be provided in each floor.
- **Sick room:** A sick room should have a comfortable bed, linen, furniture and attached toilet. Minimum of 5 beds should be provided.
- **Room for night duty nurses:** Should be in a quiet area.
- **Guest room:** A guest room should be made available.
- **Warden's room:** Warden should be provided with a separate office room besides her residential accommodation.
- **Canteen:** There should be provision for a canteen for the students, their guests and all other staff members.
- **Transport:** College should have separate transport facility under the control of the Principal. 50 seater bus is preferable.

Residential Accommodation

Residential family accommodation for faculty, should be provided, according to their marital status. Telephone facility for the principal at her residence must be provided. Residential accommodation with all facilities is to be provided to the hostel warden.

Crèche: There should be a crèche in the college campus.

Staff for the Hostel

- Warden (Female)-3: Qualification - BSc Home Science or Diploma in House keeping/Catering. Minimum three wardens must be there in every hostel for morning, evening and night shifts.
- Cook -1: For every 20 students for each shift.
- Kitchen and dining room helper-1: For every 20 students for each shift.
- Sweeper - 3
- Gardener - 2
- Security Guard/Chowkidar-3

Nursing Teaching Faculty (Tables 5 and 6)

Principal is excluded for 1:10 teacher student ratio norms
    Teacher/Tutor student ratio will be 1:10
    (For example, for 40 students intake minimum number of teachers required is 17 including Principal)

- No part time nursing faculty will be counted for calculating total no. of faculty required for a college.
- Irrespective of number of admissions, all faculty positions (Professor to Lecturer) must be filled.

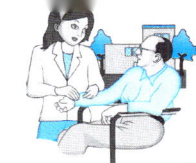

Table 5: Qualifications and experience of teachers for college of nursing

Post	Qualification	Experience
Principal cum Professor	MSc(N), PhD(N) is desirable	15 years experience with MSc(N) out of which 12 years should be teaching experience with minimum of 5 years in collegiate program.
Vice-Principal cum Professor	MSc(N), PhD(N) is desirable	12 years experience with MSc(N) out of which 10 years should be teaching experience with minimum of 5 years in collegiate program.
Professor	MSc(N), PhD(N) is desirable	10 years experience with MSc(N) out of which 7 years should be teaching experience.
Associate Professor	MSc(N), PhD(N) desirable	MSc(N) with 8 years experience including 5 years teaching experience
Assistant Professor	MSc(N), PhD(N) desirable	MSc(N) with 3 years teaching experience
Tutor	MSc(N) or BSc(N)/PB BSc(N)	MSc(N) or BSc(N)/PBBSc(N) with 1 year experience

Table 6: Faculty for nursing college

Designation	BSc (N) 40-60 (Students intake)	BSc (N) 61-100 (Students intake)
Principal	1	1
Vice-principal	1	1
Professor	0	1
Associate Professor	2	4
Assistant Professor	3	6
Tutor	10-18	19-28

- For MSc (N) program appropriate number of MSc faculty in each speciality be appointed subject to the condition that total number of teaching faculty is maintained.
- All nursing teachers must possess a basic university or equivalent qualification as laid down in the schedules of the Indian Nursing Council Act, 1947. They shall be registered under the State Nursing Registration Act.
- Nursing faculty in nursing college except tutor/clinical instructors must possess the requisite recognized postgraduate qualification in nursing subjects.
- All teachers of nursing other than Principal and Vice-Principal should spend at least 4 hours in the clinical area for clinical teaching and/or supervision of care every day.

Other Staff (Minimum Requirements)

- Ministerial
  - Administrative Officer –1
  - Office Superintendent –1
  - PA to Principal –1
  - Accountant/Cashier –1
- Upper Division Clerk –2
- Lower Division Clerk –2
- Store Keeper –1
  - Maintenance of stores –1
  - Classroom attendants –2
  - Sanitary staff- As per the physical space
  - Security Staff- As per the requirement
- Peons/Office attendants –4
- Library
  - Librarian –2
  - Library Attendants-As per the requirement
- Hostel
  - Wardens –2
  - Cooks, Bearers, Sanitary Staff -As per the requirement
  - Ayas/Peons-As per the requirement
  - Security Staff—As per the requirement
  - Gardeners and Dhobi depends on structural facilities

College Management Committee

Following members should constitute the Board of Management of the College.

- Principal — Chairperson
- Vice-Principal — Member
- Professor/Reader/Senior Lecturer — Member
- Chief Nursing Officer/Nursing Superintendent — Member
- Representative of Medical Superintendent — Member

Clinical Facilities

College of nursing should have a **100** bedded parent hospital.
- Distribution of beds in different areas/for 40 annual intake is:
  - Medical 30
  - Surgical 30
  - Obst. and Gynaecology 30
  - Pediatrics 20
  - Ortho 10
- Bed occupancy of the hospital should be minimum **75%**.
- The size of the hospital/nursing home for affiliation should not be less than **100** beds.
- Other specialities/facilities for clinical experience required are as follows:
  - Major OT
  - Minor OT
  - Dental
  - Eye/ENT
  - Burns and plastic
  - Neonatology with nursery

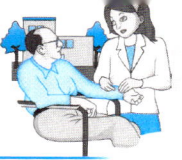

- Communicable disease
- Community health nursing
- Cardiology
- Oncology
- Neurology/Neurosurgery
- Nephrology etc.
- ICU/ICCU

* Affiliation of psychiatric hospital should be of minimum 50 beds.
* The nursing staffing norms in the affiliated hospital should be as per the INC norms.
* The affiliated hospital should give student status to the candidates of the nursing program.
* Maximum distance between affiliated hospitals and institutions:
  - Institutions generally can be in the radius of **15-30** km from the affiliated hospital.
  - In hilly and tribal area can be in the radius of 30-50 km from the affiliated hospital.
* 1:3 student patient ratio to be maintained.

If the institution is having both GNM and BSc (N) program, it would require **240** bedded parent/affiliated hospital for **40** annual intake in each program to maintain **1:3** student patient ratio.

RECOGNITION, AFFILIATION AND ACCREDITATION

Recognition is the process of granting permission and yearly approval for a particular educational program by the highest apex body on the National and State level e.g., Indian Nursing Council, Kerala Nurses and Midwives Council. etc.

Affiliation: Affiliation is the process of officially attaching, associating or connecting to an organization. It is mandatory to an educational institution and without affiliation and recognition it is not possible to conduct educational programs for example in Kerala, Nursing Colleges are affiliated to Kerala University of Health Sciences.

Accreditation is a process of granting credit or recognition for educational institutions that maintain a certain level of standards prescribed by accrediting bodies. In India, National Assessment and Accreditation Council (NAAC) is a widely recognized accreditation body of education. NAAC is an autonomous body established by UGC to asses and accredit institutions of higher education in the country. NAAC has identified criteria as curricular aspects, teaching-learning and evaluation, research consultancy and extension, infrastructure and learning resources, student support and progression, governance, leadership and management and accreditation guidelines.

Accreditation

Quality assurance and accreditation are two mechanisms that could be used to enhance the quality of nursing education. Accreditation is a status granted to an educational institution or a program that has been found to meet the defined criteria of educational quality. It has two fundamental purposes: first, to assure the quality of the nursing and midwifery institution or program, and second, to assist in improving the institution or program.

A process of review and approval by which an institution, program or specific service is granted a time-limited recognition of having met certain established standards beyond those that are minimally acceptable INC.

Organization or agency recognizes a college or university or a program of study as having met certain predetermined qualifications and standard.

Hospital accreditation is a self-assessment and external peer assessment process used by health care organization to accurately assess their level of performance in relation to established standards and to implement way to continuous service. It is a quality control measure to hospitals.

Importance of Accreditation

* Enhances quality of professional education.
* Grants recognition to hospitals and nursing education institutions.
* Improve effectiveness and efficiency of quality patient care services.
* Accreditation recognizes bench mark practices.
* Provide services by credential staff to ensure quality services.
* Promote continuous quality improvement.

Some of the hospital accreditation agencies in India are Joint Commission International (JCI), National Accreditation Board for Hospitals (NABH), Quality Control of India (QCI).

Purposes of Accreditation

* To prepare the competent individuals to serve the public.
* To guide the school/college of nursing, according to recommendation and criteria.
* To grant recognition to school and colleges.
* To prescribe the syllabus.
* To safeguard the institution from social education and political pressures.
* To help the practitioner for the broad scope of nursing practice.
* To preserve the quality of nursing education.
* To protect the autonomy of various health service programs.

Types of Accreditation Agencies

* National accrediting agency
* National professional accrediting agency
* State accrediting bodies

Each agency establishes criteria for the evaluation of institutions. It reviews the institutions periodically, and it publishes from time to time a list of those agencies which it has accredited.

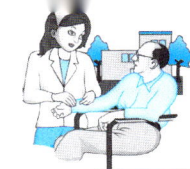

National Agencies
- National assessment and accreditation council (NAAC)
- All India council for technical education (AICTE)
- University grants commission (UGC)
- All India council for secondary education
- All India council for elementary education
- Central advisory board of education
- National professional accrediting agency
- Indian nursing council (INC) is the official accrediting agency for all programs of nursing, which include Diploma (GNM), BSc Nursing (both basic and post basic), MSc N/M.Phil (Masters) and PhD (Doctoral programs in Nursing)

Requirements for Accreditation
- Developing a statement of program mission, goals and outcomes.
- Conducting a self-study about the extent to which outcomes are being attained.
- Undergoing on-site review by an external group of peers.
- Being reviewed and the site report of the peer reviewers and makes recommendations for accreditation.

Principle Areas to be Assessed for Accreditation
- Institutional mission and objectives
- Evaluation and planning
- Organization and governance
- Program of instruction
- Special activities
- Faculty
- Student services
- Library and learning resources
- Physical resources
- Financial resources
- Advertising and publication

Criteria for Appraisal (Post Graduate Nursing Education) Outline
- Philosophy, purpose and objectives
- Organization and administration
- Faculty composition, qualification and functions
- Curriculum and instruction
- Resources, facilities and services
- Students
- Evaluation of the program

National Accreditation Board for Hospitals and Health Care Providers (NABH)

National Accreditation Board for Hospitals and Health Care Providers is a constituent Board of Quality Council of India to provide for health care organizations.

Objectives
- NABH provides accreditation to hospitals
- NABH promotes continuous quality improvement in health care system and patient safety.

NABH standards
- Access, assessment and continuity care, standards for registration, admission, discharge, transfer and referral processes are covered.
- Patient's rights and education, standard related to consent recording and archiving are important constituents of this group.
- **Care of patients:** Ensure standard delivery of clinical care across all sections of the hospital.
- **Management of medication:** Develop electronic medication, administration and reconciliation module.
- **Hospital infection control:** Standards covered in this section are CSSD and Biomedical waste management.
- Continuous quality improvement
- **Responsibility of management:** Health management information system.
- **Facilities management and safety:** Material management system.
- Human resource management.
- **Information management system:** A modern IMS needed to patients, care providers, management of the organization.

Quality Council of India

Quality council was formulated in 1997 by Government of India to provide accreditation in the field of education, health and quality in all spheres of economic and social activities.

Accrediting agencies for higher educational institutions in India include Central Advisory Board of Education, All India Council of Elementary Education, University Grant Commission, National Assessment and Accreditation Council (NAAC).

National professional accrediting agencies are Nursing Council of India, Medical Council of India, Dental Council of India etc.

National Assessment and Accreditation Council (NAAC)

NAAC is an autonomous body established by UGC in 1994 at Bangalore. NAAC evaluate the performance of universities and Colleges in India. To address the issues of quality the National Policy of Education in 1986 and Plan of Action 1992 advocated the establishment of an independent India accreditation bodies. The NAAC was established in 1994 with its headquarters at Bangalore.

Aims
- NAAC accredits higher education institutions.
- It contribute to the development of educational institutions.
- Foster global competencies among students.

NAAC has identified seven criteria for assessment of higher education institutions. They are:
- Curricular aspects

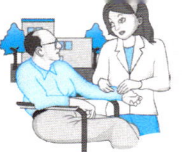

- Teaching-learning evaluation
- Research, consultancy and extension
- Infrastructure and learning resources
- Student support and progression
- Governance, leadership and management
- Innovations and best practices

NAAC function through its general council and executive committees, policy makers and senior academician from higher education.

Benefits of Accreditation

- Accreditation helps to improve quality of health care.
- Accreditation improves satisfaction of consumers of health service.
- Create a safe and clean working environment and better working condition in both hospital and educational institutions.
- Provides safety in care of patients and in professional activity.
- Enhances benchmarking.
- Improve communication and education.
- Enhances professional development of employees.
- There is opportunity for feedback services.

Limitations

- The process of accreditation is expensive.
- It is an involuntary peer reviewed procedure.
- Staff turnover create problems.
- There is difficulty in establishing an organizational culture oriented toward quality.

MANAGEMENT OF FACULTY

Faculty or academic staff of an educational institution plays an important role in the life of a student, proper direction and guidance. A faculty is an employee of the university who has instructional, advisory, evaluative, supervisory and other responsibilities.

The factors which affect the recruitment of faculty are the size of the institution, number of departments, courses offered, employment conditions in the community, working conditions, salary and other benefits, additional courses and specialization, rate of growth of the institution, plan for future expansion, cultural, economic and legal forces etc. Sources and methods of recruitment are explained in detail in Chapter 2.

Steps in Recruitment

- Determine the future needs.
- Preparation of recruitment policy and rules.
- Determine the sources of recruitment.
- Drafting the application forms and instructions to the candidate.
- Preparation of the advertisement and release in the media.
- Collection of application forms.

Selection

The selection process begins only after an adequate number of application forms have been secured through recruitment. The selection procedure is concerned with securing relevant information about an applicant. Selection process involve.

- Screening the applications, preliminary interview to scrutinize the applicants.
- Selection tests.
- Interviews.
- Checking of references.
- Provisional selection.
- Medical examination.
- Final selection and placement.

Orientation Program

Orientation is a systematic and planned introduction of employees to their jobs, their co-workers and the organization. Induction is a process by which a new employee is rehabilitated to the changed surroundings and introduction to the policies, practices and purpose of the institution.

Performance Appraisal

Performance appraisal is the process used in every organization for evaluating the performance and progress of the employees. According to Flippo, performance appraisal is a systematic, periodic and an impartial rating of employees performance and his potential for a better job. It provides feedback to employees and enhance staff development and motivate them.

JOB DESCRIPTION OF FACULTY COLLEGE OF NURSING

Job description is a broad, general and written statement of specific job based on the findings of a job analysis. Job analysis is the scientific study and statement of all the facts about a job which reveals its content and the modifying factors which surround it. It is the process of objectively determining the specific duties, responsibilities and conditions associated with specific jobs

Job description is a written record of principal duties and scope of responsibility for a particular job, together with required employee characteristics and relationship of the workers with other personnel in organizational structure.

Job description is a summary of the primary duties in a complete though not in detailed fashion.

Need for Job Description

- It assists in interpretation to the authorities of the type of person needed for the job.
- Provides a basis for orientation for the individual employees.
- Provide basis for supervision and evaluation.

Basis of Job Description
- Need of the service.
- Facilities of resources and personnel available.
- Organizational structure.
- Should be specific.
- Should arrange duties in a logical order, stating them separately, concisely and using verbs to describe the action.
- Title of the job; place of the job.
- General description of duties; working conditions.
- List of records and reports to be completed.
- List of equipment and supplies used.
- Proportion of time spend in other duties.
- Supervision given and received.
- Employee's opinion of difficulties attached to work.

Job specification is defined as a "list of various qualities that a person doing the job should possess"
- It is the final product of job analysis
- Well laid out job specification, enables the management to identify the right candidate required to do the specified job, efficiently.

Responsibilities of Principal
Principal is the administrative head of the college of nursing and is responsible for implementation and revision of curriculum, research activities of college of nursing.
- Admission of student
- Recruitment of faculty
- Maintenance of college permanent records
- Procurement of equipment and supplies (including library)
- Allocation of work to office and ancillary staff
- Planning and organizing examination schedule
- Participate in professional activity
- Preparation and presentation of report
- Review and revision of policies, rules, regulation, philosophy of college.

Responsibility Towards Teaching Faculty
- Recruitment and promotion
- Organizing workload
- Curriculum development with the help of teaching faculty
- Motivates for self development
- Encourages research/paper presentation/ongoing education
- Guidance and counselling
- In-service education
- Staff development

Responsibilities Towards Students
- Admission
- Guidance and counselling
- Planning of clinical/experience and community health field experience
- Curriculum planning and executing
- Periodic and final evaluation
- Organizes student extra curricular activities
- Overall supervision of students performance
- Supervision of student welfare and health

Maintaining High Standards of Education
- Keep abreast with latest trends in education and clinical practice
- Regular evaluation of clinical practice
- Regular evaluation/feedback/to take steps for improvement.
- Organizes workshop/conference/seminars etc.

Maintaining Desirable Public Relation
- Collaborate with other colleges
- Invite other from general education

Planning for Future Development of College/School
- Has a vision for next 20-30 years
- Plan for higher education
- Add departments of specialization (short-term courses)

In short, role of Principal can be summarized as in
- Administration
- Organizing
- Directing
- Coordinating
- Controlling
- Teaching
- Guiding

Job Specification of Vice-Principal

Administrative/Educational/Supervision
- She is directly responsible to the principal and assists her for complete administration of college and hostel
- Admission of the students
- Administration of hostel and mess
- Correspondence with INC and state nursing council and management
- Plan clinical experience for students
- Responsible to supervise other teachers and students in the college and clinical area
- Conducts incidental teaching in the hospital
- Supervises clinical teaching conducted by the teachers
- Is responsible to teach subjects assigned
- Prepares plans for periodical and final evaluation

Other Responsibilities
- She takes on any responsibility assigned to her by the principal
- Participates in 'in-service education' of clinical staff
- She is responsible for the administration of the college in the absence of principal (Therefore, the job description of the principal applies to the vice-principal when she officiates as a principal)

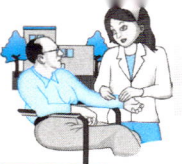

Job Specification of Lecturer/Asst Lecturer/Clinical Instructor/Demonstrator

Lecturer/asst lecturer/clinical instructor is directly responsible to the principal and in her absence to the vice-principal. Her/his working fields are nursing college and the clinical area where she/he supervises the students.

Responsibilities

Teaching

- Helps principal in planning and organizing teaching program and making plan for clinical experience of students
- Plan for teaching assignment and takes lectures using appropriate AV Aids
- Guides students in method of study and use of reference books and library
- Evaluates her teaching periodically to assess the performance of her students and effectiveness of her method of teaching.
- Plans and organizes ward teaching program in collaboration with ward sister/matron
- Plans for theory classes, demonstration and display of educational material on the notice board.
- In clinical area, assigns patients to students in consultation with ward in charge
- Conducts health teaching session in the wards
- Supervises students in clinical presentation of students in clinical area and gives and takes return demonstration on the patient.
- Evaluates each student assigned to her for clinical experience regularly and provides feed back to the principal.
- Helps students to plan nursing care for patient assigned to them methodically
- Co-ordinates with sister in creating academic atmosphere for the students in clinical area.

Student Welfare

- Assist principal in guidance and counselling of students
- Arranges health examination of students
- Organizes recreation and social program.

Maintenance of Records

- Maintains her teaching and student classroom and clinical records.
- She helps the principal in maintaining various records in the college.

General Responsibilities

- She is the key person to inculcate in students mind the values of nursing profession.
- She participates in national, state and local professional programs.
- Takes on any other responsibility assigned to her by the principal from time to time.

STAFF WELFARE

Welfare means state of living of an individual or group in a desirable relationship with the total environment Staff welfare is the voluntary efforts of the employers to establish within the existing industrial system, working and sometimes living and cultural conditions of the staffs beyond that which it is required by law, the customers of industry and the conditions of the market.

—*Encyclopedia of social services*

The report of the committee on labor welfare set up by the Govt of India in 1969 refers to welfare as broad concept, a condition of well being. It speaks the measures which promote the physical, psychological and general well being of the working population.

Objectives of Staff Welfare

- To increase the standards of living of the working class.
- To promote a positive working environment and development of high morale among staff
- To reduce stress and problems of workers in the organization as absenteeism, turnover ratio, indebtedness etc.
- To recognize human values–every person has his own personality and needs to be recognized and developed. The management employs various methods to recognize each ones worth as an individual and as an asset to the organization.
- Staff welfare improves the working relations and helps to reduce confusion.
- To improve communication and interpersonal relations

Aspects of Staff Welfare

Conditions of Work Environment

- Temperature
- Ventilation
- Lighting
- Dust, smoke, fumes
- Noise
- Humidity
- Posture–seating arrangements comfort during work etc.
- Hazards and safety devices

Environmental Sanitation and Cleanliness

- Provision of urinals and lavatories
- Provision of disposal and rubbish
- Provision of water disposal
- Cleanliness, white washing of buildings
- Care and maintenance of open spaces, roads etc.

Welfare Amenities

- Provision and care of drinking water
- Canteen services
- Lunch

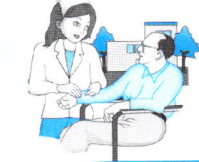

- Rest rooms
- Crèches
- Clock rooms

Staff Health Services

- Institutional health services
  - Insurance services
- Recreation as
  - Social and cultural recreation
- Leave benefits as casual leave, public holidays etc.
- Pension benefits
- **Other benefits**
  - Insurance scheme, travel allowance, increment, in-service education, promotion, transfer etc.
  - Recommendations of High power committee for staff welfare are
  - Employment
  - Job description

Working hours: 40 hours/week. Compensation for extra working hours and weekly off with all gazette holidays

  - Wages; uniform pay on the basis of posts
  - Promotional opportunity; based on merit cum seniority
  - Career development; provision for deputation for studies
- Special incentives for meritorious services
- Allowances; Dearness allowances, nursing allowances, uniform allowance and other allowances as crèche, children education etc.
- Savings as earned leave, casual leave maternity leave, commuted leave
- Health benefits; medical benefit, sickness benefit, disabled benefit, dependent benefit

STAFF DEVELOPMENT PROGRAM

Staff development programs are meant to help the nurses to develop to their highest potential. It is the process directed towards the personal and professional growth of nurses and other personal while they are employed by a healthcare agency or any other agency.

Staff development refers to all training and education provided by an employer to improve the occupational and personal knowledge, skills and attitudes of its employees. It is defined as systematized tailor-made exercise to suit the needs of a particular organization for developing certain attitudes, skills and abilities in employees irrespective of their functional levels.

Importance and Advantages of Staff Development Program

Change is a vital feature and phenomena of human life. Change is one of the ways of meeting challenges of survival. Professional roles are altered as society changes and as new knowledge and technologies emerge. Everyone has to face the challenge of change actively or the world will pass him by. Some of the changes that are taking place include shift in geographical distribution, members and ages of population, enactment of legislation designed to improve the health care, economic and educational opportunities and development of new patterns for health care.

Staff Development Program is important because there is rapid advancement in Medical Science and Technology. It also helps the nurses to update knowledge and skill which are essential to give quality of service. It also provides opportunity for nurses to grow at par with scientific advancement. These developments have an impact on the present and potential roles of nurses. Increasing public concern towards health is reflected in the growing amount of social legislation, much of which has an effect on the nature and quality of health care available to those formally unable to afford it. The changing functions of the nurses, the great variation in the nature and necessity of formal education, preparation and mobility of the nurse population, all make it necessary to conduct staff development programs regularly.

Types of Staff Development Program

Staff development includes formal and informal group and individual training and education. The goals of these programs are to assist each employee to improve performance in his or her present position and to acquire personnel and professional abilities that maximize the possibility of career advancement. It includes the following:

- **Induction training or entry training:** It is a brief, standardized introduction to an agency's philosophy, purpose policies and regulations given to each worker during her first two or three days of employment in order to ensure his or her identification with the agency's philosophy, goals and norms.
- **Job orientation and job training:** It is an individualized training program intended to acquaint a newly hired employee with job responsibilities, work place, clients and co-workers. It enables the employers to know the correct methods of handling the machines and materials at their job.

  Skills are taught through a mixture of demonstration explanation and practice, the teaching must be geared to the job, there must be a continual process of correction of errors made.
- **In-service education:** In-service education is defined as a continued program of education provided by the employing authority with the purpose of developing the competence of personnel in their functions appropriate to the position they hold, or to which they will be appointed in the service.

  It refers to an ongoing on-the-job instructions that are given to enhance, the worker's performance in their present job.

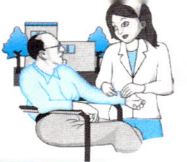

In-service education is a planned educational experience provided in the job setting and closely identified with service in order to help the person to perform more effectively as a person and as a worker. In some organization it is aimed to fill higher posts from among the existing employees. This gives encouragement to employees to work hard.

It aims at developing the ability for efficient working and the capacity for continuous learning so that one may adopt to change with judgment and produce profitable services which become an important tool for the health care of the society and nation at large. It is an agency based continuing education directed towards meeting the job related learning needs of the nurse and other personnel.

It is a planned instructional or training program provided by an employing agency in the employment setting and designed to increase competence in a specific area.

- **Continuing Education:** It is an extension of opportunities for reading, study and training to any person and adult following their completion of or withdrawal from full time school or college programs. It is the education for adults provided by specific institutions that emphasis flexible rather than traditional or academic programs. It may be voluntary, on part time or full time basis. It is the purposeful effort towards the self development of adults conducted by public or private agencies. Continuing education is a planned activity directed towards meeting the learning needs of the nurse following the basic nursing education.

Various other methods that are adopted for development program include refresher courses, conferences, seminars, workshops, departmental examination and journal club etc.

Training Guidelines

- Facilities to be given to all irrespective of their sex age and race.
- It should be based on job analysis
- Opportunities to be provided throughout the employees stay in the organization in order to meet the technological changes.
- A systematic means of assessment should be used while selecting employees for training.

ADMINISTRATION OF STUDENTS

Admission Policies

- In relation to the academic qualifications
- In relation to social and personal fitness
- Others

The methods used for selection of the students should be as objective as possible and should have proved themselves to be valuable and successful in identifying the kind of students wanted. The institution should have clearly defined selection policies.

Student Welfare Services

Student welfare services are important part of educational program. It broadly covers physical, mental and social wellbeing of students.

Student welfare services include:
- Student health services
- Recreational and cultural activities
- Counselling and guidance
- Student's associations.
- Financial Support

Student Health Services

Student health service include medical examination on admission and routine check ups, health records and student health clinic. Health room or sick room in the hostel should be provided.

Recreational and Cultural Activities

Various cultural and recreational activities are provided for students like arts, music, drama, photography, nature clubs etc. There should be adequate facilities for recreation both indoor and outdoor. The student nurses association organise sports and arts competition, exhibition, educational programs, conferences etc.

Financial Support

Stipend

For some of the nursing courses stipend is given to nursing students. During internship period also there is stipend and it is beneficial for the students.

Scholarships

Most of the colleges and professional associations like TNAI provide scholarships to students based on merit or to competent students with low socio economic status.

Guidance

Guidance is that aspect of educational program which is concerned especially with helping the pupil to become adjusted to his present situation and to plan his future in line with his interests, abilities and social needs.

—*Hamrin and Erikson*

Definition

Guidance and Counselling have a vital role in education. Now with the tremendous increase in the number of students in the institutions of higher learning, extremely wide range of course of study and job opportunities, rapidly changing health scenario

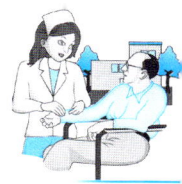

and great complexity of students need and problems, students definitely need professional help in the form of guidance and counselling. Education is the process of directing and guiding individuals to become productive members in society and guidance and counselling help the students to identify their innate potential and make plans for the future.

In education, guidance means assisting students to select courses of study appropriate to their needs and interest to achieve academic excellence and plan future career.

Guidance is a process of helping every individual through his own effort to discover and develop his potentials for his personal happiness and social usefulness.

Guidance is the systematic professional process of helping the individuals through education and interpretative procedures to gain a better understanding of his own characteristics and potentialities and to relate himself more satisfactorily to social requirement and opportunities in accord with social and moral values.

Characteristics of Guidance

- It is a process of assisting to adjust. It helps every individual in the process
- It is a continuous process. It is needed in early childhood, adolescence and old age
- Guidance is a service meant for all. It is a regular service which is required at every stage for student.
- Guidance is both generalized and specialized service
- Guidance is an organized service.
- Guidance has its roots in the educational system
- Guidance is centered around the needs and aspirations of students.

Principles of Guidance

Principles of guidance according to Crow and Crow

- All round development of individual
- Principles of individual difference
- Guidance is related to every aspect of life
- Cooperation among persons
- Guidance is a continuous and lifelong process
- Principles of elaboration
- Responsibility of teachers and parents
- Principles of evaluation
- Guidance by a trained person
- Principles of periodic appraisal

Principles of guidance according to Hollies and Hollies

- The dignity of individual is supreme.
- Each individual is different from every other individual
- The primary concern of guidance is the individual in his social setting
- The attitude and personal perceptions of individual are the basis on which he acts.
- The individual generally acts to enhance his perceived self
- The individual has innate ability to learn and can be helped to make choices that will lead to self-direction consistent with social improvement

- The individual needs the information and personalized assistance best given by competent professional personnel

Types/Areas of Guidance

Guidance means assisting students to select courses for study, to help to acquaint them with the profession to develop them and to plan future careers. The areas can be classified into:

Educational guidance

It is the guidance given to students while they are learning in a particular institution.

Educational guidance is a process concerned with bringing about between an individual with his distinctive characteristics on the one hand and differing groups of opportunities and requirements on the other a favourable setting for the individual's development or education.

—*Meyers*

Educational guidance enables each individual to understand his abilities, develop them so far as possible and relate them to the goals of life and reach that stage of mature self guidance as desirable citizen of a democratic social order.

—*Traxler*

The main objective of educational guidance is to acquaint the students with the prescribed curriculum to monitor the academic progress of the student, to assist the students in getting information about further education, to monitor the academic progress of students etc. Through educational guidance we can help the students to make curricular adjustments, help them to make plans and decisions and assess academic progress.

Educational guidance helps nursing students to develop educational plans and positive learning habits. It also helps them to make plans for career and higher education and motivate them for higher studies.

Vocational guidance

Advancement in science and technology, rapid industrialization has created new job opportunities nowadays. Vocational guidance is a process of assisting the individual to choose an occupation, preparation for it, enter up on it and progress in it.

—*National Vocational Guidance Association*

Vocational guidance assist the students in getting information about various post educational and training facilities and assist the students in developing abilities to analyze occupational information and make suitable choices by using appropriate career information effectively.

Vocational Guidance helps students in choosing an occupation and building up a successful career. Also through vocational guidance, students get opportunity to become aware of their strength and weakness. They also get opportunity to identify job placement services.

Personal guidance: Personal Guidance is the guidance given to students for the total development of personality

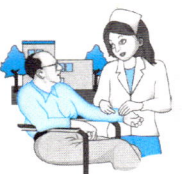

and to overcome or to solve emotional, social, ethical and moral problem. Personal guidance is the assistance given to individual to solve his emotional problems and to assist to control his emotions. Personal Guidance help students to look at himself in the right perspective.

The purpose of student guidance are to assist the students to understand and resolve their emotional problems and assist them to explore various mechanisms of adjustments.

Social guidance

Social relationship constitutes a problem area for most students and there comes the importance of social guidance. The main objective of social guidance are development of attitude and values, social adjustments, maintaining good health habits etc.

Counselling

Definition

Counselling is essentially a process in which the counselor assists the counselee to make interpretations of facts relating to a choice, plan or adjustment which he needs to make
—*Glem F Smith.*

Counselling is that interaction between two individuals to find a solution to the problems which have an emotional angle of one individual.

Counselling is the relationship between two persons in which one of them attempts to assist the other in organizing himself to attain a form of happiness, adjustment to a life situation.

Counselling is an interaction process that facilitates meaningful understanding of self and environment and result in the establishment and or clarification of goals and values for future behavior
– *Stone and Shertzer.*

Counselling is a process of enabling the individual to know himself and his present and future situations in order that they may make substantial contributions to the society and to solve his own problems through a face to face personal relationship with the counselor. In educational point of view, counselling is a process where students seek teachers help to identify and solve problems related with academic and personal matters.

Career guidance is a series of direct contact with the individual which aims to offer him assistance in changing attitudes and behavior.

Purposes of Student Counselling

Counselling in educational context centered around the needs and problems of individual students. Counselling helps:
- Students in academic and professional growth
- Develop vocational and professional maturity of students
- Developing qualities required for evidence based practice
- Acquaint students in developing a positive learning habits
- Develop leadership qualities
- Acquaint students in clinical environment
- Provide assistance to solve problems
- Counselling helps to produce changes in individual and enable students to deal with problems in an independent manner.
- Counselling helps students to know himself, get confidence
- Helps in making proper career choice
- In adapting the changing concepts of education
- Develop a positive attitude towards life and profession

The purposes of student counselling according to Dunsmoor and Miller are
- To give the student information on matters important to success
- To get information about the student which will help in solving the problem
- To establish a feeling of mutual understanding between student and teacher
- To help the student to work out a plan for solving difficulties
- To help the student know himself better his interest, abilities, aptitude and opportunities
- To encourage and develop special abilities and right attitude
- To assist the student in planning for educational and vocational choices

Skills of Counselor

- **Social skills:** The counselor requires social skills to establish working relationship and for that the counselor requires credibility, confidentiality and attention.
- **Perceptual skill:** Counsellor requires perceptual skill and perception is the way we see things.
- **Learning skills:** Counselling is a process about learning the clients situation and extending help.
- **Sensory skills:** Sensory skills refers to sensitivity with which counselor has to grasp information.
- **Cognitive skills:** Cognition is a process of learning. It is the process of reasoning to establish logical understanding of a phenomenon.
- **Reflexivity:** It is the ability to adopt to the mode of explanation of counselor
- **Observation skill:** Skill of observation is important for a counsellor. In the interaction process, words and actions are related to the articulated and observed frame of reference in a flexible manner. Observation of counselee's body language is also important.
- **Communication skill:** Communication is the core of counselling. Counsellor should be a good communicator.
- **Attention:** Attention is the most important skill required by a counselor
- **Listening skill:** The counsellor should be a good listener.

The counselor should possess certain qualities to conduct a counselling. The main qualities required by a counselor are good listener, genuine, objective, non-judgmental, confidential, creative, attentive, knowledgeable, supportive, having good pacing, calm, intelligent, experienced and pleasant.

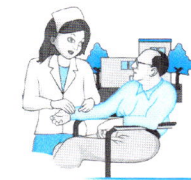

The basic qualities needed by a good counselor are: patience, interest in people, sensitive, objectivity, have good sense of humor, fairness, social intelligence, sincerity etc.

Approaches to Counsellings

The different approaches to counselling are:

Directive approach or counsellor centered approach

In this approach the counsellor plays an active role and helps students in making decisions.

Advantages
- Counsellor plays a leading role
- This approach gives emphasis to intellectual rather than emotional aspect.
- It give emphasis to problems not counselee
- The methods used in this approach are direct, persuasive and explanatory.
- This approach saves time

Disadvantages

Counselee gets over-dependent on counsellor.

Non-directive or client centered approach

In this approach, the counselor tries to direct the student's thinking by informing, explaining, interpreting and advising. Counselee is guided to use his own inner resources to solve the problems. The counselor constantly encourages the counselee to open up and reveal deeper feelings of the student problems.

Advantages
- Help individual to bring repressed thoughts on conscious level.
- Make student capable of making adjustment.

Disadvantages
- Slow and time consuming
- Depends too much on ability and initiative of counselee.
- Requires high degree of motivation

Eclectic counselling

Eclectic counselling is based on the fact that all individuals are different from one another. The counselor listens and provides knowledge, insight and a bigger picture to the client to find out solutions. The counselee is capable of thinking clearly and finding solutions. In this type of counselling the strategy arises out of the appropriate knowledge of individual behavior and is a combination of directive or other approaches.

Advantages
- Cost effective
- Flexible approach to counselling
- Is more objective approach

Disadvantages
- The role of counselor and counselee are not predetermined.

Types of Counselling (Fig. 1)

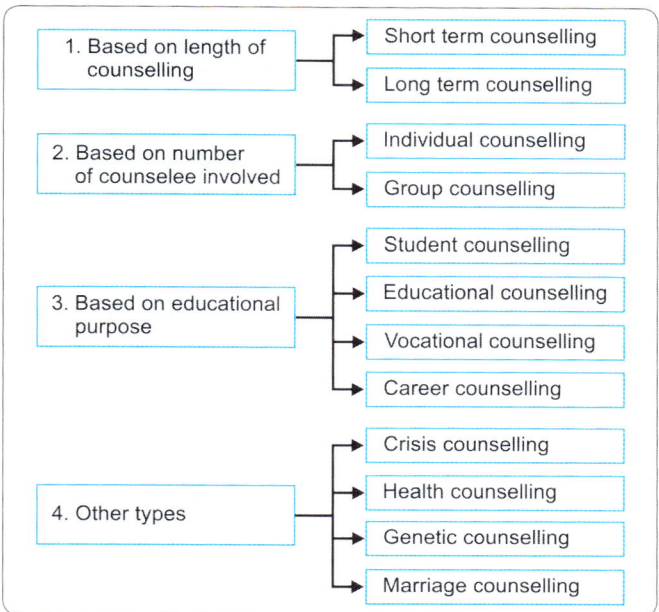

Figure 1: Types of counselling

Counselling Process/Steps

The phases of counselling include:

- **Relationship building:** The first step involves building rapport between Counselor and counselee. Good rapport building provides respect, trust and a sense of psychological comfort to Counselor and counselee. During this phase counselor introduce himself to counselee, allow counselee to sit in a comfortable position. Initially start social conversation to reduce anxiety and allow counselee to tell his problems or reasons for coming for counselling and counselor has to listen attentively and observe non-verbal communication.

- **Problem identification:** This step involves collection of information about student's life situation and his problems, both academic and personal. It is a mutual effort of the counselor and counselee to find out problems that the counselee is facing and the counselor acts as a facilitator to him. The counselor motivates counselee to provide complete information about the problem.

- **Goal setting:** Goals play an important role in giving direction. The goals should relate to the desired ends and sought by the student. The goals should be feasible and in measurable terms or stated in positive terms. Goals are set by the co-operative efforts of counselor and counselee.

- **Plan of action:** Is the planning step to achieve the desired goal and the plan must not be complex. The plan should be simple and specific to achieve the goal for successful development.

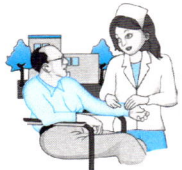

- **Intervention:** This stage is the operational phase and counselor should see whether the suggested plans are made in action in step by step process by the counselee and try to change or modify plans as and when required.
- **Termination and follow up:** This is the final stage of counselling process. Termination of counselling must be planned well ahead so that the counselee may feel comfortable to handle problems independently.

DISCIPLINE IN EDUCATIONAL INSTITUTIONS

- Discipline is training or moulding of the character of students to bring about desired behavior.
- Discipline is the treatment suited to a disciple or learner, education, development of the facilities by instructions and exercises, training whether physical, mental or moral.

—*Jane Nelson*

All educational institutions have a set of rules and regulations and policies, and violation of the same may necessitate disciplinary actions. When student's behaviour disrupts the daily functioning of institutions, disciplinary actions may become necessary.

Aims of Discipline

- To develop self-control and standards of behavior among students.
- Discipline help to control behavior of students to achieve goals of the organization.
- To promote individual growth and capacity building.
- To create a desirable teaching learning environment in the educational institution which is conducive for education.
- To promote human relations
- To maintain good communication and interpersonal relations.

Principles of Discipline

- Discipline is good standard of conduct.
- Discipline is primarily positive and constructive.
- Disciplinary measures should never interfere with the process of education.
- Discipline is always preceded by counselling.
- Use corrective disciplinary measures consistently.
- Use Discipline to strengthen student's self-control.
- Take corrective and constructive action.
- Self direct and sense of responsibility.
- Avoid favoritism and be impartial when implementing disciplinary measures.

Disciplinary Measures

In Case of Students

- **Oral Debridement:** For minor misconduct, **verbal warning** or **oral debridement** can be given. Disciplinary actions are always preceded by counselling as counselling help students to recognize their mistakes and clarify rules and regulations. Document the incident in personal records and inform parents of students.
- **Written reprimand:** For more severe misconduct, **written warning** or **written reprimand** can be given. Parents should also be informed regarding the same. Record disciplinary measures in personal records also.
- **Detention:** Temporary removal of students from class. This method of disciplinary action is taken in accordance with institutional policy.
- **Suspension:** Suspension is temporary exclusion or mandatory leave to students in the form of punishment. If the behavior of student is detrimental to the functioning of institution, suspension orders are issued in accordance with rules and regulations of the institution. Parents should also be informed.
- **Dismissal:** When all the above mentioned measures fail, students are terminated from the educational institution.

The decision for all the disciplinary measures are done by school/college discipline committee along with teachers and administrators. Proper information must be given to parents also. During admission an orientation should be given to students regarding rules and regulations of the institution and code of student's rights and conduct. To maintain good discipline, there should be written statement of policy of the organization and rules and regulations. Misconduct must be dealt with promptly. There should be provision for appeal in all disciplinary cases.

When there is any misconduct on the part of students, the faculty should collect information and document with date and time. Immediately arrange meeting with the particular student and allow the student to explain the details of misconduct and provide an opportunity for students to understand how his behavior affects the daily activities of educational institution and give suggestions regarding how to change his behavior and attitude in future.

In Case of Employees

Discipline is defined as training or moulding of character of employees to bring about desired behavior. It is a tool for promotion of growth of employee. The word discipline comes from the Latin word 'discipline' means teaching, reasoning and growing. The most effective form of discipline is self-discipline.

According to the State Human Resource Manual
The reasons for disciplinary action are:
Causes for unsatisfactory job performance

- Failure to produce work of acceptable quality, accuracy and quantity.
- Deficiencies in performance as required in work place.
- Inability to follow instructions or procedure
- Insufficient service delivery or team work
- Absenteeism, tardiness or abuses of work time
- Unsatisfactory job performance

Causes for grossly insufficient job performance.
- Death or serious body injury
- Loss or damage of govt property

Causes of unacceptable personal conduct.
- Violation of state or federal law
- Willful violation of work rules
- Conviction of a felony
- Serious disruption in work place
- Subjecting an employee or client to intentionally discriminate or harassment

Disciplinary Actions

When there is misbehavior or offence in the part of employees, the manager have the authority to take disciplinary actions and it includes

Verbal command: The administrator have to review the fact regarding violation of rule and oral reprimand can be given to minor problems. Before that arrange a meeting with employee and inform about their misconduct or behavior that altered the rules. In most of the time there is modification of behavior by verbal command.

Written reprimand: Even after oral command, if the same mistake is repeated by the employee, the manager is forced to give written reprimand. In the written command a warning regarding misbehavior is documented. In personal records, write the name of employee, the rules violated or offences with explanation given and dated signature. Both manager and employee should sign it and it should be documented in personal records.

Suspension from work: If the employee still continue misbehavior even after written reprimand, suspension or removal of employee from job for a few days, weeks or months can be done. Before giving suspension a committee appointed by organization conduct investigation of the matter. In the suspension orders mention the grounds on which decision to suspend has been taken.

Demotion: Demotion may be done for unsatisfactory job performance and grossly insufficient job performance. Demotion may be given after recipient of one or two prior disciplinary measures.

Disciplinary termination or dismissal: When all the above mentioned disciplinary measures fails the employee maybe terminated from service. Dismissal may be the result of gross misconduct or gross inefficiency in job performance. Dismissal is a serious issue as the job is often a means of livelihood for the worker.

The consequences of disciplinary action are serious so before implementing disciplinary measures the investigation team should collect facts and proceed carefully. Maintenance of discipline is a prime responsibility of nurse managers and disciplinary actions should be based on principles of justice.

ADMINISTRATION OF CURRICULUM

Master Plan

It is defined as overall plan of all the students in an institution which guide the teachers in the placement of subject matter and clinical experience, which will also give a clear picture as to how, in which year and in what stage is the subject matter going to be taught and relevant clinical experiences to be affected.

Features
- It shows the relationship between classroom teaching and clinical experience.
- The teaching and clinical experience in curriculum are organized into block in the entire program
- The teaching block will be the same but the period of clinical experience vary in length each year, but total duration is the same for all students.
- Provides teaching towards the end of each academic year for the subjects for which specific clinical experience is given in the beginning of the next year
- Each area is indicated by a code

Guidelines
- It should be prepared in accordance with requirements presented by the statutory body like INC, universities.
- It spells out the hours of planned theoretical instructions and clinical experience per week or per month of the year.
- Explain the total duration of the program (GNM – 3 ½ Years, B.SC – 4 Years)
- Total allotted time in terms of theory and practical for each course
- Mention about core content of curriculum,(nursing process approach), details of student activities like co-curricular activities, health check up, vacation, etc.

Teaching System

It is also known as study block/clinical block. It can be strategically placed at intervals throughout curriculum so that instructions related to current clinical experience and to new blocks of clinical experience for which students are to be posted, can be given.

Advantages
- The students are freed from ward responsibilities while having a concentrated period of instruction.
- Classes can conveniently be given to the whole group.
- Curriculum planning is facilitated and planning of correlated teaching made easier
- Students can have uninterrupted periods of clinical experience.
- Ward administration is made easier when students do not have to leave the ward daily to attend class.

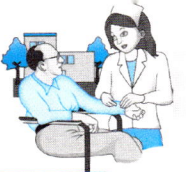

- Attention is drawn to the educational status of the student, although she does not necessarily spend any less time in the wards.

Partial Block System

In this, theoretical instruction as well as clinical experience go hand in hand. The student may attend class in the afternoon and go for postings in the morning or vice versa.

Study Day System

In this, one day or more per week is completely kept for taking classes and the other days students will be in the clinical area. Students are free from clinical responsibilities and enjoy the student status during the study day. Teaching can be more organized in a correlated manner.

Clinical Blocks

It is also known as "team nursing". All the students of the institution is posted for the clinical duty. They are fully responsible for total patient care. Final year students will act as team leader.

Master Rotation Plan

It is the overall plan of rotation of each course showing the placement of students in the program which include study block, partial block, clinical areas allotted, study leave, examination, vacation, co curricular activities.

Purposes

- It gives a clear and complete picture about student's placement either in theory or field during an academic session.
- Coordination becomes more effective when theory and practice correlates and integrity exists.
- Helps the student and the faculty to prepare themselves for working in the area.
- Enables to do modifications if required based on situations concerned.
- Evaluation of the program is effective
- Faculty and nursing staff to make tentative advance plans for leave without jeopardizing the teaching learning activities.

Guidelines

- Plan in accordance with the curriculum
- Plan for the entire course
- Plan in advance for each student in the class for all years
- Plan the activities by following the maxims of teaching
- Post the students based on their background experience/provide expected experience.
- Acquaint clinical supervisor with objectives

Nursing Program

A nursing program is identified as a single entity (program) when it can be demonstrated that all of the following criteria are met:

- It is within one governing organization that holds an appropriate institutional accreditation
- Is within the jurisdiction of one State Board of Nursing and/or other identified regulatory body
- There is one set of student learning outcomes for the program offered.
- There is one nurse administrator
- The faculty functions as a whole within a set of established faculty policies
- There is a systematic evaluation plan.
- A single degree, certificate, or diploma is offered to students
- All students are governed by a single set of policies.
- Accreditation
- Health care is undergoing rapid changes in developments in the past few years and health care awareness is also increasing, the public expect quality health care services. So it become mandatory for hospitals and nursing educational institutions to get accredited. Accreditation is found to be a strong tool in quality improvement and accreditation is needed to promote high standards in nursing service and education.

COLLEGE OF NURSING
BSc Nursing Course Master Rotation Plan

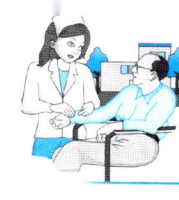

Unit 6 — Management of Nursing Educational Institutions

Months	August	September	October	November	December	January	February	March	April	May	June	July	August
Weeks	1 2	3 4 5 6	7 8 9 10	11 12 13 14 15	16 17 18 19	20 21 22 23 24	25 26 27 28	29 30 31 32	33 34 35 36	37 38 39 40	41 42 43 44 45	46 47 48 49 50	51 52

Ist Year

	T	P
Anatomy	60	
Physiology	60	
Microbiology	60	
Biochemistry	30	
Nutrition	40	20
Psychology	60	
Sociology	60	
Nursing Foundation	465	450
English	30	
Computer	25	25
Total	**910**	**475**

IInd Year

	T	P
Medical Nursing	115	480
Surgical Nursing	120	560
Community	100	165
Pharmacology	45	
Pathology	30	
Total	**410**	**1205**

IIIrd Year

	T	P
Medical Nursing II	100	400
Child Health Nursing	140	420
Mental Health Nursing	120	360
Nursing Research	50	80
Total	**410**	**1260**

IVth Year

	T	P
Obstetrics	90	480
Gynecology	30	160
Community	100	320
Nursing Education	80	120
Management of Nursing		
Service and Education	70	120
Total	**370**	**1200**

Keys

- Orientation
- Holidays
- Theory
- Obstetrics and Gynecology
- Model Exam
- Nursing Foundation Practical
- Preparatory Holidays
- Education Practical
- Child Health Nursing
- Mental Health Nursing
- Sessional Exam
- Nursing Management Practical
- Nutrition and Computer Practical
- Nursing Research
- University Exam
- Community Health Nursing II
- Community Health Nursing I
- Medical Surgical Nursing I
- Medical Surgical Nursing II

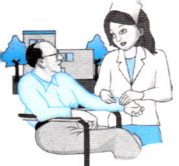

Suggested Reading

- Sudha R. Nursing Education-Principles and Concepts. Jaypee Brothers Medical Publishers (P) Ltd. Haryana. 1st edition. 2013
- Basavanthappa. BT. Nursing Administration. 2nd edition. New Delhi. 2009
- www.Ncbi.nlm.nih.gov.pubmed/11291003
- www.Indian Nursing Council.org.
- Lynne E Young, Barbara L Paterson. Teaching and Learning – Developing a Student-centered Learning Environment. Lippincott Williams and Wilkins. 2007.
- Elakuvana Bhaskara Raj. Textbook of Nursing Education. Jaypee Brothers Medical Publishers.
- R. C. Goyal. Hand Book of Hospital Personnel Management. Second Edition. Pp. 217-222.
- Chatterjee SS. An introduction to Management its Principles and Techniques. 3rd ed, 1963, page no. 209-216. The World Press Private Ltd. Calcutta.
- Heidgerken LE. Teching and Learning in Schools of Nursing Principles and Methods, 3rd ed. 1965 JB Lippincott Company Pp. 213-219.
- Discipline. Available from URL-www.discipline.google.com
- Ann Marriner. Nursing Management and Leadership. 5th edn Mosby.
- Ref: http://en.wikipedia.org/wiki/schooldiscipline
- http://files.nc.gov/ncoshr.dtatehuman resourcesmanual.oct.2017

Assess Yourself

LONG ANSWERS

1. Describe the guidelines for the establishment of new school of nursing/college of nursing.
2. Explain the job description of faculties of an educational institution.
3. Describe about the institutional records and reports. Describe the equipment and supplies needed to establish nursing educational institutions.
4. Discuss the principles of budgeting. Explain the role of administrator in planning budget for a college of nursing with annual intake of 50.
5. Define curriculum. Explain the steps in curriculum revision. Discuss the role of administrator in curriculum revision.
6. Define organization. Explain the principles of organization and prepare the organization chart of school of nursing.

SHORT NOTES

1. Budgeting of an educational institution
2. Student health programs
3. Student welfare programs
4. Master rotation plan
5. Faculty staff development program
6. Public relations
7. Student evaluation
8. Student orientation program
9. Staff evaluation
10. Job analysis
11. Staff welfare
12. Performance appraisal
13. Transcript
14. Job description of principal

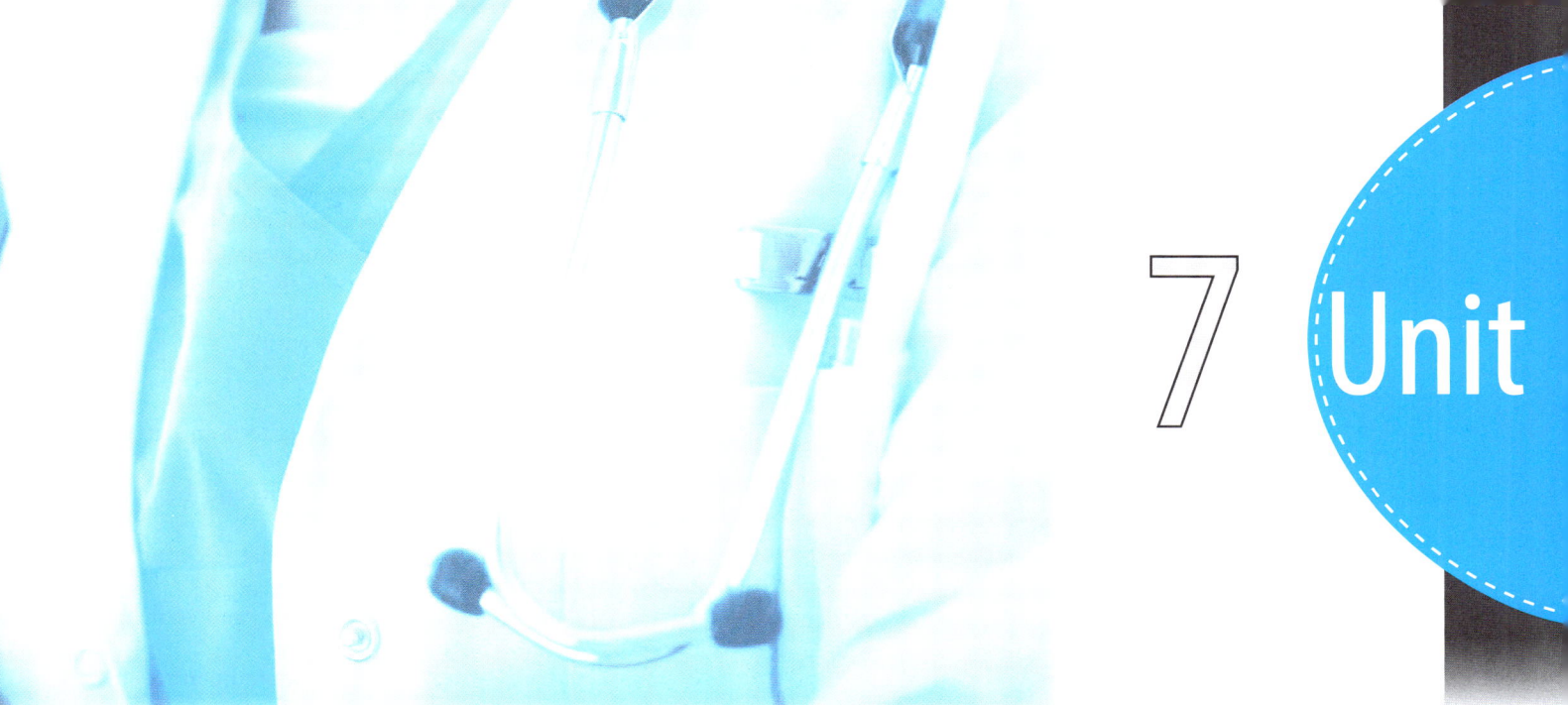

Unit 7

NURSING AS A PROFESSION

Unit Outline

- Profession
- Nursing as a Profession
- Regulatory Bodies
- Issues and Challenges in Nursing Management
- Ethical and Legal Aspects in Nursing
  - Ethical Principles
  - Code of Ethics
  - Standards for Nursing Practice/Code of Professional Conduct
- Patient's Bill of Rights
- Consumer Protection Act
- Redressal Agency
- Legal Aspects in Nursing
- Legal Safe Guards in Nursing Practice
- Ethical and Legal Issues in Nursing
- Legal Responsibilities of Nurses
- Hospital Ethics Committee

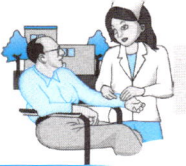

PROFESSION

A profession is a paid occupation especially one that involves prolonged training and a formal qualification.
—*Oxford dictionary*

Profession is any type of work that needs special training or a particular skill, often one that is respected because it involves high level of education. —*Cambridge dictionary*

Common Characteristics of Profession

- A profession has a well-defined body of knowledge that provides the framework for practice.
- A profession provides a specific service.
- A profession has standardized formal higher education.
- A profession is an ethic that is binding on the practitioner.
- Profession controls practice through professional standards and code of ethics.
- A profession has a set of skills.
- A profession has a recognized setting in which it is practiced.
- Members practicing a profession have autonomy in decision making and practice.
- It is a theory of social benefits derived from ideology.

Criteria of Profession

The different criteria which explain profession are given below:

Abraham Flexner's Criteria

- It is basically intellectual and is accompanied by a high degree of individual responsibility.
- It is based on a body of knowledge that can be learned, refreshed and refined through research.
- It is practical in addition to being theoretical.
- It can be taught through a process of highly specialized professional education.
- It has a strong internal organization of members and a well developed group consciousness.
- It has practitioners who are motivated by altruism (desire to help) and who are responsive to public interests.

Bixler and Bixler Criteria for Profession (1945)

According to him the criteria of profession are:

- A profession when utilized in its practice is a well-defined and well-organized body of knowledge, which is at the intellectual level of the higher learning.
- A profession constantly enlarges the body of knowledge, its uses and improves its techniques of education and service by the use of scientific methods.
- A profession entrusts the education of its practitioners to institutions of higher education.
- A profession applies its body of knowledge in practical services, which is vital to human beings and social welfare.
- A profession works autonomously in the formulation of professional policy and in control of professional activities there by.
- A profession attracts individual of intellectual and personal qualities, who exalt service above personal gain and who can recognize their chosen profession, lifelong.
- A profession strives to compensate its practitioners by providing freedom of action, opportunity for continuous professional growth and economic security.

Kelly's Criteria (1981)

Kelly reiterated and expanded Flexner's criteria in her 1981 listing of a profession.

- The services provided are vital to humanity and the welfare of the society.
- There is a special body of knowledge that is continually enlarged through research.
- The service involves intellectual activity, and individual responsibility (accountability).
- Practitioners are relatively independent and control their own policies and activities (autonomy)
- Practitioners are motivated by service (altruism) and consider their work as an important component of their lives.
- There is a code of ethics to guide the decision and conduct of practitioners.
- There is an organization (association) that encourage and support high standards of practice.

Richard H Hall's Criteria (1968)

Richard described a professional model that classified attribute such as educational qualification, professional organization and a sense of calling. He identified five indicators of an individual attitude toward professionalism.

1. Use of a professional organization is a primary point of reference.
2. Belief in the value of public service.
3. Belief in self-regulation.
4. Commitment to profession that goes beyond economic incentives.
5. A sense of autonomy in practice.

NURSING AS A PROFESSION

Nursing is an art and science. It requires the understanding and application of specific knowledge and skills, and it draws on knowledge and technique derived from the humanities as physical, mental, medical and biological sciences. —*WHO*

Within the total health care environment, nurses share with other health professions and those in other sectors of public service, the functioning of planning implementation and evaluation to ensure the adequacy of the health system.
—*ICN*

The definition of nursing by American Nurses Association (2004) is the protection, promotion and optimization of health and abilities, prevention of illness and injury, alleviation of sufferings through the diagnosis and treatment of human

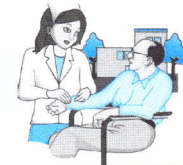

response and advocacy in the care of individuals, families, communities and population.

Nursing is an integral part of the health care delivery system. The fundamental role of a nurse is to promote health, prevent disease and provide curative and rehabilitative care in all settings. It is a profession that uses specialized knowledge and skills to care for people in both health and illness and in a variety of practice setting. Nursing passed through many phases and it has its own independent origin. Currently nurse practitioners have demonstrated the ability to deliver high quality health care economically without compromising care quality.

To prepare for nursing in future, we must have an understanding of events in past and also changing trends and technology in the field of health system. Factors affecting changes in the field of nursing are—increased scientific knowledge, increased demand for quality nursing care, changing roles of nurses and the concept of hospital being a social institution that provide services to all community members. Also nurses have an ethical and legal obligation to provide safe patient care, to maintain competence and identify those situations.

Nursing is a noble profession which has a well-defined body of knowledge, service orientation, recognized by professional organization, had code of ethics (ICN and INC) and there is facility for ongoing research and autonomy.

Criteria of Nursing Profession

- **Specialized body of knowledge:** Nursing has developed a specialized body of knowledge which forms the theoretical basis and applies its body of knowledge for the practice in nursing.
- **High intellectual level of functioning:** Nursing is a profession which needs individuals of high intellectual and personal qualities to provide quality, care.
- **High level of individual responsibility and accountability:** Nurses must be accountable and are responsible to the service they provide to clients. Responsibility refers to being entrust with a particular function and accountability means being responsible and accountable to self and other behaviors and outcomes included in one's professional value.
- **Evidence-based practice:** Nursing profession practices nursing, in which care and interventions are based on data available from research.
- **Autonomy:** Nursing is a profession which provides freedom for action and opportunity for continued professional growth and economic security.
- **Service to society:** Nursing has been associated with service to others. Professionals service to society requires integrity and responsibility for ethical practice and a lifelong commitment.

Characteristics of Nursing Profession

- Nurses make contributions to society and have relationship to the society, its culture and institutions.
- In nursing profession, there is a body of knowledge that is continually enlarged through research and applies this knowledge in nursing practice.
- Nursing profession uses nursing theories as a basis for practice.
- The nursing services involve responsibilities and intelligent decisions and care.
- Nursing practitioners are relatively independent and control their own policies and activities.
- In nursing profession, there is code of ethics to guide nursing practice.
- Nursing profession provides its practitioners freedom of action and opportunity for personal and professional growth.
- In nursing service, there are professional organization as Trained Nurses Association of India (TNAI) which encourages high standards of nursing practice.

Qualifications of Professional Nurse

According to Arther Corney (1955) the good nurse should:
- Have faith in the fundamental values that underlie the democratic way of life
- Have a sense of responsibility for understanding those with whom they work or associate.
- Have faith in the reality of spiritual and esthetic values and awareness of the value in the pleasure of self-development
- Have the basic skills and knowledge necessary to apply to present day social problems realistic, incisive and well ordered.
- Have skill in using written and spoken language.
- Understand and appreciate the importance of good health
- Like hard work and possess a capacity for it.
- Appreciate high standards of workmanship.
- Really try to accept and understand people of all sorts, regardless of race, religion or color.
- Know nursing so thoroughly that every person will receive excellent care.

Qualities of a Nurse

Nursing is a profession focused on the care of individuals, families and communities, so they may attain, maintain or recover optimal health and quality of life. The aim of nursing is to ensure quality health care for all, while maintaining code of ethics, standards and competencies and continuing their education. The qualities of nurses are:
- **Sense of caring:** Nurses must have competencies to provide comprehensive nursing care to patients, families and communities. Nurses help clients and families to regain their health.
- **Critical thinking:** Critical thinking means purposeful, informed, outcome of focused thinking that requires careful

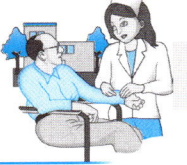

identification of key problem and issues. It helps nurses to judge the situation and take appropriate decisions.
- **Emotional stability** in dealing with different situations.
- **Ability to judge:** It means ability to take accurate and suitable decisions and actions.
- Nurses must have **problem solving skills**.
- **Responsible** nurses must be able to perform all duties and responsibilities scientifically.
- Nurses must **respect** people.
- **Flexibility:** Be flexible with regard to nursing service and other responsibilities.
- **Empathy to patients:** Empathy is the capability to share patients' emotions and feelings. Empathetic approach to nursing care are the keys of quality patient care.
- Nurses should be **self-disciplined and obedient**.
- **Honesty** and **loyalty**
- **Good listener** and a **keen observer.**
- Have **leadership skills**.
- **Good communication skill:** Nurses should have ability for communication with clients and family, between nurses and with other members of health team.
- They should be **enthusiastic.**
- They should Nurses should have good **interpersonal relations** with member of health team.

Responsibilities of a Professional Nurse
- Care giver
- Decision maker
- Client advocate
- Manager
- Communicator
- Educator
- Safety agent
- Accountability
- Integrity
- Holistic care.

REGULATORY BODIES

Regulatory body is a public authority and Government agency responsible for exercising autonomous authority over some areas of human activity in a regulatory or supervising capacity. Regulatory bodies help to ensure the public's right to quality care services, to support and assist professional members, set and enforce standards of nursing practice, monitor and enforce standards of nursing education and practice.

Major regulatory bodies are International Council for Nurses, India Nursing Council, State Nursing Council, etc.

International Council for Nurses (ICN)

ICN was founded in 1899 by Mr Bedford Fenwick. Headquarters of ICN is at Geneva in Switzerland. It is a federation of nonpolitical and self-governing National Nurses Association. The main purpose of ICN is to provide means through which the National Association can share their interests in the promotion of health and care of the sick.

The goal of ICN is to influence health and social policies, raise professional and socio-economic standards, world wide.

Objectives
- To promote the development of National Nurses Association.
- To assist National Nurses Association to improve the standards of nursing education and practice.
- To improve the status of nurses within their countries.

Activities
- Professional nursing practice
  - Advance nursing practice
  - Primary health care
  - Family health
  - Women's health
- Nursing regulations
  - Code of ethics
  - Standards and competence
  - Continuing nursing education
- Socio-economic welfare for nurses
  - Occupational health and safety
  - Career development

Indian Nursing Council (INC)

INC is the supreme governing body of nursing practice and nursing education in India. It is an autonomous body under Government of India, Ministry of Health and Family Welfare. It was constituted by the central government under section 3(1) of the Indian Nursing Council Act, 1947 of Parliament. It was established in 1949 with the aim to provide uniform standards in nursing education and reciprocity in nursing registration in the country.

Aims and Objectives
- To recognize the qualification of nurses for the purpose of registration and employment in India and abroad.
- To establish uniform standards of training for nurses, midwives and health visitors.
- To prescribe syllabus and regulations for nursing program.
- To improve quality of nursing education program.
- To advice the State Nursing Councils, Examining Board, State and Central Government in matters regarding nursing education and practice in the country.

Functions
- Provide uniform standards of nursing education and reciprocity in nursing registration.
- Regulation and maintenance of standards of training in nursing profession.
- Authorize State Nursing Council and Examination Board to issue qualifying certificates.

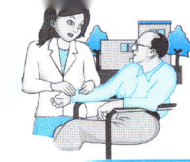

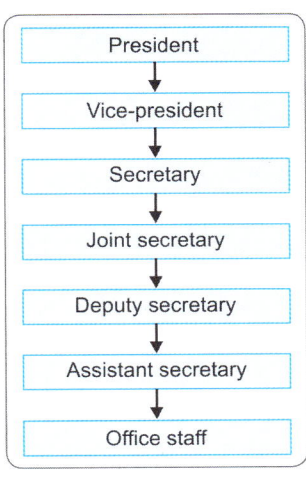

Figure 1: Organization pattern of Indian Nursing Council (INC)

- Prescribe syllabus and regulations for various nursing courses.
- Inspection of schools and colleges of nursing and examination centers to maintain uniformity and the requisite standards of nursing education in the country.
- INC authorizes State Nurses Registration Councils and Examination Board to issue qualifying certificates.
- Advice State Nursing Councils, State and Central Government authorities in various matters regarding nursing profession in the country.
- To regulate policies and programs in the field of nursing.
- Promote research in nursing.
- Prescribe code of ethics and professional conduct.

Organization (Fig. 1)

There are different committees as executive committee of the council, finance committee, purchase committee, nursing education committee, equivalence committee, vigilance committee, departmental promotion committee, etc. and various other sub-committees.

State Nursing Registration Council

State nursing registration council is an autonomous body under State Government. Registration in a regulatory board is important as it serves as a legal protection to the nurses and also to the public as it prevents incompetent nurses to practice nursing. In all states of India there are State Nursing Registration Council which are affiliated to INC. The council maintains a record of all registered nurses.

Functions

- Establish and maintain uniform standards of nursing education in the state.
- Registration of nurse and midwives in their states.
- To renew registration of nurses and midwives periodically.
- Inspection and recognition of nursing institutions in the state.
- Conduct examination for GNM, ANM and diploma courses in specialty nursing.
- Developing policies, standards and rules of conduct.
- Prescribing syllabus and curriculum for nursing courses.
- Regulation of training program by conducting periodical inspection and if necessary surprise inspection of nursing education institutions.
- Maintain registers and records.

ISSUES AND CHALLENGES IN NURSING MANAGEMENT

Technology has taken us faster and further than we ever thought possible and health care has become more technical and complicated. The role of nurse managers is becoming more difficult and they require experience, skill and ability to foresee future.

Issues in Nursing Management

- No separate department of nursing as Directorate of Nursing.
- Shortage in number of nurses and nursing supervisors.
- Nurse managers were not involved in planning and policy making at government level.
- Lack of coordination between nursing service and nursing education.
- Written nursing policies and manuals are not available in all health care centers.
- No proper job specification/job descriptions for different nursing caders.
- Renewal of nursing registration.
- Different pay structure in different health care centers.
- Role ambiguity among nurse administrators.
- Lack of adequate facilities/resources for providing patient care.
- Evaluation of nursing service is not followed correctly.
- Professional organization fails to upgrade the standard of nursing service.
- Lack of regular staff development program.
- Nursing audit system is not properly implemented in many hospitals.
- Lack of adequate evidence-based practice and not utilizing facilities for nursing research.

Issues Recognized by Indian Nursing Council

Indian Nursing Council recognized that there are issues in nursing profession as:

- Renewal of nursing registration
- Diploma vs degree in nursing for registration to practice as nurse nursing
- Specialization in clinical area
- Nursing care standards
- Staffing pattern/nurse patient ratio

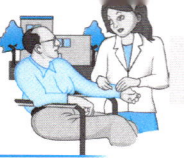

- Conduct of nursing research
- Nursing audit
- Higher education for senior positions in nursing
- Independent nurse practitioners

To combat these issues INC recommended various solutions to improve overall scenario of nursing service in India as:

- Strengthen involvement of nurses in health and nursing policy formulation and planning.
- Empower nursing leaders
- Develop and implement a quality assurance system for nursing service.
- Ensure nursing work force management as an integral part of human resource planning and health system development.
- Enhance nursing autonomy in practice.
- Enforce implementation of recommended norms on nurse patient ratio.
- Produce advanced skill having practice nurses.
- Ensure appropriate facilities and adequate equipment and supplies.
- Promote evidence-based practice and nursing research.
- Establish a continuing nursing education system.
- Improve pay scales, incentive systems and working conditions.
- Ensure quality of nursing education by strengthening nursing programs, increasing qualified nurse educators and allocate appropriate resources to maximize efficiency and effectiveness.

Challenges in Nursing Practice

The challenges forced by nurses are because of following reasons:

- Advancements in medical technology
- Changing trends in disease pattern
- Quality patient care
- Independent nurse practitioner
- Evidence-based approach in care/nursing research
- Rising cost of health care
- Nursing informatics

ETHICAL AND LEGAL ASPECTS IN NURSING

Ethics is a group of standards that a society places on itself which helps and guides the behavior and actions. Ethics usually focus on the quality of the society and its long-term survival. The word 'ethics' is derived from the Greek word 'ethos' means character habit customs ways of behavior etc. Ethics is a branch of philosophy and it is the study of values and guidelines by which we live.

Code of ethics is a formal statement of groups ideas and values. It is concerned with determining what is good or valuable for all people. Code of ethics is a set of ethical principles which are accepted by all members of the profession. It is a written list of professional values and standards of conduct. Values are written standards, ideals or concepts that give meaning to a person's life. Values exist at many levels. Each and every individual have personal values that are commonly derived from societal norms, religion, tradition culture etc. When they interact with other groups or profession they accept the values of that particular organization. The values of a profession are outlined in a code of ethics.

Ethics refers to the moral code for nursing and is based on the obligation to service and respect to human life

—*Melanie and Evelyn*

Bioethics is a systematic study of moral dimensions—including moral vision, decisions, conduct and policies of the life sciences and health care, employing a variety of ethical methodologies in an interdisciplinary setting.

—*Warren Reich*

ETHICAL PRINCIPLES

Ethical principles guide nurses when confronted with ethical issues.

- **Autonomy:** An autonomy is the right of self-determination and freedom. Autonomy refers to the rights of patients to make health care decisions for himself. Patients are enabled to take decisions about their care and they should have control over their lives and entitled to decide what they may be. Nurses respect the client's right to make decisions even when choices seems not to be in the client's best interest and when patients wants to be involved in treatment decisions they can make final decision about treatment. For that patient should be given adequate information about treatment options and get informed consent.
- **Beneficence:** The principle of beneficence refers to doing good. Nurses are obliged to do good things for patient's that is to implement actions that benefits clients and their caregivers for example while giving care to a patient who is at risk of fall, put side rails of bed to prevent fall.
- **Justice:** Justice is the obligation to be fair to the patients. Justice refers to fairness or equity in dealing with service and care.
- **Nonmaleficence:** Nonmaleficence is avoiding harm to others. Nurses should recognize that each client is unique has the right to choose personal goals.
- **Fidelity:** Fidelity is health care personnel's faithfulness or loyalty to agreements and responsibilities as part of their practice in profession. Nurses should be faithful in fulfilling duties and obligations. Being professional caregivers nurses have responsibility to patients, employers, society and to themselves and they should not give promise to any patients something that she cannot be able to provide.
- **Veracity:** Nurses should tell the truth to patients and never mislead them. Be honest with patients and families. Veracity guides nurses to practice truthfulness.

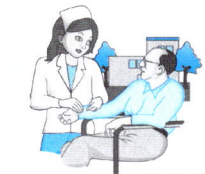

- **Accountability:** Nurses are accountable to patients, their family members, employees, nursing profession, society and the organization in which they are working.
- **Confidentiality:** It is the rights of individual patients to have their personal and health care information as diagnosis, prognosis etc to be kept in confidence. Nurses should maintain confidentiality while caring patients.
- **Responsibility:** Ability of professionals to perform nursing care activities scientifically and thoughtfully.

CODE OF ETHICS

Code of ethics for nurses act as a guide in carrying out good quality nursing care and ethical obligations to the profession. Code of ethics are expected standards of moral behavior of a particular group, philosophical ideas of right or wrong behavior. It is expected as each nurse should assume obligation to uphold and adhere to the code of her professional society.

Code of ethics provides a framework for decision making for a profession and should be oriented toward the day to day decisions made by members of a profession. A code of ethics is a set of ethical principles that is shared by members of a group, reflects their moral judgments overtime and serves as a standard for their professional actions.

The code of ethics of the American Nurses Association (ANC), International Council for Nurses (ICN) and Indian Nursing Council (INC) provide guideline for safe and compassionate nursing service to public.

Purpose

Code of ethics provide standards for behavior of nurse and general guidelines for nursing action:
- It serves as a formal guidelines for professional actions.
- It protects the rights of individual, families and community.
- Code of ethics contribute to quality nursing care.
- It provides information to the public in understanding professional nursing conduct.

Indian Nursing Council Code of Ethics and Code of Professional Conduct

- **The nurse respects the uniqueness of individual in provision of care**—Nurse:
    - Provides care of individuals without consideration of caste, creed, religion, culture, ethnicity, gender, socio-economic and political status, personal attributes, or any other grounds.
    - Individualizes the care considering the beliefs, values and cultural sensitivities.
    - Appreciates the place of individual in the family and community and facilitates participation of significant others in the care.
    - Develops and promotes trustful relationship with individual(s).
    - Recognizes uniqueness of response of individuals to interventions and adapts accordingly.
- **The nurse respects the rights of individuals as partner in care and helps in making informed choices**—Nurse:
    - Appreciates individual's right to make decisions about their care and therefore gives adequate and accurate information for enabling them to make informed choices.
    - Respects the decisions made by individual(s) regarding their care.
    - Protects public from misinformation and misinterpretations.
    - Advocates special provision to protect vulnerable individuals/groups.
- **The nurse respects individual's right to privacy, maintains confidentiality and shares information judiciously**—Nurse:
    - Respects the individual's right to privacy of their personal information.
    - Maintains confidentiality of privileged information except in life-threatening situations and uses discretion in sharing information.
    - Takes informed consent and maintains anonymity when information is required for quality assurance/academic/legal reasons.
    - Limits the access to all personal records written and computerized to authorized persons only.
- **Nurse maintains competence in order to render quality nursing care**
    - Nursing care must be provided only by registered nurse.
    - Nurse strives to maintain quality nursing care and upholds the standards of care.
    - Nurse values continuing education, initiates and utilizes all opportunities for self-development.
    - Nurses values research as a means of development of nursing profession and participates in nursing research adhering to ethical principles.
- **The nurse is obliged to practice within the framework of ethical, professional and legal boundaries**—Nurse:
    - Adheres to code of ethics and code of professional conduct for nurses in India developed by INC.
    - Familiarizes with relevant laws and practices in accordance with the law of the state.
- **Nurse is obliged to work harmoniously with members of the health team**—Nurse:
    - Appreciates the team efforts in rendering care.
    - Cooperates, coordinates and collaborates with members of the health team to meet the needs of people.
- **Nurse commits to reciprocate the trust invested in nursing profession by society**—Nurse:
    - Demonstrates personal etiquettes in all dealings.
    - Demonstrates professional attributes in all dealings.

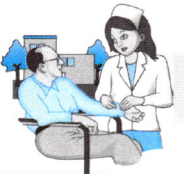

Code of Professional Conduct for Nurses in India

- **Professional responsibility and accountability**—Nurse:
  - Appreciates sense of self-worth and nurtures it.
  - Maintains standards of personal conduct reflecting credit upon the profession.
  - Carries out responsibilities within the framework of the professional boundaries.
  - Is accountable for maintaining practice standards set by INC.
  - Is accountable for own decisions and actions.
  - Is compassionate.
  - Is responsible for continuous improvement of current practices.
  - Provides adequate information to individuals that allows them informed choices.
  - Practices healthful behavior.
- **Nursing practice**—Nurse:
  - Provides care in accordance with set standards of practice.
  - Treats all individuals and families with human dignity in providing physical, psychological, emotional, social and spiritual aspects of care.
  - Respects individuals and families in the context of traditional and cultural practices, promoting healthy practices and discouraging harmful practices.
  - Presents realistic picture truthfully in all situations for facilitating autonomous decision-making by individuals and families.
  - Promotes participation of individuals and significant others in the care.
  - Ensures safe practice.
  - Consults, coordinates, collaborates and follows up appropriately when individuals' care needs exceed the nurse's competence.
- **Communication and interpersonal relationships**—Nurse:
  - Establishes and maintains effective interpersonal relationships with individuals, families and communities.
  - Upholds the dignity of team members and maintains effective interpersonal relationship with them.
  - Appreciates and nurtures professional role of team members.
  - Cooperates with other health professional to meet the needs of the individuals, families and communities.
- **Valuing human being**—Nurse:
  - Takes appropriate action to protect individuals from harmful unethical practice.
  - Considers relevant facts while taking conscience decisions in the best interest of individuals.
  - Encourages and supports individuals in their right to speak for themselves on issues affecting their health and welfare.
  - Respects and supports choices made by individuals.
- **Management**—Nurse:
  - Ensures appropriate allocation and utilization of available resources.
  - Participates in supervision and education of students and other formal care providers.
  - Uses judgment in relation to individual competence while accepting and delegating responsibility.
  - Facilitates conductive work culture in order to achieve institutional objectives.
  - Communicates effectively following appropriate channels of communication.
  - Participates in performance appraisal.
  - Participates in evaluation of nursing services.
  - Participates in policy decisions, following the principle of equity and accessibility of services.
  - Works with individuals to identify their needs and sensitizes policy makers and funding agencies for resource allocation.
- **Professional advancement**—Nurse:
  - Ensures the protection of the human rights while pursuing the advancement of knowledge.
  - Contributes to the development of nursing practice.
  - Participates in determining and implementing quality care.
  - Takes responsibility for updating own knowledge and competencies.
  - Contributes to core of professional knowledge by conducting and participating in research.

CODE OF ETHICS

International Council for Nurses Code of Ethics

An international code of ethics for nurses was first adopted by the ICN in 1953. It has been revised and reaffirmed at various times and most recently with the reviews and revisions was completed in 2012.

The ICN Code of Ethics for Nurses has four principal elements that outline the standards of ethical conduct.

Elements of the Code

1. **Nurses and people:** The nurse's primary professional responsibility is giving nursing care to the people. In providing care, the nurse promotes an environment in which the human rights, values, customs and spiritual beliefs of the individual, family and community are respected. The nurse ensures that the individual receives accurate, sufficient and timely information in a culturally appropriate manner on which to base consent for care and related treatment. The nurse holds in confidence personal information and uses judgement in sharing this information. The nurse shares with society the responsibility for initiating and supporting action to meet the health and social needs of the public, in particular

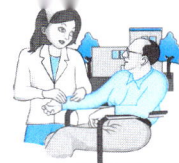

those of vulnerable populations. The nurse advocates for equity and social justice in resource allocation, access to health care and other social and economic services.

The nurse demonstrates professional values such as respectfulness, responsiveness, compassion, trustworthiness and integrity.

2. **Nurses and practice:** The nurse carries personal responsibility and accountability for nursing practice, and for maintaining competence by continual learning. The nurse maintains a standard of personal health such that the ability to provide care is not compromised. The nurse uses judgement regarding individual competence when accepting and delegating responsibility. The nurse at all times maintains standards of personal conduct which reflect well on the profession and enhance its image and public confidence.

The nurse, in providing care, ensures that use of technology and scientific advances are compatible with the safety, dignity and rights of people. The nurse strives to foster and maintain a practice culture promoting ethical behavior and open dialogue.

3. **Nurses and the profession:** The nurse assumes the major role in determining and implementing acceptable standards of clinical nursing practice, management, research and education. The nurse is active in developing a core of research-based professional knowledge that supports evidence-based practice. The nurse is active in developing and sustaining a core of professional values. The nurse, acting through the professional organization, participates in creating a positive practice environment and maintaining safe, equitable social and economic working conditions in nursing.

The nurse practices to sustain and protect the natural environment and is aware of its consequences on health. The nurse contributes to an ethical organizational environment and challenges.

4. **Nurses and coworkers:** The nurse sustains a collaborative and respectful relationship with coworkers in nursing and other fields. The nurse takes appropriate action to safeguard individuals, families and communities when their health is endangered by a coworker or any other person.

The nurse takes appropriate action to support and guides coworkers to improve ethical conduct.

The American Nurses Association Code of Ethics (2001 and 2015 versions)

- The nurse in all professional relationships practices with compassion and respect for the inherent dignity, worth and uniqueness of every individual, unrestricted by considerations of social or economic status, personal attributes, or the nature of health problems.
- The nurse's primary commitment is to the patient, whether an individual, family, group or community.
- The nurse promotes, advocates for and strives to protect the health, safety and rights of the patient.
- The nurse is responsible and accountable for individual nursing practice and determines the appropriate delegation of tasks consistent with the nurse's obligation to provide optimum patient care.
- The nurse owes the same duties to self as to others, including the responsibility to preserve integrity and to maintain competence and to continue personal and professional growth.
- The nurse participates in establishing, maintaining improving healthcare environments and conditions of employment conducive to the provision of quality health care and consistent with the values of the profession through individual and collective action.
- The nurse participates in the advancement of the profession through contributions to practice, education and knowledge development.
- The nurse collaborates with other health professionals and the public in promoting community, national, international efforts to meet health needs.
- The profession of nursing, as represented by associations and their members, is responsible for articulating nursing values, for maintaining the integrity of the profession and its practice, and for shaping social policy.

Amendments of 2015

- The nurse practices with compassion and respect for the inherent dignity, worth, and personal attributes of every person without prejudice.
- The nurses primary commitment is to the patient, whether an individual, family, group, community, or population.
- The nurse promotes, advocates for, and protects the rights, health and safety of the patient.
- The nurse has authority, accountability, and responsibility for nursing practice, makes decisions, and takes action consistent with the obligation to provide optimal care.
- The nurse owes the same duties to self as to others, including the responsibility to promote health and safety preserve wholeness of character and integrity, maintain competence, and continue personal and professional growth.
- The nurse through individual and collective action, establishes, maintains, and improves the moral environment of the work setting and the conditions of employment, conducive to quality health care.
- The nurse, whether in research, practice, education, or administration, contributes to the advancement of the profession through research and scholarly inquiry, professional standards development, and generation of nursing and health policies.
- The nurse collaborates with other health professionals and the public to protect and promote human rights, health diplomacy and health initiatives.

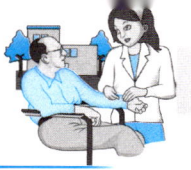

- The profession of nursing, collectively through its professional organizations, must articulate nursing values, mar the integrity of the profession, and integrate principles of social justice into nursing and health policy.

STANDARDS FOR NURSING PRACTICE/ CODE OF PROFESSIONAL CONDUCT

Professional Responsibility and Accountability

- Nursing care is based on quality assurance model:
    - Demonstrate an understanding of the concept of quality assurance.
    - Analysis and identifies needs and problems.
    - Uses relevant tools and procedures to evaluate care.
    - Takes appropriate action to improve quality.
- Nursing care is professionally managed and ethically justified:
    - Demonstrate knowledge of current ethical issues in health care.
    - Adhere to the code of ethics and professional conduct for nurses in India.
    - Participate effectively in ethical decision making.
    - Demonstrate managerial skills.
    - Demonstrate a humanistic approach to management.
- Nursing care is provided within the legal framework:
    - Describe the legal framework for practice and its implications.
    - Performs activities that are authorized within the legal boundaries.
    - Recognizes breach of law related to practice and reports to appropriate authorities.
- Nursing care is documented accurately and completely:
    - Demonstrate an understanding of the values and implications of maintaining records
    - Maintain legible, complete and accurate records
    - Keep record systematically and safely
    - Maintains confidentiality of records
- Nurse accepts responsibility and accountability for own action:
    - Recognizes the scope of nursing practice and own competence.
    - Assumes and delegate responsibility within the scope of nursing practice and competence.
    - Consults other members of nursing team when requisite nursing care beyond own competency.
    - Consults other health care professionals as and when required.

Nursing Practice

- Nursing care reflects that practice standards are being adhered to:
    - Demonstrate understanding of standards of nursing practice.
    - Demonstrate adherence to satisfactory level of practice standards.
    - Maintain records of care that are congruent with practice standards.
- Delivery of nursing care reflects nursing process approach:
    - Conducts systematic, comprehensive and accurate nursing assessment of individuals and groups.
    - Formulates a plan of care based on prioritized needs.
    - Collaborates with individuals and groups in formulating the plan of care.
    - Implements the care as per plan.
    - Evaluate the outcome of actions taken and revises the plan of care.
- Nursing care is provided in a safe environment:
    - Ensures safe and therapeutic environment in care settings.
    - Adheres to standard safety measures.
    - Follow guidelines for biomedical waste management.
    - Sensitizes coworkers, individuals and groups about the importance of safe environment.

Communication and Interpersonal Relationship

- Nurse fosters effective interpersonal relationship with individuals and families:
    - Establishes and maintains rapport with individuals and groups.
    - Demonstrates effective communication skills.
    - Demonstrate ability to listen attentively and patiently.
    - Respond empathetically and constructively to concerns expressed by individuals/groups.
    - Fosters a conducive environment of communication.
    - Engages in ethically justifiable communication.
    - Maintains interpersonal relationship within professional boundaries.
- Nurse initiates strategies to promote the learning of individuals and groups:
    - Identifies learning needs of individuals and groups.
    - Optimizes learning opportunities for individuals and groups.
    - Conducts planned and incidental teachings.
    - Evaluate outcome of teaching learning process.
- **Valuing human beings:**
    - Nursing care enhances the dignity, individuality and self-esteem of individuals and groups:
        - Conveys respects to individuals in all dealings.
        - Promotes and supports self-awareness, self-esteem and self-determination among individuals.
    - Nursing care reflects active pursuit for rights of all individuals and in particular the vulnerable groups:
        - Describe the constitutional and legal rights of individuals.
        - Informs and educates individuals about their rights.

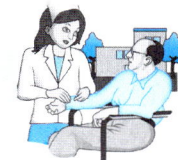

- Seeks consent of individuals after giving adequate and factual information.
- Respects the rights of individuals and families to refuse care after ensuring that they understand the consequences of refusal as per policy.
- Mobilizes support of health team members, families, and communities for protection of rights of vulnerable group.
  - Nursing care reflects gender sensitivity toward the needs of women related to their health:
    - Describes cultural, social, economical and political context in which women live.
    - Promotes and supports self-awareness, self-esteem and self-determination among women.
    - Enhances the dignity of women as reflected in dealing with them.
    - Promote health seeking behavior in women.
    - Mobilizes support for educating health team members, families and communities for rights of women.

Management

- Management of nursing services reflects effective management techniques:
  - Demonstrate understanding of different management techniques.
  - Applies appropriate management techniques based on situational analysis.
  - Initiates activities for enhancement of own managerial skills.
- Management of nursing service reflects use of quality assurance model:
  - Appreciates the significance of quality assurance program for quality nursing care.
  - Demonstrates an understanding of quality assurance program and role in implementation.
  - Involve team members in development and implementation of quality assurance program.
- Management of nursing services organizes and utilizes resources efficiently:
  - Asses the essential requirements of resources for delivery of quality nursing care.
  - Demonstrate an understanding of the system for procuring, utilizing and monitoring of resources.
  - Delegates responsibilities to appropriate team members for inventory control.
  - Ensure preventive maintenance of equipments.
- Management of nursing services contributes to development and implementation of institutional policies in conformity with statutory regulations:
  - Demonstrate an understanding of institution policies and statutory regulations.
  - Contributes to framing and renewing the institution policy as per the statutory regulations.
  - Communicates the policies, rules and regulations to concerned persons and ensure compliance.
- Management of nursing services develops and implements staff development and welfare program:
  - Prepares a plan for staff development program and welfare.
  - Facilitates implementation of staff development and welfare activities.
  - Participates in ongoing training activities.
  - Assesses the effectiveness of staff development activities.
  - Advocates the interest of the nurses for welfare measures.
- Management of nursing ensures disaster preparedness.
  - Participates in institutional plan for disaster preparedness.
  - Organizes training and drill for the members of the disaster management.

Professional Advancement

- Nursing care reflects the commitment to ongoing education and professional growth of self and others:
  - Participates in continuing education program.
  - Reviews current literature.
  - Participates in professional meetings.
  - Seeks new information.
  - Related to nursing practice from professional colleagues.
  - Assesses own learning needs and identifies areas of further training.
  - Contributes to professional growth of others.
  - Contributes to professional journals.
- Nursing care includes activities which focus on the advancement of profession:
  - Identifies the need for change in scope of nursing practice.
  - Participates in research activities.
  - Conducts nursing research and disseminates findings.
  - Interprets and utilizes research findings in nursing practice.
  - Share information regarding advancement in nursing with administration, professional and policy makers.

PATIENT'S BILL OF RIGHTS

Patient's bill of rights is the first bioethical statement showing the rights of patients. It makes health care workers aware of patient's rights and to use them appropriately during patient care services.

In 1973, American Hospital had adopted a **'Patient's bill of rights'** as national policy statement. The 12 rights of patients are:

- A patient has the right to considerate and respectful care.
- Patient has the right to obtain from his physician complete current information concerning his diagnosis, treatment and prognosis in terms of the patient can be reasonably expected to understand.

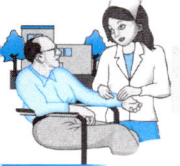

- Patient has the right to receive from the physician, information necessary to give informed consent prior to the start of any procedure and treatment (except in emergency) and patient also has the right to know the name of the person responsible for the procedure and treatment.
- Patient has the right to refuse treatment to the extent, permitted by law and to be informed of the medical consequences of his action.
- Patient has the right to every consideration of his privacy concerning his own medical care program. Case discussion, consultation, examination and treatment are confidential and should be conducted discreetly.
- Patient has the right to expect that all communication and records pertaining to his case should be treated as confidential.
- Patient has the right to expect that within its capacity a hospital must make reasonable response to the request of the patient for service.
- The patient has the right to obtain information as to any relationship of his hospital to other health care institutions as his care is concerned.
- Patient has the right to be advised if the hospital proposes to engage in or perform human experimentation affecting his care or treatment. Has patient the right to refuse to participate in such project?
- Patient has the right to expect reasonable continuity of care.
- Patient has the right to examine and receive an explanation of his bill regardless of the source of payment.
- Patient has the right to know what hospital rules and regulations apply to his conduct as a patient.

The rights of an individual have been emphasized by various agencies and organizations. But an individual when he gets ill can claim more rights as a patient.

He can expect:
- That he will at all times receive the nursing care which is necessary to help him regain or maintain his maximum degree of health.
- That all the nursing personnel who are working for him are well qualified through education, experience and have ability and personality to carry out the services for which, they are responsible.
- That all nursing personnel, who care for him, are sensitive to all his feelings and responsive to all his needs.
- That doctor will explain to the patient and his family about the illness he is suffering from. Hence the patient, with the help of his family may help himself and maintain his health.
- That all nursing personnel will carefully assist in keeping adequate records and reports of his illness, and will treat with great confidence all his personal matters that intimately relate to him.
- That possible efforts to adjust his surroundings so that he will be able to maintain his health.
- That even at the time of his discharge necessary plans will be made with him and his family to follow-up and thus provide him with nursing services and other facilities throughout the period of his need and requirement.

CONSUMER PROTECTION ACT

Aims of Consumer Protection Act (CPA) 1986
- To safeguard the rights of consumers.
- To make provisions for establishment of consumer councils and other authorities.
- To provide speedy and sound remedy to the consumers.

Consumer Protection Act 1986 is a social welfare legislation which was enacted as a result of widespread consumer protection movement. The Act provides for better protection of the interest of consumers or to protect consumers from exploitation:

A Consumer is Any Person Who
- Buys any goods for a consideration which has been paid or will be paid.
- Hires or avail any service for a consideration which has been paid or will be paid.
- It does include a person who obtains goods for resale or any commercial purpose.

A consumer in a medical profession is:
- A patient who pays to get service from hospital.
- Any patient who pays for the patient, legal heirs, representatives of patients.
- In case of death of a patient who is a consumer, the legal hires of deceased will be considered as a consumer.
- If the payment has been made by any person who is not a legal heir of the deceased too will be considered as a consumer.

Rights of a Consumer
- Rights to safety to be protected against marketing of goods and services.
- Right to be informed about quality, quantity, potency, purity, standard, and price of goods and services.
- Right to be heard and to be assured that consumers interests will receive due consideration at appropriate terms.
- Right to redressal against unfair trade practices.
- Right to consumer education.

REDRESSAL AGENCY

- **District forum:** District forum is established by State Government with at least one forum in each District. Each forum has three members: District Judge as the President, a person of eminence in the field of education, trade or commerce and a lady social worker. District forum shall have jurisdiction to entertain complaints where the value of goods or services and the compensation if any, claimed which does not exceed ₹20 lakhs.

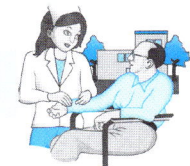

- **State commission:** It shall have jurisdiction to entertain complaints where the value of goods and services and compensation if any does exceed ₹1 crore and appeals against the order of any district forum within the state.
- **National commission:** It is situated at New Delhi. It shall consists of a person who is or has been a Judge of the Supreme Court. It takes up all cases exceeding the value of one crore rupees.

LEGAL ASPECTS IN NURSING

Nursing is a profession rendering services to patients and society. Nursing is a vital aspect of health care and nursing department forms one of the largest departments of the hospital. As nurses are accountable for their professional judgment and actions, they must be aware of the basic legal concepts and issues.

In our country, legal system is there to control individual behavior and it include laws, legislations, rules and judicial system. It also helps to safeguard the fundamental rights of people in the society.

Law is a system of rules that are created and enforced through social or governmental institutions to regulate behavior. It is a set of rules, enforceable by the courts, which regulates the government of the state and govern the relationship between the state and its citizens and between one citizen and another.

Definition

Nursing law is defined as that body of status and executive orders, regulations, rules and legal precedents which have their objective, promotion and protection of individual and community by nursing service.

Functions

- Law acts a framework for nursing action.
- Law helps to maintain standards of nursing practice.
- It differentiates nurse's responsibilities from those of other health professionals.
- Law helps to protect the nurses from liability.

Types of Law

Public Law

Public law is concerned with the relationship between the state and its citizens. Public law is comprised of:

- **Constitutional law:** Constitutional law is the judgmental law of the country. It governs the relationship between the judiciary, the legislature and the executive with the bodies under its authority. All people irrespective of race, religion, caste and sex have the right to approach the High Court or Supreme Court for the enforcement of their fundamental rights.
- **Administrative law:** Administrative law regulates bureaucratic managerial procedure and defines the powers of administrative agencies. This law consists of rules and regulations established by administrative agencies that have been made as executive branches of government. This law regulates international trade, manufacturing, taxation etc.
- **Criminal law:** Crime is an act that indicates violation of duty or breach of law, punishable by the state by fine or imprisonment. Criminal law is concerned with providing misdemeanors which are minor criminal offences and felonies/the major criminal offences. An individual who commits a crime is called defendant. Health care individuals may also be involved in criminal offences during their practices. For example, Illegal diversion of narcotics is a criminal offence. Criminal law deals with the actions against the safety and welfare of public, e.g: homicide, theft, etc.

Civil Law or Private Law

It is the body of law that deals with the relationship among person and protection of a person's right, i.e. violation of one's right by another person. Civil laws are categorized into contract law and tort law.

- **Contract law:** A contract law is a legally binding exchange of promises or agreement between parties that the law will enforce.
- **Tort law:** It is a wrongful act committed against a person or his/her property independently of a contract.

Tort

A tort is some kind of wrongful act that causes harm to someone else or it is a wrong committed against a person or person's property.

Four essentials of tort are:

- **Act or emission:** In order to make a person liable for a tort, he must not have done some acts which he/she is expected to do or he must have failed in his duties.
- **Wrongful act** or omission must be recognized by law.
- **Legal damage:** Legal damage means infringement of a legal right.
- **Legal remedy:** It must give rise to legal remedy in the form of action or damage.

Classification

Tort may be classified as intentional tort and unintentional tort.

Intentional Tort

Intentional tort refers to willful acts that violate another person's right or property.

Types of intentional tort

- **Battery:** Battery is the actual or unwarranted contact with another person without his/her consent. It is one of

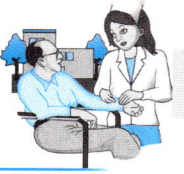

the common tort seen in nursing practice, e.g. starting an intravenous line without asking consent of the patient. But if it is done in an emergency situation where patient's life is at risk, it will not be considered as battery.

- **Assault:** Assault is the unjustifiable attempt against another person. It is touching of another person without his/her consent, or it is a threat that causes the person to feel reasonable apprehension about imminent, harmful or offensive contract, for example, threatening to take medicines to a patient if he/she does not comply with treatment.
- **False imprisonment:** False imprisonment is the confinement without legal authority. It is the unlawful restrain of an individual's personal liberty. Unnecessarily restraining a patient may constitute false imprisonment. So while restraining a patient's movement, select an appropriate restraining device to protect him from additional hazard.
- **Fraud:** Fraud is the willful, purposeful misinterpretation of self or an act that may cause harm to a person or property. Fraud can be committed through many methods including mailing, through phone and others internet sources.
- **Defamation of character:** This include false communication or communication resulting in injury to a patient's reputation by means of written statement (libel) or oral statement (slander). It is the act of holding up of a person to ridicule, scorn or contempt within the community. Defamation injures a person's reputation, diminishing the self-esteem, respect or confidence that others have for the person. Slander is spoken communication that harms a person's reputation. Libel is the written communication in which a person uses statement that harms another person's reputation.
- **Invasion of privacy:** It means trespass upon his body or personality. Legal obligations of nurses include responsibilities for protecting the right to privacy, getting consent for treatment, keeping confidentiality for patient information etc. Although some degree of exposures may be necessary in caring of the sick and injured, all care givers are expected to maintain privacy of patients. Privacy includes:
  - **Organizational privacy:** This is concerned with the privacy where Governmental agencies and other organizations keep their activities or secrets from being revealed to other organizations or individuals.
  - **Informational privacy:** It refers to privacy related to data or information. One has to maintain the confidentiality of protecting the dignity of the patient. Confidentiality is a legal protection and assurance of right to privacy to the fullest extent allowable by state law.
  - **Workplace privacy:** Employers might choose to monitor employees activities using CCTV camera or record their activities while using institutional owned computers or telephones.

Unintentional Torts

Unintentional tort is a type of unintended accident that leads to injury, property damage or financial loss. Negligence and malpractices are examples of unintentional torts that can occur in health care settings.

Negligence

It is the failure to act as a reasonably prudent person the way he could have acted in a specific circumstances. Negligence is defined as omission of an act that a reasonable and prudent person would perform in a similar situation or something a reasonable person would not do.

Nursing negligence occurs when a nurse who is fully capable of caring patients does not give care and as a result patients suffer unnecessarily. For example, failing to read medication label, incorrectly calculated dosages, failure to put up side rails of bed for a confused patient are also considered as negligence. For a negligence suit, the complaints must contain the following four distinct elements:
1. A duty was owed to the client.
2. The professional violation of the duty.
3. The professionals failure to act was the proximate cause of injury or death.
4. Actual injury resulted from breach of duty.

Malpractice

Malpractice is the negligence that occurred while the nurse is performing care, e.g. injury to patient while giving care.

Medical malpractice is an act or omission by a health care provider which deviates from accepted standards of practice in the medical community and which causes injury to the patient. Medical malpractice is professional negligence that causes an injury. When a nurse commits a negligent act that result in injury it is known as malpractice.

Malpractice is more serious than negligence because it indicates professional misconduct or unreasonable lack of skill in performing professional standards of care and a deviation from that standards of care.

Some examples of common malpractice allegations are failure to maintain safety of patient, improper technique or treatment, failure to monitor and report, leaving a foreign object inside the body during surgery, failure to observe and assess a patient as directed, failure to obtain informed consent.

Elements of malpractice

Four elements must be met to prove guilty of malpractice:
1. **Duty:** Nurses responsibility to give care in an acceptable manner.
2. **Breach of duty:** Failed to provide care in an acceptable manner.
3. **Injury or (damages):** Harm due to nursing action/care.
4. **Proximate cause:** Reasonable cause and effect can be shown between omission and commission and the harm.

To prevent the risk of malpractice, nurses should know and follow **State Nurse Practice Act**. Maintain good interpersonal relationship between members of health care team. Communicate clearly with patients and family. Document all nursing services done for the patient and if necessary report to higher authority.

Some of the common acts of negligence/malpractice on the part of nurses are burns caused by use of hot water bags or sitz bath, fall from bed due to improper securing of patient in bed or improper application of restrain to patient; injury due to defective apparatus; injury due to administration of wrong medicines; wrong dosage and concentration, assault and battery; failure to report accident to authority; failure to follow standards of care; failure to use equipment in a responsible manner, failure to communicate or document; failure to follow standards of care or to adhere to standard protocols, policies and procedures, failure to use aseptic technique where required; leaving a foreign object in a patient's body.

LEGAL SAFE GUARDS IN NURSING PRACTICE

It is important for nurses to know the legal rights so as to protect themselves from unhappy incidences. The following safe guards are worth mentioning (Fig. 2):

- **Good Samaritan law** provides rules that govern how a citizen in a state can by law act in lending assistance to another citizen. It has been enacted in almost every state and province so as to encourage healthcare provider to give assistance to people in distress or to provide help in an emergency situation by providing reasonable care.

  To become citizens to be good Samaritans, most states enacted legislation releasing a good Samaritan from legal liability for injuries caused even if the injuries are resulted from negligence of the person offering emergency help.
- **Standards of care:** A standard is a descriptive statement of a desired level of performance. A nursing care standard is a statement of desired quality nursing care which is necessary to achieve desirable care and treatment to patients.

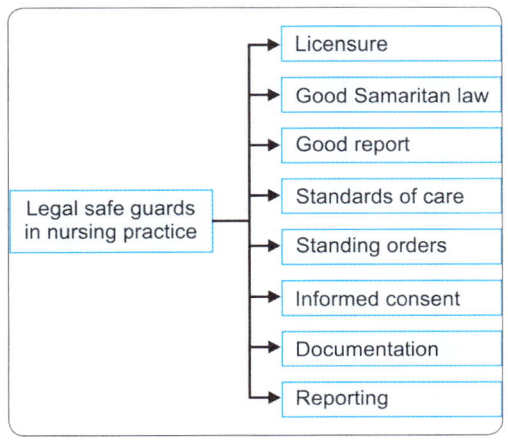

Figure 2: Legal safe guards in nursing

Through establishment of standards of practice the nurses can work and practice safely. The standards are often used to evaluate the quality of care provided by health care providers, for example ANA's standards of clinical practice. Standard provides direction for the provision of nursing care. Standards are written statements that define the acceptable level of performance in a profession. Standards provide a set of expectation that can be consistently applied to evaluate nursing care practice.

- **Licensure:** It is a process by which a competent authority/ council grants permission for a qualified individual to offer his/her skills and knowledge to the public in a particular jurisdiction where such practice would be unlawful without a license. The primary purpose behind it is to protect the public from injury by unqualified practitioners. Licenses are issued to registered nurses who have successfully completed course of studies in a school/college accredited by the State Board, passed the examination of recognized authority with a score that is acceptable to the board and paid the required fee.
- **Registration** is a process by which an applicant provides specific information to the state agency administrating registered process. The state board provides registration to practice.
- **Informed consent:** It is legal document. Consent includes details of invasive procedure to be done on the patient and the risk and benefits of the procedure and it also states that the content of the informed consent have been read and clearly understood by the patient, before obtaining his/her signature with date and time. An informed consent must contain:
  - Information regarding type and nature of treatment
  - Possible alternative treatment methods
  - Potential risk and benefits involved in treatment

  Informed consent is necessary before doing any invasive procedure for diagnostic or therapeutic purposes, e.g. before surgical treatment, diagnostic services as lumbar puncture etc. As it is the most important legal document, explain the purpose and importance of treatment to patients and relatives. Allow them to read clearly and explain the risk involved during the procedure or treatment. Clarify their doubts and allow them to sign the consent form with date and time.

  It is an agreement by a patient to accept a procedure or a course of treatment after being provided complete information including the benefits and risks of treatment. The consent must be given voluntarily by a mentally competent adult. The patient must understand exactly what he is consenting to. The consent is usually written to provide a record of transaction and should include risks to the procedure. Consent to treatment of a minor is usually given by the parent or the legal guardian. Health care providers who performs a procedure on a patient without informed consent may be held liable for committing battery.

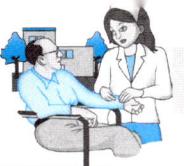

- **Documentation:** Medical records are legal documents that can be produced in court as evidence. So keep accurate and complete records. Inaccurate assessment and documentation can cause legal issues. Failure to keep proper records constitute negligence and may be the basis for tort liability.

ETHICAL AND LEGAL ISSUES IN NURSING

- **Collective bargaining:** In collective bargaining the management and representatives of labor union/trade association of a professional organization negotiate employment. Conditions as working hours, leave and wages of employees through written agreement between employer and employees. When there is a problem in collective bargaining, the mutual agreement cannot be satisfied and may lead to dispute between employees and management that may even lead to strike.
- **Informed consent:** Usually in hospitals before doing any procedure it is the responsibility of doctor to get consent signed. It is the nurse's duty to verify that clients are informed and nurses should get consent before doing nursing procedures. Before obtaining consent, the health care providers should explain in detail the need and nature of treatment, side effects, risk and hazard of treatment. Consent should be obtained from individuals who have the capacity and competence to understand. A competent adult person over 18 years of age, who is oriented and competent can give consent. In case of minors, a parent or guardian can give consent. Patients who are unconscious or those who are mentally ill or severely injured are not capable of giving consent. Minor is a person who has not attained the age at which he/she is considered to have the rights and responsibility of adults. Consent must also be witnessed by another person. Violation of the above mentioned is a legal issue.
- **Misuse of controlled substances:** It is the responsibility of nurses to keep the controlled substances like narcotics, depressants, hallucinogens etc. under safe custody. Misuse of such may lead to criminal penalties.
- **Confidentiality:** It is the responsibility of health care personnel to maintain confidentiality of patients and the details of treatment. Failure to maintain confidentiality is legal liability. Health Insurance Portability and Accountability Act 1996 (HIPPA) set rules and limits on who can look at and receive health care information.
- **Invasion of privacy:** Invasion of privacy includes unnecessary exposure of body parts, disclosure of patient details etc. Such acts leads to legal liability.
- **Negligence and malpractice:** Negligence is an unintentional tort.
- **Assault and battery:** Assault is an attempt or threat to another person unjustifiably and battery is the willful touching of a person without consent. Both are legal issues.
- **Death and related issues:** Legal issues related with death include euthanasia, autopsy, organ donation etc. Nurses who are responsible should be very conscious to avoid legal liabilities.
- **Witnessing will** is also one of the legal issues in nursing.
- **Medical research:** Medical research is an essential component of nursing profession for evidence-based practice. A number of ethical issues need to be considered when doing research. Institutional ethical committee are to be formulated for the same. The Genetic Information Non-Discrimination Act passed in 2008 helps health care professionals in the use of genetic information.
- **Organ transplantation:** Organ transplantation is a group decision and there is involvement of health care professionals from various medical specialties and public, both donor recipient and their family. Similarly the cost is also very high and it involves many ethical and legal issues.
- **Euthanasia:** It means taking a positive movement to kill a person in order to end his sufferings. It is the practice of killing or permitting the death of a hopelessly sick or injured patient in a relatively painless way for reason of mercy.
- **Quality control:** Nurses have a legal obligation to ensure the quality of health care in a hospital.
- **Records and reports:** Accurate recording of care and proper reporting of incidents or events to the higher authority is essential.

LEGAL RESPONSIBILITIES OF NURSES

In order to avoid legal issues, the nurses must observe the following:

- **Licensure:** License allows nurses to practice. License is a legal permit to engage in practice and the purpose of licensing is to ensure the public that they are protected from unqualified practitioners.
- Registration is a legal framework for nursing practice in India. It is a must for practicing in nursing according to State Nursing Practice Act. Registration is mandatory for practice and periodic renewal is essential. Registration can be suspended by State Board of Nursing if there is any legal issue.
- Good Samaritan Act protect nurses from legal issues. Good Samaritan Act is law that has been designed for health care providers to protect him from legal liability.
- As a nursing care provider, the nurse should ensure that patients are receiving competent and comprehensive nursing services. Competent nursing practice is a major legal safeguard for nurses.
- Nurses should follow 10 rights while administering drugs as: Right patient, right drug, right dose, right time, right route, right education, right to refuse, right assessment, right evaluation and right documentation.
- **Follow standards and protocols of hospital:** Standards are used to evaluate the quality of nursing service and they are legal guidelines for nurses.

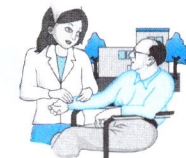

- Nurses should know the job description, responsibilities, rules and regulations, legal responsibilities, legal and ethical issues and laws that are protecting them. Knowledge is essential to become safe from legal issues.
- **Practice safety and competency while implementing care:** Protect patients from accidents or falls. Nurse administrators should frequently check whether all equipment are functioning well. Repair or replace defective hospital equipments.
- **Effective communication and interpersonal relations:** Develop a caring relationship. Establish and maintain rapport with the patients through accurate and open communication. Maintain good inter personal relations with coworkers, superiors and subordinates. Care patients and families with respect.
- **Use restraints whenever necessary:** Use only safe devices. Take measures to protect patients from fall.
- Enhance skill and competency by participating in continuing nursing education programs and skill training.
- **Documentation:** Medical records are important documents that can be produced before court in case of legal liability so keep them under safe custody. Unusual or unexpected incidence should be reported and a copy of incidental report should be kept in patient's record. Nurses have legal responsibility for accurate reporting and recording of patient's conditions, treatment and responses to care. Nurses should document all events and nursing care with date, time and signature.
- **Report to higher authority as and when incidents occur:** Keep information confidential. The best possible way to prevent law suit is to provide competent nursing care to patients.
- **Legal responsibility for death and dying:** There are chances of arising of many issues related with the event of death of a patient. So nurses should check all legal aspects of death and handover body to relatives. Document all events related with death and care.
- Laws are rules of conduct established and enforced by authority which prohibits extremes in behavior so that one can live without for oneself or ones' property

—Sullivan and Decker

HOSPITAL ETHICS COMMITTEE

Hospital ethics committee is constituted by majority of hospitals with the aim to review, approve and monitor biomedical and behavioral research involving humans with the aim to protect the rights and welfare of the research subjects.

Ethics committee is needed:
- To protect the rights, dignity and welfare of human subjects during clinical research.
- To have a formal procedure to monitor and assess the ethical standards for clinical research.
- To review independently and to ensure that research meets the ethical standards.

Structure of Hospital Ethics Committee

The composition of ethics committee is based on Indian Council of Medical Research (ICMR) guidelines. The members of ethics committee include Chairperson, member secretary, one or two person from basic science areas, 1–2 clinicians, one legal experts, one social scientist/representative of NGO, one philosopher, one lay person from community and subject expert if required.

Functions

The functions of institutional ethics committee include review of procedures, decision making process and documentation. Some of the specific roles of ethics committee include:
- Clarify ethical problems arising from the project or research.
- Ensure that informed consent has been properly obtained.
- Periodic follow-up of institutional projects, approved.
- Documentation is important and it must be kept confidential.

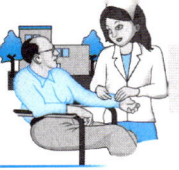

Suggested Reading

- Billing MD, Halstead JA. Teaching in Nursing: Guide for Faculty 3rd ed. Philadelphia: Saunders Elsevier Publishers; 2009.
- Kozier B, Erb G, Berman A, et al. Fundamentals of Nursing - Concepts, Process and Practice, 7th ed. Philadelphia: Pearson Education; 2007. Pp. 201-03.
- Stanhope M, Lancaster J. Foundations of Nursing in the Community, 2nd ed. Philadelphia: Mosby; 2006. Pp. 606.
- Kishore J. Health Programs in India, 7th ed. New Delhi: Century Publications; 2007. Pp. 486-87.
- Lindeman CA, Mc Cathie M. Fundamentals of Contemporary Nursing Practice. Philadelphia: Saunders; 1999. Pp. 465.
- Rosdahl CB, Kowalski MT. Textbook of Basic Nursing, 9th ed. Philadelphia: Lippincott W and W; 2008. Pp. 1597.
- Nettina SM. Manual of Nursing Practice. Philadelphia: Lippincott W and W; 2006. Pp. 20-21.
- Stone SC, Mcguire SL, Eigsti DG. Comprehensive Community Health Nursing, 5th ed. USA: Mosby; 1998. Pp. 724-25.
- Hood LJ, Leddy SK. Conceptual Basis of Professional Nursing, 6th ed. Philadelphia: Lippincott W and W; Pp. 415.
- http://www.cdacmohali.in S_Telenursing.aspx
- http://wwww.crnns.ca/documents/telenursingpractice2008.pdf.
- Potter PA, Perry AG, Fundamentals of Nursing, 6th ed: 2006; Mosby an imprint of Elsevier; Pp. 477-87.
- www.americatelemed.org
- Colmer Malcom R. Moroney's Surgery for Nurses, 16th edn. Churchill Livingstone: Pearson Professional Limited; 1995. Pp. 110-12.
- Trained Nurses' Association of India, 2007, Pp. 61-62.
- Basavanthappa BT. Nursing Adninistration. 2nd edition. New Delhi; Jaypee Brothers Medical Publisher Pvt. Ltd.
- Marquis BL, Huston CJ. Leadership Roles and Management Functions in Nursing—Theory and Application, 6th edition. Philadelphia: Lippincott William and Wilkins Publications; 1996.
- Joseph T. Catalano. Nursing Now, 7th Edn. Jaypee Brothers and Medical Publishers.

 ## Assess Yourself

LONG ANSWER

1. Define profession. List down the characteristics of nursing profession. Discuss the current trends and issues in nursing profession.

SHORT NOTES

1. Legal issues in nursing practice
2. Consumer Protection Act
3. Code of professional conduct
4. Professional ethics
5. Torts

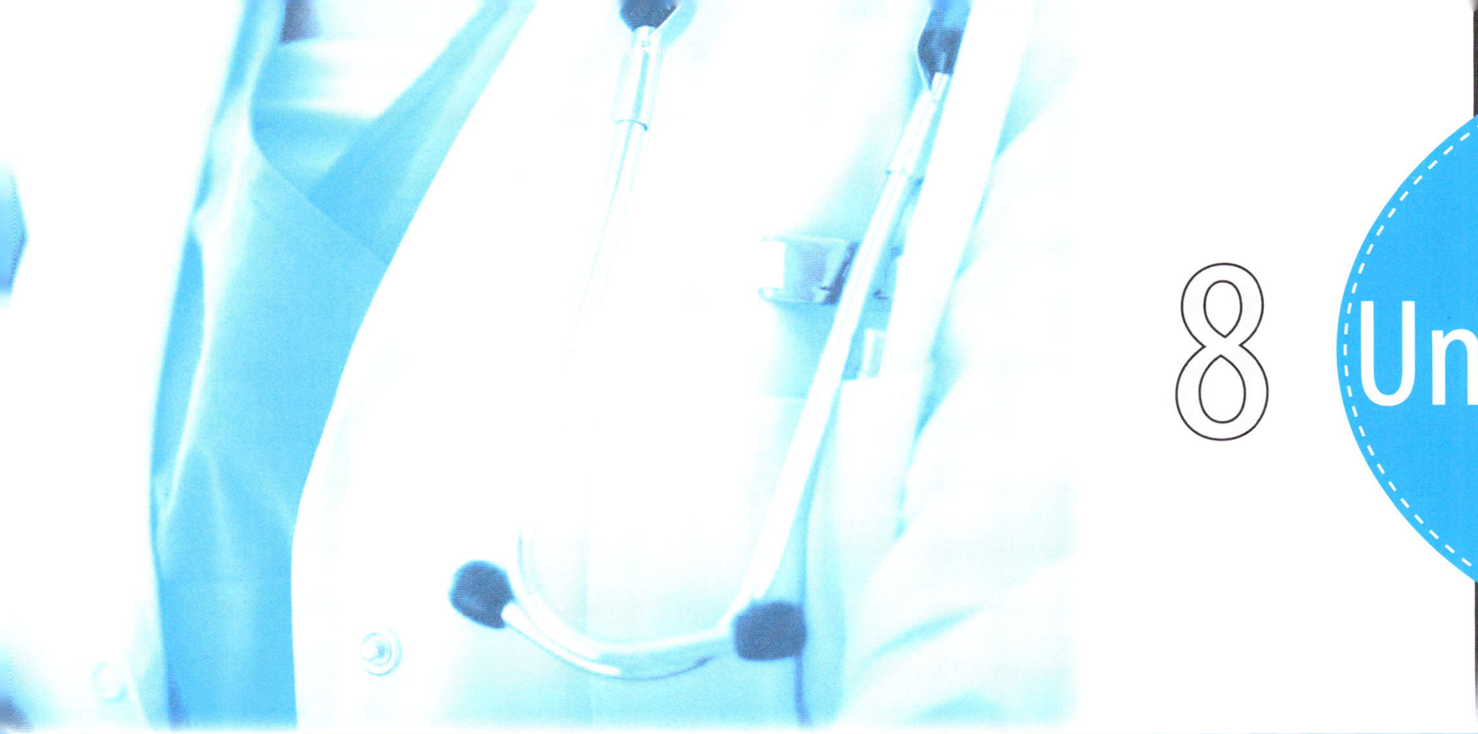

Unit 8

PROFESSIONAL DEVELOPMENT

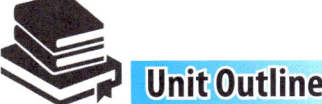

Unit Outline

- Career Development in Nursing
- Career Opportunities in Nursing
- Scope of Nursing Career
- Membership with Professional Organization: National and International
- Professional Organization at National Level
- Nursing Informatics
- Management Information System
- Application of Nursing Informatics

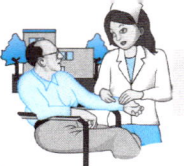

CAREER DEVELOPMENT AND CAREER OPPORTUNITIES IN NURSING

Career is defined as the sequence and variety of occupations which are undertaken throughout a life time. Career opportunities are the processes which involve the completion of variety of actions geared to help individuals to determine the desired life directions.

Career development is the planning and implementation of career plan and it can be accomplished through assessment, job analysis, job search and work experience. Career development is an ongoing process of attaining knowledge and improving skills that will help individuals to make career plan.

Objectives of Career Development

- To attract qualified and efficient employees in organization
- To reduce employee attrition
- To maintain communication and harmonious organizational relations
- To promote maximum utilization of resources
- To make employees adaptable to changes

CAREER DEVELOPMENT IN NURSING

The International Council of Nurses (ICN) believes that career development is a major contributing factor in the advancement of nursing profession worldwide and is directly linked with the maintenance of high quality health care delivery. ICN also mentioned that career development must be supported and maintained by means of articulated educational system, recognized career structures flexible enough to provide career mobility and access to nursing intra/entrepreneurship and/or independent practice opportunities. ICN also mentioned that appropriate incentives and provision for continuing education should be available to all nursing personnel.

Within the nursing education and practice system, ICN and National Nurses Association are committed to the responsibilities of developing, promoting and facilitating a comprehensive integrated framework for profession which will support the recruitment and retention of qualified nurses to provide nursing care. The nurses organizations play a major role in determining satisfying patterns of career development in nursing, creating national and international database, professional development and protection of nurses and public.

CAREER OPPORTUNITIES IN NURSING

For ANM

Works as a multipurpose health worker; male and female at sub centers. With experience and training can be promoted to Lady Health Inspectors (LHI) and Lady Health Supervisor (LHS). For career development, they can do diploma in nursing.

For GNM

- Diploma nurse may work as a registered nurse in different departments of the hospital.
- Diploma nurse may upgrade himself/herself to BSc Nursing and become a graduate Nurse
- Diploma nurse may upgrade himself/herself to Speciality Nurse by completing the certificate courses on different specialities like dialysis, ICUs, neonatology, neurology, Cardiology and palliative care etc.

BSc Nursing

As graduate nurse he/she may work in the following settings:

Hospital Settings

- As a registered nurse or Nursing Officer in the different departments of the hospital
- Can work as Nurse educator, Quality control nurse, Infection control nurse etc.
- He/she may work as nurse supervisor/Assistant Nursing Superintendent/Deputy Nursing Superintendent/Nursing Superintendent based on the experience

Community Settings

- As a Community health nurse, works in the community and is involved in the promotion of health and prevention of diseases at all levels.
- He/she may work as an industrial nurse, school health nurse, Geriatric nurse, Hospice nurse and Palliative care nurse etc.
- He/she may work as a researcher in the community settings.

Other Areas

- He/she may work as a Nursing Tutor/Clinical Instructor in schools of Nursing for teaching the students in ANM, and GNM courses.
- He/she may work as a Nurse Expert in healthcare related organizations.
- He/she may work as a Nurse assessor in health insurance organizations.
- He/she may upgrade with certificate courses in nursing to become specialized in interested field.
- He/she may upgrade with MSc Nursing course in nursing to become expertise in specialized field.

MSc Nursing

Teaching

- Post graduate nurse may work as a lecturer in college of nursing to teach various subjects of nursing and thereby promoted to Assistant Professor, Associate Professor and Professor as per the experience in the college of nursing
- Postgraduate nurse may be promoted to various posts like Vice Principal and Principal based on their experience.

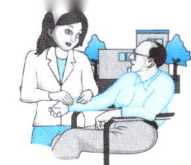

Hospital Settings

- As a Registered Nurse or Nursing Officer in the different departments of the hospital
- Can work as Nurse educator, Quality control nurse, Infection control nurse etc.
- He/she may work as nurse supervisor/Assistant Nursing superintendent/ Deputy Nursing superintendent/Nursing superintendent based on the experience.
- He/she may work as Nursing Director, Chief Nursing Officer etc.

Community Settings

- As a Community health nurse, works in the community and is involved in the promotion of health and prevention of diseases in all levels.
- He/she may work as an Industrial nurse, School health nurse, Geriatric nurse, Hospice nurse and palliative care nurse etc.
- He/she may work as Nurse practitioner and midwife.
- He/she may work as a researcher in the community settings
- He/she can further pursue M Phil or PhD in nursing.
- He/she can act as a counsellor in the community services.

SCOPE OF NURSING CAREER

The scope of nursing profession is increasing in all parts of the country and in the world due to changes in population trends, advancement in technology, globalization, changes in climate, increasing numbers of elderly population advancement in nursing research etc.

Clinical Nurse Specialist

Clinical nurse specialists are advanced practice registered nurses who functions in nursing's areas of specialists. They are expert in a particular field of clinical practice like community health, geriatric health, mental health etc. They may provide direct care to patients, teach in a variety of health care settings and work as research consultants and as nurse managers.

Work Areas

Community, hospitals, industries, nursing homes, private homes, private practice settings, public health departments, research centers and schools.

Requirements

Registered nurse with MSN.

Licensed Practical Nurse

Licensed Practical Nurse provides basic nursing care. Supervise nursing assistants and maintains patient records.

Work Areas

Community health clinics, hospitals, long term care facilities, mental health institutions, nursing homes, physician's office, public health departments, research centers and schools.

Nurse Practitioner

They are qualified to handle a wide range of health problems in speciality areas as family care, geriatric care etc. Nurse practitioner assesses health condition, identifies and diagnoses problems and develops plans, prescribe medication and formulate treatment plans to improve health care outcomes.

Work Areas

Community, hospitals, industries, nursing homes, private homes, private practice settings, public health departments, research centers and schools.

Certified Registered Nurse Anesthetist (CRNA)

Nurse anesthetist has to complete masters program and administers anesthetic drugs, monitor the patient's vital signs and other medications to assure optimal patient safety and comfort.

Working Areas

Operation theatres, obstetrical delivery centers, dental clinics, hospitals and pain clinics.

Nurse Midwife

Nurse midwife provides care for women, before, during and after child birth. They assist in newborn care and counsel mothers on infant growth and future pregnancies.

Working Areas

Birth centers, clinics, hospitals, public health departments.

Qualification

Bachelor's degree with current nursing licence and minimum of one year experience as registered nurse.

Registered Nurse

Registered nurse provides care to patient's. They provide treatment, education and rehabilitation measures.

Work Areas

Community, hospitals, industries, nursing homes, private homes, private practice settings, public health departments, research centers, prisons, rehabilitation centers and schools.

Nurse Educator

Registered nurses work in areas of schools and colleges of nursing, who teach various degree and diploma program in nursing.

Infection Control Nurse

Assess the incidents of infection and conduct comprehensive review to ensure prompt and accurate treatment.

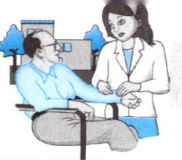

Quality Management Nurse

Assess compliance of the institution with established standards, ensures that patients' services are consistent with standard through chart review and ongoing interaction with the staff.

Others

- Intravenous team nurse
- Ostomy nurse
- Nurse educator
- Nurse Coordinator
- Hospice nurse
- Informatics nurse specialist
- Occupational nurse specialist
- Quality manager
- Case manager
- Flight nurse
- Forensic nurse
- School nurse
- Travel nurse
- Parish nurse
- Clinical nurse leader

MEMBERSHIP WITH PROFESSIONAL ORGANIZATION: NATIONAL AND INTERNATIONAL

Professional nursing organizations are an effective tool for the nursing profession to influence health care policies, protect and educate nurses and provide the highest quality care possible to the public. There are many nursing organizations that support the interest of the nurse members.

Mission

Each professional has a mission statement, which clearly indicates the organization's primary purposes and drives the development of several priority objectives for that specific organizations.

A professional association is usually a non-profit organization seeking to further particular profession, the interests of individuals engaged in that profession, and the public interest.

Professional Organizations in Nursing

Nowadays there are a large number of international professional organizations and national professional organizations in the field of nursing profession to promote safe and ethical environment and to improve quality health care.

The membership in professional organizations are important as it.

- Helps to focus career in a better way and in important manner for the professional development of nurses
- Helps to protect interests of nurses
- Members get access to know the current trends and issues in nursing profession in regard to both service and education.
- Participate in activities and conventions organized by professional organizations
- Provide facilities for networking opportunities
- Helps to get idea about new approaches and initiatives and there were opportunities to exchange ideas and challenges.
- Many professional organizations are offering certificate programs in speciality
- Can get involved in the continuous nursing education programs organized by professional bodies which provide a venue to disseminate the research evidences.
- Get access to organization's website and gets carrier assistance
- Opportunities for educational, personal and professional development through professional journal, seminar etc.
- Facilitate leadership development
- There is provision for networking opportunities

Important professional nursing organizations at International Level are:

American Nurses Association (ANA): It is the oldest and largest professional organization founded in 1896. It was initially known as the Associated Alumina of Trained Nurses of United States and Canada. The headquarters of ANA is United States.

The aim of ANA is establishing standards of nursing practice, protecting the rights of nurses on the workplace and advancing the economic and general welfare of nurses. It also helps to protect the quality of health care.

The publications of ANA are American Nurse Today, The American Nurse, The online Journal of Issues in Nursing. The members of ANA also get opportunity to use online library and free access to magazines and journals.

National League for Nursing

National League for Nursing (NLN) is the first professional organization founded in 1893 and it was initially named as the American Society of Superintendents of Training Schools for Nurses and later was known as NLN. It is the premier organization for nursing faculty and leaders in nursing education and it promotes excellence in nursing education. The publication is "Nursing perspectives – the NLN research Journal"

The mission of NLN is to promote excellence in Nursing education to build a diverse nursing workforce. NLN provides access to networking, continuous nursing education and activities related to professional development.

International Council of Nurses

The International Council of Nurses was founded in 1899 by Mrs. Bedford Fenwick. It is federation of non-political and self-governing national nurses association. ICN is the global

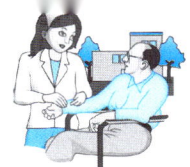

voice of nursing. The main purpose of ICN is to provide the means through which the national associations can share their interests in the promotion of health and care of the sick.

Objectives of ICN

- To promote the development of the strong national nurses association.
- To assist national nurses association in improving standards of nursing education and practice.
- To serve as the authoritative voice for nurses and nursing internationally.

Activities

- The ICN has published the **Code for Nurses**
- It makes the policy statement on health and social issues.
- It also maintains and improves the status of nurses and standard of nursing around the world.
- The council works to improve the nursing education and practice by publishing the guidelines for National Nurses Association.

The governing body of the ICN is the Council of National Representatives, which is made up of the ICN honorary officers and the presidents of the national member associations.

ICN publishes the **International Nursing Review** and the **News Letter**, which gives the news of the ICN and the National Member Association.

Sigma Theta Tau International

Sigma Theta Tau International is the second-largest nursing organization in the world with approximately 135,000 active members.

Membership is by invitation to baccalaureate and graduate nursing students, who demonstrates excellence in scholarship, and to nurse leaders exhibiting exceptional achievements in nursing. 61% of active members hold master's and/or doctoral degrees; 56% have a specialty certification; 48% are clinicians; 40% have more than 15 years of work experience; 21% are administrators or supervisors, and 20% are educators or researchers. In addition to English, members are fluent in 20 other languages including Spanish, Dutch and Finnish.

Student Membership Criteria

Graduate Students (Master's and Doctorate) must have completed ¼ of the nursing curriculum; achieved academic excellence (at schools where a 4.0 grade point average system is used, this equates to a 3.5 or higher); and meet the expectation of academic integrity. They must also be in the top 35 percentile of their nursing program.

Nurse Leader Membership Criteria

Nurse Leader Candidates must be legally recognized to practice nursing in his/her country; have a minimum of a baccalaureate degree or the equivalent in any field; and demonstrate achievement in nursing.

International Confederation of Midwives

To strengthen Midwives Associations and to advance the profession of midwifery globally by promoting autonomous midwives as the most appropriate caregivers for childbearing women and in keeping birth normal, in order to enhance the reproductive health of women, their new-borns and their families.

PROFESSIONAL ORGANIZATION AT NATIONAL LEVEL

Indian Nursing Council

Indian Nursing Council (INC) was authorized by the Indian Nursing Council Act of 1947. It was established in 1949 to provide uniform standards in nursing education and reciprocity in nursing registration throughout the country.

Functions

- It provides uniform standards in nursing education and reciprocity in nursing registration.
- It has authority to prescribe curriculum for nursing education in all states.
- It has authority to recognise program of nursing education or to refuse recognition of a program if it did not meet the standards required by the council.
- It registers the foreign nurses.
- It also maintains the Indian Nurses Register.
- INC authorises State Nurses Registration Council and examine boards to issue qualifying certificates.

Trained Nurses Association of India

Trained Nurses' Association of India (TNAI) is a national organization of nurse professionals at different levels. It was established in 1908 and was initially known as Association of Nursing Superintendents. The Government of India has recognized TNAI as a service organization in 1950. A similar recognition by all the State Governments has been an asset to the promotion of its objectives.

Objectives

- To maintain dignity and honor of the nursing profession,
- Promoting a sense of espirit de corps among all nurses,
- To advance professional, educational, economic and general welfare of nurses.

Functions

- To enunciate standards of Nursing Education and implement these through appropriate channels.
- To establish standards and qualifications for nursing practice.
- To enunciate standards of Nursing Service and implement these through appropriate channels.
- To establish a code of ethical conduct for practitioners.

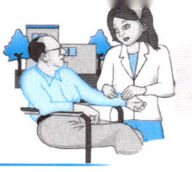

- To stimulate and promote research designed to enhance the knowledge for evidence-based nursing practice.
- To promote legislation and to speak for nurses in regard to legislative action.
- To promote and protect the economic welfare of nurses.
- To provide professional counseling and placement service for nurses.
- To provide for the continuing professional development of practitioners.
- To represent nurses and serve as their spoke person with allied national and international organizations, governmental and other bodies and the public.
- To serve as the official representative of the nurses of India as a member of the International Council of Nurses.
- To promote the general health and welfare of the public through the association programs, relationships and activities, e.g. disaster management.
- To render care as per the changing needs of the society.

Membership

A life member is a person who is a registered Nurse and Midwife (equivalent of midwifery training in case of male nurse), trained from an institution recognised by the Indian Nursing Council/State Nursing Council and holds a certificate of training issued by a Nursing Registration Council or Board of Examinations recognised by the Indian Nursing Council.

Activities

- **Publications:** The TNAI brings out a monthly journal—The Nursing Journal of India which was founded in 1910 as its official organ. This is the main link between the members of the Association, the Headquarters and State Branches on all important matters.
  - **Issuance of the railway concession:** Since 1991, Railway is granting concession to the TNAI members and the association was authorized to issue certificates to members for getting 25% concessions in second classes.
  - **Affiliation with government committees and councils:** TNAI is involved in all governmental endeavors in the field of nursing and are given the opportunity to put across its points of views on all matters of consequence (Bhore committee, Central Council of Health).
  - **Affiliation with other organizations:** TNAI is affiliated with all governmental and nongovernmental/National and International organizations.
- **Collaboration in research activities:**
  - HIV/AIDS project in collaboration with the American Nurses' Association (1994).
  - UNICEF Reproductive Child Health project on "Strengthening System Support to ANMs and Health Supervisors, females' capabilities for implementing Safe Motherhood Practices in the Reproductive and Child Health Program." (2001).
  - Feasibility of study in collaboration with European Commission on improving healthcare for safe motherhood services of independent private practice by unemployed and under-employed ANMs in India (2002).
  - TNAI/ Swedish International Development Corporation Agency/Indian Institute of Management, Ahmedabad, project on improving midwifery and emergency obstetric services in India (2005)
  - TNAI in collaboration with The Association of Women Health, Obstetric and Neonatal Nurses (AWOHNN, US-based organization) is in the process of preparing the guidelines for newborn skin care as per the Indian perspective.
- **Socio-Economic Welfare (SEW) Programs**
  TNAI Being committed to provide socio-economic welfare to nurses in the country, a Socio-Economic Welfare (SEW) Committee was formed in 1963. TNAI conduct surveys to study the socio-economic welfare problems of nurses in India and recommended appropriate reforms and solutions.

Student Nurses Association of India

Student Nurses Association (SNA) organised in 1929 is associated under the jurisdiction of the TNAI, in addition to providing a means of personnel and professional development for the nursing students. It serves as a source of membership for the parent organization. In addition the TNAI serves as the advisor for the SNA.

Functions of SNA

- To help the student nurses learn how the professional organizations serve to uphold the dignity and the ideals of the nursing profession.
- To furnish student nurses, in the courses of study leading to professional qualification.

Christian Medical Association of India

The Nurses League of the Christian Medical Association of India (CMAI) was founded in 1930.

Objectives

- To promote cooperation and encouragement among Christian nurses.
- To promote efficiency in nursing education and services.
- To secure the highest standard possible in Christian Nursing Education through the Christian Schools of Nursing

Nurses League of CMAI

The Nurses League of the CMAI was started for the nurses in the year 1930. Christian Nurses in India strengthen the noble profession of nursing and demonstrate care and compassion as part of the Healing Ministry. The Nurses League of CMAI,

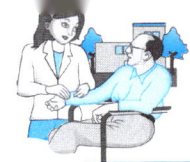

with over 6,100 current members, focuses on building nurse leadership for the country through reaching over 700 nurses annually.

Objectives

- Promotion of cooperation and support among nurses in India.
- Advocates the productiveness in nursing education and services.
- Secures the best attainable standard in Nursing Education through the Christian Schools of Nursing.
- Examines the individual work and problems of Christian nurses working throughout the country.

Activities

Conducting leadership conferences, seminars, workshops, retreats and meetings regularly in different parts of India.

National Research Society of India

National Research Society of India (NRSI) was established in the year 1987. It is the first premier research organization for nursing in India. Society organizes research presentation opportunities for the nurse scientists throughout the country to promote nursing research activities. It consisted of more than 1700 members including 35 international members on its roll.

It promotes researches to be conducted by the nurses, disseminating the research findings by conducting conferences and publications. It renders the best practice evidence for nursing services and positively modifies the quality of nursing services in India. The society is growing steadily larger and stronger.

Society of Community Health Nurses of India

Society of Community Health Nurses of India (SOCHNI) is a professional organization recognized as the primary voice for Community Health Nursing activities in India, leading the way to protect all Indians and their communities from preventable, serious health threats and striving to assure community-based health promotion and disease prevention activities.

Indian Society of Psychiatric Nurses

Indian Society of Psychiatric Nurses (ISPN) was started in the year 1991 with a motive of:
- Enhancing the advanced knowledge and skills in the field of Mental Health/Psychiatric nursing.
- To provide platform for discussion and deliberation on evidence based practice.
- To create awareness and to translate the research findings in Mental health/Psychiatric nursing practice.

Membership

- Fellow of Indian Society of Psychiatric Nurses
- ISPN Life Members
- Associated Life Members
- Indian registered nurses association
- Indian registered nurses association is a nonpolitical, nongovernmental, not for profit organization; tries to resolve the existing difficulties and exploitations faced by the largest healthcare work force and to bring about considerable improvement in the working environment.

The Society of Indian Neuroscience Nurses

The Society of Indian Neuroscience Nurses (SINN) is the first professional organization for nurses working in neurological settings aimed for the promotion of neuroscience nursing in India.

Objectives

- Promotes high quality care in Neurological and Neurosurgical Nursing in India.
- Exchanges views and disseminates knowledge and practice in the field of neuroscience nursing across India.
- Facilitates interaction among neuro nurses within and outside India.
- Encourages research in Neurological and Neurosurgical Nursing.

Activities

Conducts annual scientific conference for neuronurses, along with the annual meeting of Neurological Society of India (NSI).
- Oration by the nurses will be organized during annual conference.
- Awards to best scientific paper, model, poster, neuroquiz, essay and elocution. Dr AD Sehgal's Oration Award.

Other Associations

- Asian Cardiac Nurses Association
- Indian Association of Neonatal Nurses (IANN)
- Oncology Nurses Association of India, Mumbai

NURSING INFORMATICS

Nursing service system is progressing rapidly with advancements in technology in the field of medicine. Nursing Informatics is a new trend in the field of nursing. Nursing informatics is the use of computer technology in collection, storage and use of data to improve quality of nursing service. Nursing informatics is the integration of Nursing information and information management with information processing and communication technologies to support health efforts.

—*ICN 2006*

It is concerned with the study of nursing information and manipulation via computer based tools–health care information and management systems of society.

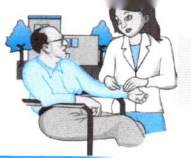

The ANA (1994) defines nursing informatics as the development and evaluation of applications, tools, processes and structures which assist nurses with the management of data in taking care of patients or supporting the practice of nursing.

So nursing informatics is an integration of computer science, Information Science and nursing science combining computer technology with hospital information system.

According to Hebde, nursing informatics is the use of computer technology to support nursing including clinical practice, administration, education and research.

The goal of nursing informatics is to use technology to improve quality of nursing service and to help nursing administration in planning, organization and decision making functions.

Importance

- Nursing Informatics use computer technology in improving quality nursing care services
- It enables prompt delivery of evidence based care by the use of technology
- Facilitate nursing management functions

Advantages

- Health management information are readily available. In a well organized system patients data are readily available to health care providers.
- Nursing administration function as decision making, staffing, scheduling are made easy with help of computer technology.
- There is organized method of documentation.
- Evaluation of nursing service can be made easy.
- Data can be utilized for research.
- Help to create nursing care plan to follow nursing process approach in giving nursing care.

Purpose

- To improve quality of nursing service
- To help nurse administrators in management functions as resource management, problem solving and decision making.
- Use of computer technology will enhance nursing service in areas of nursing management, nursing education and research.
- To improve accuracy of documentation

Challenges and Issues

- Confidentiality of clinical data of patients
- Security of information stored.
- Training of staff in computer application
- Technical issues
- Licence issue with teleconference
- Copyright of articles on the web

Issues

Legal and Ethical issues are:
- Confidentiality
- Informed consent
- Licence issues
- Copyright of materials on web

MANAGEMENT INFORMATION SYSTEM

Information technology is the management of information with the assistance of computer technology. The main goal of IT is to improve quality of healthcare, improve patient care services, promote safety of patients, reduce medical errors, improve documentation and strengthen interaction. Also it can be applied in the areas of nursing practice, decision making, nursing administration and research. It is increasingly being used in many organization.

The management Information System (MIS) is a system of collecting, processing, and disseminating data needed to carry out management functions in the form of informatics. It is a computer based information system which is concerned with processing of data for effective management of the organization.

MIS provides information needed to support planning, organizing and control function of nursing management. It also helps nurse managers to organize, evaluate and manage different departments of the hospital and also help in personal and resource management.

MIS refers to computer-based system that provides managers with the tools to organize, evaluate and efficiently manage departments in the organization.

—*Subbalekshmi Joshi*

MIS is an array of components designed to transform a collective set of data into knowledge that is directly useful and applicable in the process of directing and controlling resources and applications to the achievement of specific management objectives. —*Hanson 1982*

MIS is a formal system of gathering, comparing, analyzing and dispensing information internal and external to the enterprise in a timely, effective and efficient manner.

—*Koontz Harnold*

Objectives of MIS

- Provide information's to monitor progress, measure or evaluate performance of employees
- To provide data to take administrative decisions
- Planning systematically and coordinating activities
- To support organization's goals and direction
- Help to enhance communication and interpersonal relations among workers

Importance of MIS

- MIS support management functions as planning, organizing, coordinating etc
- MIS provides information to manage organizations effectively
- It provides information necessary for decision making
- It helps to plan comprehensive patient care
- Improves interdepartmental communication
- Enhances evidence based practice
- Enhances nursing education and research
- It provides indicators for monitoring and evaluation of performance

Essentials of Good Information System

- **Accuracy:** The information must be accurate and available in time
- **Adequacy of data:** Collect as much data as needed by various levels
- **Design tools** according to needs of the organization
- **Relevance:** The information must be relevant
- **Integrated system:** In MIS, information should flow smoothly from one system to another without interference
- **The system should be dynamic** and designed to meet the challenges of health system

Advantages

- MIS provides timely information which support and enhance decision making
- MIS is cost effective when implemented properly as a large number of work gets automated and it saves related costs
- Less time consuming. It helps in quick decision making
- Helps in administrative functions as planning and control
- Improves patient satisfaction
- It enhances easy availability of patient information
- Helps to keep data safe with minimum retrieval time
- Effective utilization of human resources
- Enhancescommunication between departments in hospital
- Helps in monitoring of hospital activities and evaluation of nursing service

Hospital Management Information System

Hospital Management Information Systems (HMIS) are information systems used to manage the medical, administrative, financial and legal aspects of hospital service. HMIS are large complex computer systems which have division as nursing—Laboratory, radiology, pharmacy, and administrative departments.

The HMIS is an information system specially designed to assist in the management and planning of health programs as opposed to delivery of care (WHO).

The HMIS is a system which deals with collection, utilization, analysis and transmission of information for providing health service, training and research.

Objectives

- To provide reliable health information at all levels of people
- To formulate hospital policies and procedures based on feedback
- To improve efficiency and quality in health management
- To provide adequate information for planning of health care
- To provide data necessary for evaluation and appraisal

Components

- Nursing management information system
- Clinical information system
- Laboratory information system
- Pharmacy information system
- Radiology information system etc.

Nursing management Information System is a network of computer systems that manages clinical data and makes it available to help nurses in improving nursing care to patients.

Nursing information systems use computer technology to manage clinical data. Nurse managers can use data to analyse, plan and make decisions.

Nursing information systems are computer systems that collect, store, process, retrieve and communicate information needed in nursing practice, education, administration and research —*Malliarou 2006*

According to Lippeveld, nursing information systems contribute to an integrated effort to collect, process, report and use health information and knowledge to influence policy making, program action and research.

NIS is a part of health care information system that deals with nursing aspects, particularly the maintenance of nursing record. —*Currell. 2003*

It is a part of health care information system that deals with nursing management.

NIS can be used to provide better quality care and also help in nursing administrative functions as human resource management, planning and organizing, budgeting, decision making and evaluation of nursing services. Also helps in nursing auditing and analyzing quality assurance information.

Benefits

- Facilitate better planning of care. All departments of hospitals are interconnected and informations are easily accessible for quick decision making.
- Nurses can spend more time with patients and nursing care as time spent for creating care plan and documentation are reduced.
- It can be used to generate staff schedule.
- It reduces paper work.
- NIS provide accurate and complete information.
- NIS help to reduce medication errors and improve patient safety.
- Improve satisfaction of consumers of care.
- Quality of service can be improved.

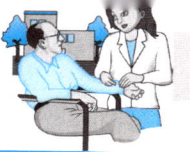

- It enables staff education and used to evaluate performance and outcome of nursing care services.
- Enhance continuity of care.

APPLICATION OF NURSING INFORMATICS

Management information system is not a new aspect in the field of nursing but the use of computer is new. Computerization has added the dimensions as speed, accuracy accessibility and use of increased volumes of data. For nurse managers use of informatics provide information's for decision making, planning, organizing, controlling etc. Its applications are summarized below.

- **Nursing service:** Through nursing information's system helps nurses to:
    - Enter and retrieve data related to patients. Nurses can use computer system to enter data regarding patient assessment values of vital signs, laboratory investigations, nursing care problems and can generate nursing care plans.
    - Update day to day progress and treatment and thereby modify care plans
    - Use information system for patient education
    - Uses system for communication between health care professionals and other departments.
    - Document and store data and retrieval of previous records
    - Provide access to current information and standards
- **Nursing administration:** Management information system provide information plan, organize and control the nursing services department of the hospital.
    - Able to create policy, procedures and nursing manual that guide administration
    - Used for intending and stocking
    - Information can be used for quality management
    - Nursing information system can used for staff scheduling, preparation of budget plan, master rotation plan, staff rotation plan etc.
    - Conduct teleconferencing to improve quality of care
    - NI can be used in quality management plan and patient instructional programs.
    - Plan and schedule in-service education programs
    - Help in continues evaluation of nursing service system
- **Nursing education:** In the field of nursing education, nursing information system can be used for
    - Computer assisted instruction, educational instructions, educational presentations and programs.
    - Teleconferencing and distance education
    - Organize simulation laboratories
    - Web based education
    - Online access to library and online publication
- **Nursing research:** In nursing research management information system helps for
    - Identification of nursing needs and problems
    - Search literature and current research findings
    - Search research design and tools
    - Data collection
    - Research analysis through descriptive and analytical statistics
    - Presentation of data – Tables and figures

Suggested Reading

- Barbara C, Susan RJ. Contemporary Nursing: Issues Trends and Management. 4th ed. St. Louis: Mosby Elsevier; 2008.
- Diane L Huber. Leadership and Nursing Care Management. 3rd ed. Saunders, Elsevier, 2000
- Joglekar S. Kamal. Professional Adjustments and Trends in Nursing. 2nd edition. Bombay: Vora Medical Publications; 1993.
- Jeanette Lancaster. Nursing Issues in Leading and Managing Change. 3ed ed. St Louis: Mosby Publishers; 1999.
- Katherine W Vestal. Nursing management: Concepts issues. 2nd ed. Philadelphia: JB Lippincott Company; 1995.
- Patricia S Yoder Wise. Leading and Managing in Nursing. 2nd ed. St Louis: Mosby publishers; 1995.
- Russell C Swansburg and Richard J Swansburg. Introduction to Management and Leadership for Nurse Managers, 3rd ed. Boston, Jonesand Barelett; 2002.
- Warren R Plunkett, Raymond F Attner and Gemmy S. Allen. Management: Meeting and exceeding customer expectations. 9th ed. South 1Western-cengage learning. Canada 2008.

Assess Yourself

LONG ANSWER

1. Write in detail about the membership with professional organizations.

SHORT NOTE

1. Career opportunities in nursing

Index

Please refer page number followed by 'b' as box, 'f' as figure and 't' as table, respectively.

A

ABC analysis 83t
    classification 84
    matrix of 84f
Abraham
    Flexner's criteria 194
    Maslow's need hierarchy
        theory 11, 29, 143
Accountability 97, 199
Accounting 51
Accreditation 100, 178
Accuracy 45, 108, 219
Acquirable qualities 10, 28, 135
Actualization 37
Adam's equity theory 145
Adequacy
    of data 219
Adjourning 148
Administer 13
Administration 13, 14, 59
    of
        curriculum 189
        versus management 13
Administrative 90
    class 8, 26
    educational/supervision 181
    law 205
    level 3
    planning 20
    responsibility 79
    theory 27
    theory: Henry Fayol 9
Admission
    and
        orientation 96
        management 14t
    nursing assessment 107
    policies 184
    selection committee 172
    strength 173
    terms and conditions 172
Adult
    ego state 133
    learning 161
    cycle 162
Advanced
    nurse practitioner 80
Advantages of a
    bureaucratic structure 9, 26
    appropriate placement 40
    bench marking 49
    centralization 33
    decentralization 33
    internal recruitment 38
    line organization 31
    nursing audit 119
    organizational charts 34
    performance appraisal 115
    planning 21
    POMR 106
Aims 179
    of
        CPA 19, 86 204
        discipline 188
        hospital planning 62
        in-service education 156
        material management 81
Ambulatory care 80
Amendments of 2015 201
American Nurses Association 214
    code of ethics (2001 and 2015
        versions) 201
ANA quality assurance model
    (Dr Norma Lang) 102
Annual reports 151
Anticipated
    accuracy 21
Antisocial 9, 27
Appraisal 40
    parameters 116
Area of hostel block 167
Arrange follow up meeting and
    take corrective actions 113
Assault 206
    and battery 208
Assessment 159
    of
        needs 80
        needs and problems 96
        resources 59
Assistant Director of Nursing
    Service 78
Assumptions 11, 28, 136
    of
        theory X 145
        theory Y 145
Attention 186
Audit 101, 118
    committee 118
    cycle 118
    reports 118
Auditorium 168, 175
Authority 33
    and
        responsibility 7, 24
    level principle 86
Autocratic 139
Autocratic/authoritarian
    style 138
    model 129
Autonomy 195, 198

B

Bargaining
    outcomes 153
    phase 152
Barriers
    in
        process of delegating 88
        delegate 88
        the delegator 88
        the situation 88
    of communication 132
    to TQM 105
Basic (Vertical chart) 34
Battery 205
Bed
    distribution 65
    planning 65
Bedside clinic 94
Behavioral
    science theory 10, 27
    theory 11, 28, 136
Bench marking 49
Beneficence 198
Benefits 219
    of
        accreditation 180
        delegation 86
        EMR 112
        good organizational
            structure 31
        in-service education
            program 159
        skill training 157
        TQM 105
        transactional analysis 134
Biomedical research 61
Bixler and Bixler criteria for
    profession 194
Blind self (Blind area) 134
Brain storming 149
Branches of classical theory 26
Breach of duty 206
BSc nursing 212
Budget 19, 50, 171
    committee 51
    for college of nursing 51
    planning 50f
Budgeting 6
Buffer stock 85
Bulletin board 151
Bureaucracy 8, 26
Bureaucratic structure 8, 25
Business policies 51

C

Canteen 170, 176
Capital
    and revenue budget 52, 81
Career
    day programs 39
    development in nursing 212
    opportunities in nursing 212
Caregiver 79
Case management 107
Categorization
    of hospital and space
        requirements 63
Centralization 7
    and decentralization 33
Centralized
    in-service education 158
    orientation 157
Central
    sterilization and supply
        department 65, 68
Certification 100
Challenges
    for organizational
        behavior 131
    in nursing practice 198
Channels of communication 132
Characteristics of
    adult learners 162
    a good in-service education
        program 159
    a sound organization 24
    Gantt chart 46
    guidance 185
    leadership 135
    MMT 13, 30
    neo-classical theory 10, 27
    nursing profession 195
    nursing standards 91
    planning 19
    strategic and operational
        plans 20
Check list 90
Child ego state 133
Christian Medical Association of
    India 216
Civil law
    or private law 205
Classical theory 8f, 25
    branches 26
Classification of
    activities/tasks 25
    budget 52
    disasters 120
    hospital 61
    nursing theories 8

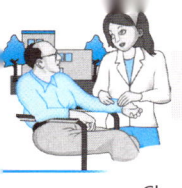

Class rooms 168, 174
Clayton Alderfer's ERG theory 144
Climate 163
Clinical
   audit 101
   blocks 190
   data repository 111
   facilities 177
   laboratory 64
   nurse specialist 80, 213
Closing phase 95
Code of ethics 199, 200
Code of professional conduct for nurses in India 200
Cognitive
   approach 129
   evaluation theory 146
   skills 186
Collective bargaining 152, 208
   issues 153
   process 152
College management committee 177
Collegial model 130
Command group 148
Commanding 6, 9
Common
   characteristics of profession 194
   delegation errors 87
   rooms 169, 175
Communication 5, 43, 117, 131
   and interpersonal relationship 200, 202
   process 131, 132f
   skill 15, 186
   management 131
Communicative 90
   skills 11, 28, 136
Communicator 80
Community
   based disaster management 122
   health nursing field practice area 172
   practice laboratory 168
   relations 151
   settings 212, 213
Components of
   orientation 157
   planning 19
   ward unit 68
   in-service education 157
Computerized
   medical records 111
   patients record 111
Computer laboratory 168
Concept of
   in-service education 156
   supervision 88
   management 3
   organizational behavior 128

Conclusion phase 95
Concurrent review 118
Conduction phase 95
Constitutional law 205
Consumer Protection Act (CPA) 204
Contingency theory 13, 30, 137f
Continuing education 158, 184
Continuous
   integrated triage 120
   quality improvement (CQI) 104
Contract
   law 205
   staffing 39
Control chart 103f
Controlling 5, 6, 9
Control over
   costs 46
   employees 45
   methods and manpower 46
   organization 45
   research and development 46
   policies 45
Coordination 6, 9, 122
Counselling 151, 186
   process/steps 187
   types 187f
Crèche 170
Credentialing 100
Credit system 173
Criminal law 205
Critical
   incidents method 114
   path method 48, 49f
   thinking 195
Crossed transactions 133
Cumulative record 173
Custodial model 129

D

Daily progress note and discharge summary 106
Database 106
Davis' OB model 129
Death and related issues 208
Decentralized
   approach 158
   orientation 157
Delayed decisions 32
Delegation 69, 85
   of authority 31
Delphi technique 150
Deming model (PDCA) 102f
Democracy 9, 26
Democratic 139
Demotion 189
Donabedian model of QA 102f
Departmental EMRs 111
Dependent variables 130
Depersonalized work 9, 27

Deputy director of nursing services 79
Design
   and planning 160
Design tools 219
Desirable items 84
Detention 188
Didactic interactions 150
Dietary serviced 67
Digital medical record 111
Directing 5, 42
Directional planning 20
Direction
   initiates action 42
   integrates employee's effort 42
Disadvantages of
   decentralization 33
   planning 21
   the nursing audit 119
Disaster
   management 110, 120, 123
   mitigation 122
   nursing 123
   preparedness 121
Discharges 42
Disciplinary
   Actions 189
   Measures 188
Discipline
   in educational institutions 188
Discussion phase 152
Dismissal 188
Disposal 82
Disseminator 15
Distribution
   of beds 171
District nursing officer 78
Disturbance handler 15
Documentation 105, 208, 209
Donabedian model (Dr Donabedian) 102
Donated time 153
Double line
   of commands 32
Downward
   and sideward delegation 86
   communication 132
   responsibilities 91
Dr CB Gupta 3
Due diligence 41
Duty roster 73

E

Early warning systems 122
Eclectic counselling 187
Economic
   feasibility 45
   make or buy 82
   order quantity (EOQ) 85

Educational
   design 163
   functions 75
   guidance 185
   responsibilities 74
Edward Deming 98
E-hiring 40
Electronic
   client records 112
   health care record 111
   medical records 111
   meetings 150
   patients record 111
Elements
   affecting organizational behavior 128f
   of
      a hospital 66
      bureaucracy 26
      malpractice 206
      the code 200
      TQM 104
      direction 43
Emergency
   department 67
   room 64
Emotional intelligence (EQ) 142b
Empathy 10, 28, 135
Empirical standards 92
Employee-production orientation 139
Employment exchanges 39
Empowerment and autonomy 41
End standards 92
Entrepreneur 15
Environment 128
Environmental
   barriers 132
   sanitation and cleanliness 182
Equipment planning 63
Equity 7
ERG theory 144f
Esprit de corps 7
Essay 114
Esteem needs 12, 29, 143, 144
ET for Gantt chart 46
Ethical
   and legal aspects in nursing 198
   and legal issues in nursing 208
   principles 198
Ethics
   and code of conduct 62
Euthanasia 208
Evaluation methods 160
Existence
   needs 144
Expectancy 145
Exploitative device 9, 27

Index

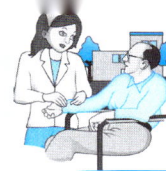

Extended
   and expanded role of nurse 79
External
   benchmarking 49
   lead time 85
   lecturers 170
   recruitment 38, 39
   sources 38
Extramural education 158
Extrinsic motivation 142

F

Factors
   affecting
      adult learning 162
      good ward management 69
      group behavior 148
      in-service Education 158
      recruitment policy 38
      ward design 68
   evaluation system 70
   influencing
      budget planning 51
      the quality patient care 72
False imprisonment 206
Faulty transmission 132
Favorable reciprocal relations 82
Fayol's six 27
Functions of management 9
Fidelity 198
Fiedler's contingency model 140f
Field review method 114
Films 151
Financial
   planning 62
   support 184
Finer's principles of administration 7f
Fire extinguisher 169, 176
Five rights of delegation 86
Fixed
   and flexible budgets 52
   budget 52
   ceiling budget 52
Flexibility 196
Flexible budget 52
Florence Nightingale 98
Flow sheets 107
Fluid balance record 108
Forecasting 51
   and planning 6, 9
Foreign Nationals 172
Forge authentic connections 41
Formal
   communication 132
   groups 147
   leadership 148
   or informal delegation 86

Forming 148
Forms
   of organizational structures 31
Formulation of
   derivative plan 20
   goals 59
   operational goals and objectives 19
Fraud 206
Frederick Herzberg's motivation hygiene theory 29, 144
Frederick Winslow Taylor 9
Free
   online ads 39
   response report 114
FSN analysis 84
Functional
   benchmarking 49
   method 71
      of work assignment 71f
   organization 32
Functions of
   budget in nursing 53
   management – POSDCORB 4f
   management by Henri Fayol 6
   management 4
   material management 82
   SNA 216
   supervision 90
   the hospital/hospital services 60

G

Games analysis 134
Gantt chart 46, 47f
General
   or specific delegation 86
George, Veigas and Isaac, 1984 98
Goal setting theory of Edwin Locke 146
Good Samaritan law 207
Grand theory 8
Graphic record 107
Great man theory of leadership/charismatic leadership theory 138
Group
   cohesiveness 149f
   composition 149
   decision making techniques 149
   development 148
   dynamics 147
   process 149
   structure 148
Guidance 184
Guidelines
   and minimum requirements to establish BSc (N) college of nursing 173

   minimum requirements to establish school of nursing 166
   for establishment of new BSc (N) college of nursing 173
   for preparation of budget 50
Guiding principles 8, 25

H

Head nurse 75
Health services 173
Henri Fayol 6f
Henri Fayol's
   principles of management 6f
Hezberg's two-factor theory 12f, 29f
Hierarchy 8, 26
   of material management 82
Histogram 104f
HML analysis 84
Home health care 79
Horizontal chart 34
Hospice and
   palliative care nursing 80
Hospital
   building 65
   commissioning 65
   departments 66
   design 65
   EMRs 111
   ethics committee 209
   infection control 179
   information system 61
   inpatient service 68
   level 63
   management information system 219
   planning 62
   settings 212, 213
   ward 68
Hostel
   block 167, 176
   facilities 169, 176
   room 176
Human
   relations 10, 28, 135, 140, 150
      theory 10
   resource
      department 68
      management 36
   philosophy 37
   skills 15
Hursey-Blanchard's situational model 141
Hypothetical
   construct of PERT 47

I

Impersonality 9, 26
Impersonal relationships 8, 26
Implications 12, 30, 144

   for management 12, 29, 143
Importance of
   accreditation 178
   benchmarking 49
   control 44
   direction 42
   human resource management 37
   leadership 135
   management 3
   MIS 219
   planning 18
   organizing 24
Improper delegating 87
Independent variables 130
Indian Nursing Council 196, 215
   code of ethics and code of professional conduct 199
Indian Society of Psychiatric Nurses 217
Indian Trade Unions Act 1926 152
Indirect supervision 89
Individual
   and group conference 90
   evaluation methods 113
   factors and turnover 41
   level variables 130
Induction
   training or entry training 183
Infection control nurse 213
Informal
   communication 132
   groups 147
Information
   management 122
      system 179
Informed consent 207, 208
Initiating structure 139
Innate qualities 135
In-service education 156, 158, 183
   benefits 159
   concept 156f
   components 157
   methods 160
   sample 160t
Institutional records 173
Integrated system 219
Integration 45
   versus disintegration 25
Integrative function 43
Intelligence 10, 28, 135
Intensive care unit 64, 67
Intentional tort 205
Interacting group 150
Inter-departmental
   EMR 111
   harmony 82
Interest arbitration 153
Inter-hospital EMRs 111
Internal
   lead time 84

223

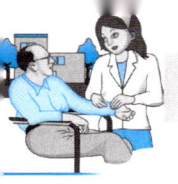

benchmarking 49
recruitment 38, 39
sources 38
International
benchmarking 49
confederation of midwives 215
council for nurses 196
council for nurses code of ethics 200
council of nurses 214
nursing review 215
Interpersonal
and communication 31
relations 196
role 15
skills 15
Interrelated functions 8, 25
Intervention 188
Interviewing 40
Intrinsic
motivation 142
Introduction phase 95
Invasion of privacy 206, 208
Inventory
carrying cost 85
control 82, 83
Involuntary separation 42
Ishikawa/fish bone diagram 104
Issues
and challenges in nursing management 197
in nursing management 197
leading to collective bargaining 153
recognized by Indian Nursing council 197

J

JIT (Just in time) 85
Job
analysis 73f
enrichment 146
orientation/training 183
responsibilities of different categories of nursing personnel 74
Johari window 134f
Journals 151

K

Kardexes 107
Kelly's criteria 194
Knowles'
4 principles of andragogy 162
5 assumptions of adult learners 162
Kootz and O'Donell 5

L

Laissez faire 139
Lateral
or horizontal Communication 132
Leadership 5, 43, 135
and management development 157
as a continuum 139
based on behavioral approach 138
based on situational approach 140
behavior styles 141
position power 140
skills 141
styles 138, 139t 140, 141
Lead time 84
Lean methodology 103
Learner 163
Legal
aspects in nursing 205
damage 205
nurse consultants 80
prudence 108
remedy 205
responsibilities of nurses 208
responsibility for death and dying 209
safe guards in nursing practice 207
Legibility 108
Lewin's leadership styles 138
Liaison role 15
Licensure 100, 207, 208
Likert's
management system 140
leadership styles 140f
Line organization 31f
Lines of authority 51
Long
range Vs short range planning 21
term and short term budget 52f
Luther Halsey Gullick 4f

M

Management 2
functions 4f
level 4f
Malpractice 206
Maslow's hierarchy of needs 12f, 29
Mass resignations 153
Master
and functional budget 52
Plan 189
for staffing pattern 59
Rotation plan 190, 191f
Material management 61, 81

hierarchy 82f
system 82
planning (Demand estimation) and budgeting 82
resources and facilities 163
Matrix organization 32
of ABC and VED items 84f
McClelland's theory of needs 144, 145
McGregor theory 11, 28, 136f
Means standards 92
Measurement
of patient classification system 70
Media relation 151
Medical
records department 68
research 208
Medication administration form 108
Meritocracy 37
Meta theory 8
Middle
level management 4
range theories 8
Mixed stroke 134
Modern
approach 30
theory 12
Modified nightingale ward 68
Motivation 5, 43, 142
factors 12, 29, 146f
theories 11, 29
Multipurpose AALL 175

N

National accreditation board for hospitals and
health care providers (NABH) 179
National
agencies 179
assessment and accreditation council (NAAC) 179
commission 205
council of state boards of nursing, resources section 97
League for nursing 214
Research Society of India (NRSI) 217
Negative
motivation 142
strokes 134
Negligence 206
and malpractice 208
Neoclassical theory 10, 27
Nightingale ward 68
Nominal group technique (NGT) 150
Nonmaleficence 198
Non-verbal communication 132
Normative standards 92

Norming 148
Norms 36
Norms of staffing (S I U- Staff Inspection Unit) 36
Nurse
advocate 80
educator 80, 213
entrepreneur 80
managers 80
midwife 80, 213
practitioner 213
researcher 80
league of CMAI 216
Nursing audit 101, 117
cycle 118f
Nursing
care plans 107
education 220
informatics 217
manuals 93
program 190
research 220
rounds 94
service 58, 76, 220
superintendent 76

O

Objectives 19, 58, 112, 161, 173, 179, 196, 215, 216, 217, 219
of
assignment planning 70
career development 212
collective bargaining 152
disaster management 123
ICN 215
in-service education 156
leadership and management development 157
material management 81
MIS 218
quality assurance 98
staffing in nursing 35
staff welfare 182
supervision 89
hospital 60
ward management 96
Objective structured clinical examination (OSCE) 157
Objective structured practical examination (OSPE) 157
Open
ended budget 52
house 39
self (public area) 134
system view 13
Operational budget 81
planning 20
Operation theater 64, 67, 74
Optimistic time 48
Oral debridement 188

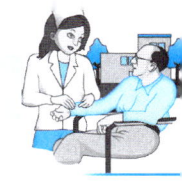

Index

Organizing 5
Organization
    nature 24f
    of hospital 60
    process 25
    theories 25
Organizational charts 33, 35
    example 35f
    types 34
Organ transplantation 208
Orientation 41
Orientation program 157, 180
Outcome
    audit 119
    standards 92
Outpatient department 66
Overdelegating 87

P

Para verbal communication 132
Parent ego state 133
Pareto chart 103f
Partial block system 190
Path-goal model of
    leadership 138, 141
Patient
    bill of rights 203
    care 96
    classification system (PCS) 70
    method/case method 70
    record system
        documentation 105
Peer review 100
    method 115
Performance
    appraisal 112
    budget 52
    checklist 114
    feedback 162
    methods 113
    process 113
    sample 116
    standards 113
    system 113f
Permanence 108
Persecutors 134
Personal health record 111
PERT 46, 47, 48f
Pessimistic time 48
Peterson, Kovel- Jarboe 99
Phases
    of disaster 120f
Pitchfork effect 116
Placement 40
Plan each day's program 69
Planning 5, 18, 159
    hierarchy 21f
    methods 46
    steps 19f
    time 96
    types 20

Policies 19
Positive
    motivation 142
    strokes 134
Potential 37
Power 3
Prebargaining stage 152
Predictability 9, 21, 26
Preparation phase 95
Principles of guidance
    according
    to
    Crow and Crow 185
    Hollies and Hollies 185
Problem oriented medical
    records 106
Process
    audit 119
    theories of motivation 145
Procurement cost/ordering
    cost 85
Production budget 52
Productivity 130
Profession 194
Program 19
Programmed budget 52
Program planning 163
Progressive patient care (PPC) 72f
Progress notes 108
Project organization 32
Prototype evaluation system 70
Public
    law 205
    relations 150
Purchasing 82
Pyramid
    structure of classical theory 25f

Q

Quality
    assurance 98
        cycle 99f
        model 101, 102f
    control 98, 208
    council of India 179
    management 62
Quits 42

R

Radio 151
Ranking method 114
Rating scale 91, 115
Realistic time 48
Recognition 146, 178
Recommendations by SIU 36
Record 8, 26
    and report 60, 117, 163, 208
    keeping 44
    room 169, 175
Recruitment 37
    methods 39

    process 39f
Rederick Herzberg's motivation
    hygiene theory-or-Herzberg's
    two factor theory 12
Redressal agency 204
Red tape 9, 26
Registration 207
Regulatory bodies 196
Reinforcement theory 146
Relevance 219
Reporting 6
Rescuer 134
Resignation 42
Retention 40
Retirements 42
Retrospective view 118
Revenue budget 52
Reverse triage 120
Richard H Hall's criteria 194
Rigg's ward 68
Rigidity 9, 26
Robbin OB model 130
Roll over budget 52

S

Sample
    in-service education plan 160
    of recording 109
    performance appraisal for ward
        incharges 116
Scalar chain 7
    of command 7f
Scatter diagram 103f
Scholarships 184
SDE analysis 84
Selection 40, 180
Self-actualization 12, 29, 144
Self-appraisal 114
Self-concept 162
Separation 42
Short-term budget 52
Sick room 176
Sigma Theta Tau
    International 215
Simple ranking method 114
Simple triage 120
Situational variables 140
Six Sigma 102
Skill training program 157
Society of Community Health
    Nurses of India 217
Socio-economic Welfare (SEW)
    Programs 216
Source-oriented records 105
Specialization 9, 26
Staff development 156
    program 183
Staff Health Services 183
Staffing 5, 35, 172
    process 37

Staff
    inspection unit 36
    management 61
    nurse 74
    organizational structure 31
    training and development 40
    welfare 182
Standardization 82
State commission 205
State Nurse Practice Act 206
State Nursing Registration
    Council 197
Statistical information 51
Steps in
    budget planning 51
    budgetary process 80
    construction of Gantt
        charts 46
    control process 45
    critical pathway method 48
    delegation 87
    developing in-service
        program 159
    organizational structuring 30
    PERT 47
    planning duty roster 73
    planning nursing service
        unit 59
    planning process 19
    recruitment 180
    setting of standards 92
Stipend 184
Store room 169, 175
Storming 148
Strategic planning 20
    and operational plans 20t
Strikeouts 153
Structural mitigation 123
Structure audit 119
Structure of
    hospital ethics committee 209
    PERT chart 48f
    process and outcome
        standards 92
    standards 92
Student health services 184
Student Nurses Association of
    India 216
Student
    patient ratio 171
    welfare 182
    services 184
Study day system 190
Subordinates maturity 141
Sunset budget 52
Supportive
    model 129
    services 60
Suspension 188
System theory 13, 30f

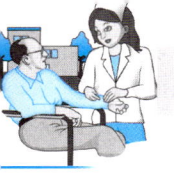

T

Taylor's
　philosophy in a nutshell　27
Teaching　182
　system　189
Team
　method of work
　　assignment　71f
Technology　128
Tele education　110
Telehealth care　110
Telemedicine/Tele health　109
Telenursing　110
Television　151
The decision making model　130
Theo Haimann　6
Theories of
　leadership　10, 27, 135
　motivation　142
　nursing management　7
　organization　25
Theory
　X　11, 28, 136
　X and Theory Y of Douglas
　　McGregor　145
　Y　11, 28, 136
The Society of Indian Neuroscience
　Nurses　217
Tort　205
　law　205
Total quality management
　(TQM)　104
Trained Nurses Association of
　India　215
Trait
　rating scale　115
Theory　135
　of leadership　10, 27
Transactional analysis　132
　complementary　133f
　crossed　133f
　ulterior　133f
Transcript　173
Transport　170, 176
Types of
　accreditation agencies　178
　bench marking　49
　budget　51
　budgetary process　81
　clinical audit　101
　communication　131
　counselling　187
　delegation　86
　EMRs　111
　groups　147
　intentional tort　205
　law　205
　motivation　142
　organizational chart　34
　planning　20
　PCS　70
　separation　42
　staff development
　　program　156, 183
　standards　92
　supervision　89
　transactions　133
　ward　68

U

Ulterior transactions　133
Unacceptable personal
　conduct　189
Undemocratic　9, 27
Underdelegating　87
Unintentional torts　206
Union　152
Unit philosophy　22
Unity of
　command　7, 24, 86
　direction　7
Unknown self (Dark area)　134
Unpsychological　9, 27
Unrealistic　9, 27
Unsolicited applicants/
　walk-ins　40
Update PERT chart　47
Upwards communication　132
Uses of
　PERT　48
　telemedicine　109
　transcript　173
　vision and mission　22

V

Valuing human beings　202
Variables　139
　dependant　139
　independent　139
VED analysis　84
　matrix　84f

Veracity　198
Verbal
　command　189
　communication　131
　　barriers　132
　　vision　21
　　and mission　22t
Vital Items　84
Vocational
　guidance　185
　Separation　42
Vroom's expectation theory　145

W

Ward management　74
　role of head nurse　96
Wards　64
Welfare amenities　182
Witnessing will　208
Working areas　213
　phase　95
Workplace privacy　206
Work schedules　41
Written or oral delegation　86
Written
　repridment　189
　reprimand　188
　warning　188
　wrongful act　205